Passport to a Healthy Pregnancy

Dr Gita Arjun

westland ltd
Venkat Towers, 165, P.H. Road, Maduravoyal, Chennai 600 095
No. 38/10 (New No. 5), Raghava Nagar, New Timber Yard Layout, Bangalore 560 026
Survey No. A - 9, II Floor, Moula Ali Industrial Area, Moula Ali, Hyderabad 500 040
23/181, Anand Nagar, Nehru Road, Santacruz East, Mumbai 400 055
4322/3, Ansari Road, Daryaganj, New Delhi 110 002

First published by westland ltd 2009

Copyright © Dr Gita Arjun 2009

All rights reserved.

10 9 8 7 6 5 4 3
ISBN: 978-81-89975-68-5

Book Designed and Formatted by Malvika Mehra
Printed at : HT Media Ltd., Noida

This book is sold subject to the condition that it shall not by way of trade or otherwise, be lent, resold, hired out, circulated, and no reproduction in any form, in whole or in part (except for brief quotations in critical articles or reviews) may be made without written permission of the publishers.

Dedicated to the women in my life

Dr E.V. Kalyani, who by her surgical skills made possible my very existence,

>Vanajakshi Padmanabhan, my mother, who in her own gentle way taught me to be fearless,

Padma Rajagopalan, my mother-in-law, who with immense generosity gave me the freedom to succeed,

>Dr T. Tharabai and Dr S. Neela, my aunts, who, as amazing obstetricians, have been my lifelong role models,

And to all the women who have allowed me the privilege of sharing their joy during their pregnancies.

For Arjun, Ashvin and Kavita
without whom life would be leached of all its colours.

CONTENTS

INTRODUCTION

SECTION 1 — KNOWING YOUR PREGNANCY

CHAPTER 1	How pregnancy happens	10
CHAPTER 2	Pre-pregnancy counselling	16
CHAPTER 3	Am I pregnant?	20
CHAPTER 4	A visit to your obstetrician	26
CHAPTER 5	The first trimester (0-13 weeks)	32
CHAPTER 6	The second trimester (14-27 weeks)	40
CHAPTER 7	The third trimester (28-40 weeks)	48
CHAPTER 8	Eating healthy in pregnancy	56
CHAPTER 9	Exercising in pregnancy	62
CHAPTER 10	The role of the father-to-be	66

SECTION 2 — HOW IS THE BABY DOING?

CHAPTER 11	Tests in pregnancy: how do I know my baby is normal?	74
CHAPTER 12	Ultrasound scans in pregnancy	80
CHAPTER 13	Special tests in pregnancy	86
CHAPTER 14	Birth defects	90

SECTION 3 — LABOUR AND DELIVERY

CHAPTER 15	Preparing for labour	96
CHAPTER 16	Planning for labour	100
CHAPTER 17	Labour and delivery	104
CHAPTER 18	Augmentation and induction of labour	114
CHAPTER 19	Forceps delivery and vacuum-assisted birth	120
CHAPTER 20	Pain relief in labour and delivery	124
CHAPTER 21	Monitoring the baby's well-being during labour	130
CHAPTER 22	Complications in labour	134
CHAPTER 23	Caesarean section	138

SECTION 4 — AFTER THE DELIVERY

CHAPTER 24	After-delivery care	146
CHAPTER 25	Breastfeeding	152
CHAPTER 26	Diet and exercise after delivery	158

SECTION 5 — WHEN THINGS GO WRONG

CHAPTER 27	Miscarriage (abortion)	166
CHAPTER 28	Bleeding in pregnancy	172
CHAPTER 29	Premature or preterm labour	178
CHAPTER 30	Postdated pregnancy	182
CHAPTER 31	Breech delivery	186
CHAPTER 32	Twin pregnancy: double trouble?	190
CHAPTER 33	High blood pressure in pregnancy	196
CHAPTER 34	Diabetes in pregnancy	202
CHAPTER 35	The Rh factor: how can it affect pregnancy?	208
CHAPTER 36	Pregnancy after thirty-five	212
CHAPTER 37	Handling pregnancy loss	216

SECTION 6 — COMMON ILLNESSES IN PREGNANCY

CHAPTER 38	Fever in pregnancy	222
CHAPTER 39	Urinary tract infection and vaginal infection	226
CHAPTER 40	Medical disorders in pregnancy	230

SECTION 7 — BEING A PARENT

CHAPTER 41	Preparing your child for the arrival of the new baby	238
CHAPTER 42	Your new baby	242

SECTION 8 — BIRTH CONTROL

CHAPTER 43	Methods of birth control	258
CHAPTER 44	Emergency contraception	268

FOR YOU 271

ACKNOWLEDGEMENTS 281

INDEX 282

INTRODUCTION

Pregnancy is a time of great joy. The drama of a new life is unfolding within you. However, for some couples, pregnancy can be tinged with worry and plagued with anxiety. Being pregnant is a life-altering event that every woman looks forward to. At the same time, having heard numerous anecdotes from friends and relatives, many women are apprehensive once they discover that they are pregnant.

Passport to a Healthy Pregnancy has been specifically written to disseminate valuable information about the processes involved in going through a pregnancy in the 21st Century. With technology and an array of investigations available today to the modern obstetrician, pregnancy has been made safer for mother and child. At the same time, nothing can replace the empathy and compassion a pregnant woman requires and expects from her family, friends and obstetrician.

Most of the worry is caused due to the lack of knowledge about pregnancy or, worse still, due to misinformation, myths and misplaced beliefs. **Passport to a Healthy Pregnancy** will place all the facts before you and help you go through your pregnancy with confidence. We want you to enjoy every moment of your pregnancy, armed with correct facts, specific information and essential details.

In my years of practising obstetrics, I have had the privilege of interacting with thousands of pregnant women. I have been allowed into their lives and have shared their joy, their tears, their deepest feelings, their hopes and their despair. The one thing that strikes me is the fact that no two women will react in the same way to different aspects of pregnancy. Every woman has her own take on her pregnancy. I have found that there are two ends of the spectrum: some women are calm while there are others who are over-anxious and behave as if they are the first ever to get pregnant. Fortunately, the majority take an active, cheerful interest in their pregnancies. With the help of their husband, other members of the family and an empathetic obstetrician, they are able to get the correct perspective on their pregnancy.

In the Indian cultural setting, husbands have traditionally been relegated to the background since pregnancy is perceived as the sole domain of women. The pregnant woman's mother, mother-in-law and other female members of the family play a more active role than the husband himself. However, with nuclear families having become the order of the day and more couples living by themselves, Indian husbands too have started taking the responsibility of steering their wives through a comfortable and supported pregnancy. **Passport to a Healthy Pregnancy** has a chapter defining the role of husbands in helping their wives through pregnancy and delivery.

Sometimes, a pregnancy does not follow the normal, expected path. Things can go wrong. **Passport to a Healthy Pregnancy** helps you understand what causes mishaps and complications in a pregnancy. This knowledge will help you withstand unexpected setbacks, be they minor or major, and help you go on.

Come, learn about your pregnancy and prepare yourself for a woman's greatest experience - you deserve to have a wonderful, healthy pregnancy!

Dr. Gita Arjun

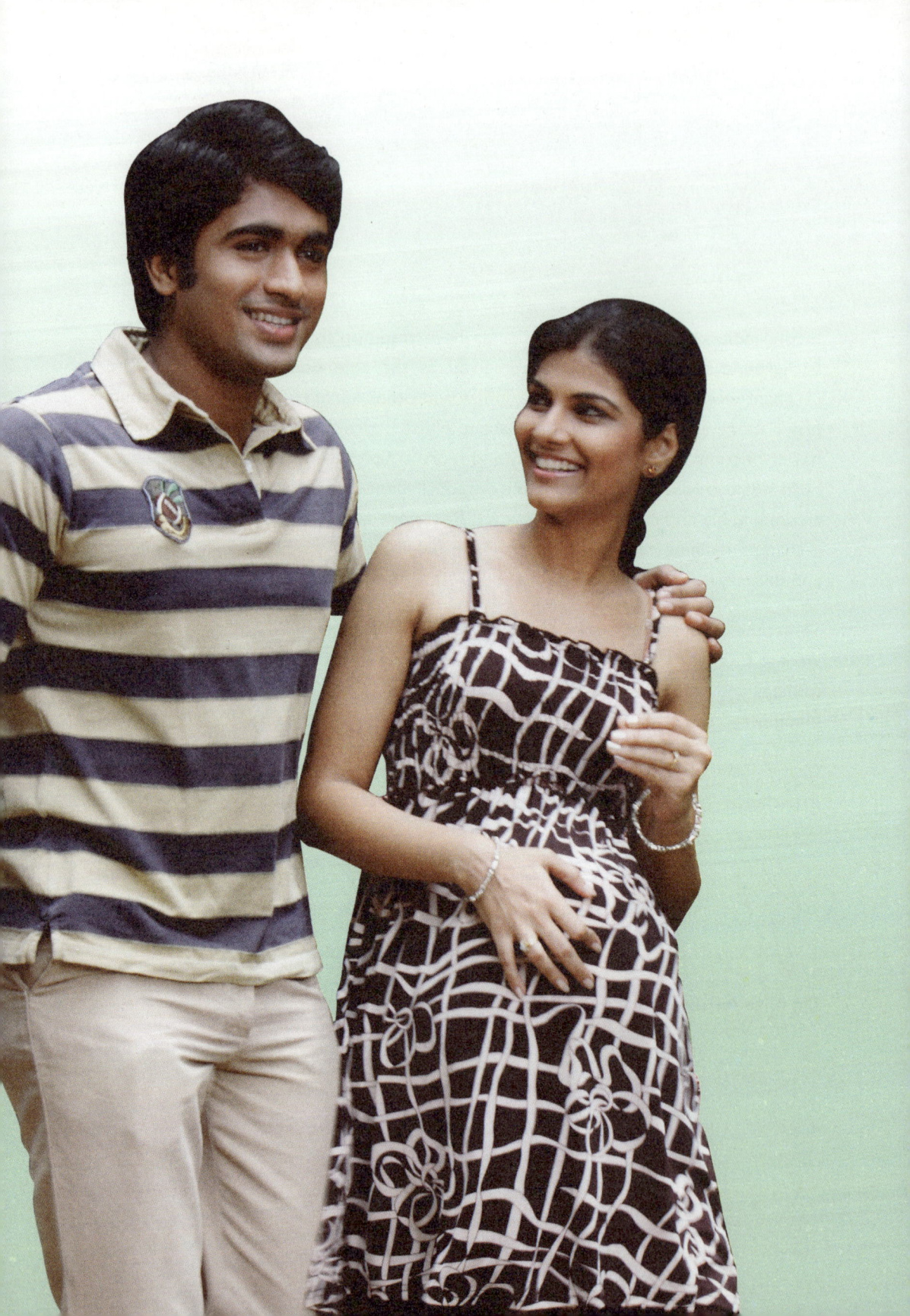

Knowing your pregnancy

CHAPTER 1

How pregnancy happens: fertilisation, implantation and foetal development

Sadhana and Girish are excited about the pregnancy. Their baby! They can't believe that a life is growing inside her. How miraculous that their love has created a new being. They are curious about how their baby is developing in the womb.

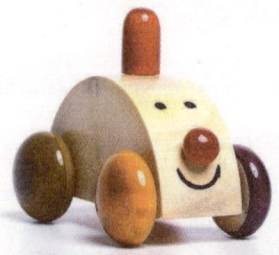

1 How pregnancy happens:
Fertilisation, implantation and foetal development

Stages of foetal development

Life begins with the fertilisation of the egg by the sperm. This possibly represents one of the most important processes in human biology. The fertilised egg then progressively develops into a blastocyst, an embryo and then a foetus.

The process of fertilisation

During each normal menstrual cycle, one egg (ovum) is usually released from one of the ovaries, about 14 days before the next menstrual period. This process is called **ovulation.** The Fallopian tubes have finger-like projections (fimbriae) which pick up the egg and transport it into the funnel-shaped end of the tube.

At ovulation, the mucus in the cervix becomes thinner and watery, facilitating the entry of sperm into the uterus. Within a short time, usually minutes, the sperm may swim rapidly from the vagina through the cervix into the uterus and into the Fallopian tube — the usual site of fertilisation. If fertilisation does not occur, the egg degenerates and passes through the uterus with the next menstrual period.

Fertilisation occurs if a sperm penetrates the egg. Once fertilisation occurs, the egg starts dividing to form a **zygote,** a solid ball of cells. Tiny hair-like cilia lining the Fallopian tube propel the zygote through the tube toward the uterus.

The cells of the zygote divide repeatedly as the zygote moves down the Fallopian tube. The zygote enters the uterus in 3 to 5 days. In the uterus, the cells continue to divide, becoming a hollow ball of cells called a **blastocyst.**

Development of the blastocyst

Between six and seven days after fertilisation, the blastocyst gets attached to the lining of the

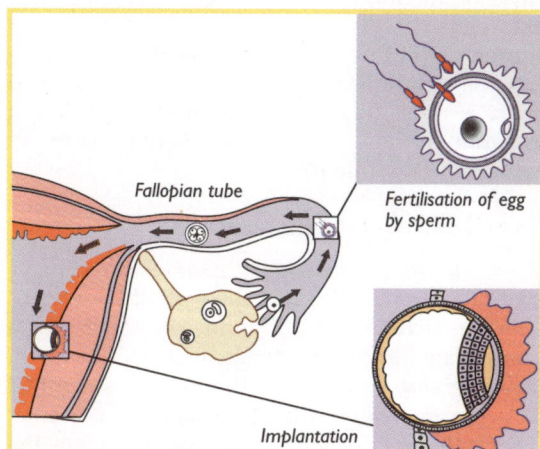

The process of fertilisation and implantation

uterus, usually near the top, called the fundus of the uterus. This process, called **implantation,** is completed by Day 9 or 10. There is a small window of about four days, when the lining of the uterus (endometrium) is receptive to the blastocyst and allows the blastocyst to adhere and burrow into the uterine lining.

The wall of the blastocyst facing the uterine cavity is one cell thick. The part of the blastocyst which penetrates the uterine wall is three to four cells thick. The inner cells in the thickened area develop into the **embryo,** and the outer cells burrow into the wall of the uterus and develop into the **placenta.** The placenta links the mother and foetus: it carries oxygen and nutrients from the mother to the foetus and waste materials from the foetus to the mother.

One of the important functions of the placenta is the production of hormones that help maintain the pregnancy. For example, the placenta produces **human chorionic gonadotropin (hCG),** which prevents the ovaries from releasing more eggs. This stops menstruation and stimulates the

---

If more than one egg is released and fertilised, the pregnancy results in more than one foetus, usually two (twins). Such twins are called fraternal. When one fertilised egg separates into two embryos after it has begun to divide, identical twins are formed.

ovaries to produce the hormones **estrogen** and **progesterone** continuously.

The wall of the blastocyst becomes the outer layer of membranes called **chorion,** surrounding the embryo. An inner layer of membranes (amnion) develops by about Day 10 to 12, forming the **amniotic sac.** The amniotic sac is filled with a clear fluid called **amniotic fluid** and expands to envelop the developing embryo, which floats within it.

Development of the placenta

As the placenta develops, it extends tiny finger-like projections (villi) into the wall of the uterus. The projections branch and re-branch in a complicated tree-like arrangement. This arrangement greatly increases the area of contact between the wall of the uterus and the placenta. The villi are constantly in contact with the mother's blood so that nutrients and waste material can be exchanged. At delivery, the placenta weighs about 500 grams.

Development of the embryo

The next stage in development is the **embryo.** The embryonic period extends from the 5th week to the 10th week of your pregnancy. This stage is characterised by the formation of most internal organs and external body structures. Organ formation begins about three weeks after fertilisation, when the embryo is first recognisable as having a human shape. Shortly thereafter, the area that will become the brain and spinal cord (neural tube) begins to develop. The heart and major blood vessels begin to develop by Day 16 or 17. The heart begins to pump fluid through blood vessels by Day 20, and the first red blood cells appear the next day. Beyond the 10th week, this growing mass of cells with a human shape is called a **foetus.**

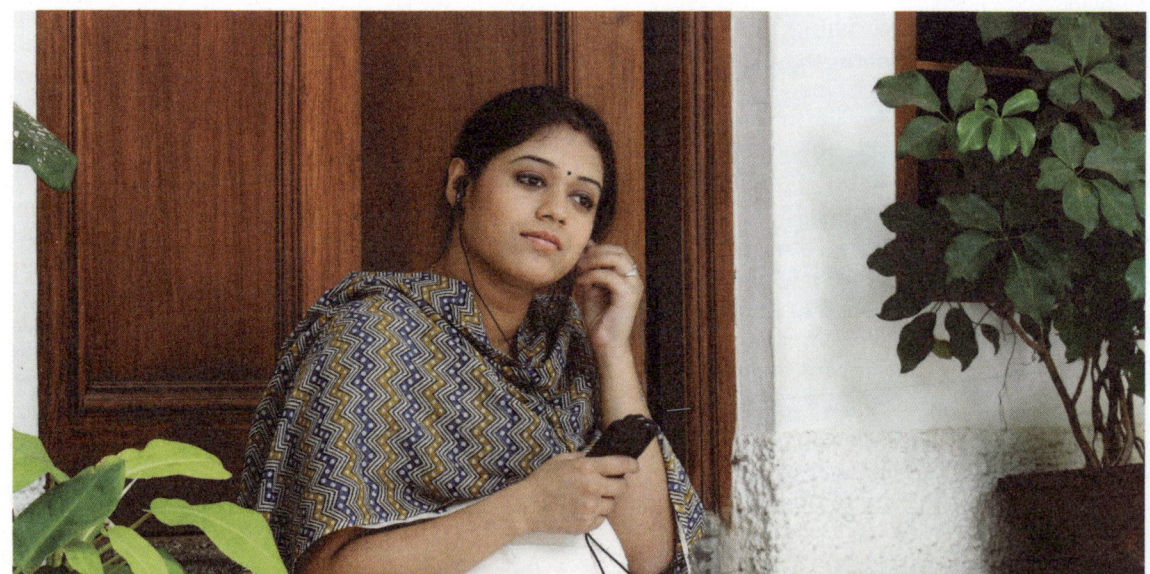

How many weeks pregnant am I?
Your obstetrician will count the number of weeks of your pregnancy from the first day of the last period. For example: if your last period was on May 1, then on June 12, you will be six weeks pregnant ('gestational age'). If you actually counted from the day of fertilisation, it will be four weeks ('ovulation age').

| By the end of 6 weeks | - all major systems and organs begin to form
- the embryo looks like a tadpole
- the neural tube (which becomes the brain and spinal cord), the digestive system, the heart and circulatory system begin to form
- the beginnings of the eyes and ears are developing
- tiny limb buds appear (which will develop into arms and legs)
- the heart starts beating |
|---|---|
| By the end of 8 weeks | - all major body systems continue to develop and function, including the circulatory, nervous, digestive and urinary systems
- the embryo takes on a human shape, although the head is larger in proportion to the rest of the body
- the mouth develops tooth buds (which will become baby teeth)
- the eyes, nose, mouth and ears become more distinct
- the arms and legs are clearly visible
- the fingers and toes are still webbed but can be clearly distinguished
- the main organs continue to develop
- the bones begin to develop and the nose and jaws rapidly develop
- the embryo is in constant motion but these movements cannot be felt by the mother |
| From embryo to foetus | After 10 weeks, the embryo is now referred to as a foetus

Although the foetus is only 2.5-3.5 cm long at this point, all major organs and systems have been formed |
| During weeks 10-12 | - the external genital organs are developing
- fingernails and toenails appear
- eyelids are forming
- foetal movement increases
- the arms and legs are fully formed
- the voice box (larynx) begins to form in the trachea |

Egg to embryo: a miraculous journey

Once a month, an egg is released from an ovary into a fallopian tube. After sexual intercourse, the sperm move from the vagina through the cervix and uterus to the Fallopian tubes, where one sperm fertilises the egg. The fertilised egg (zygote) divides repeatedly as it moves down the fallopian tube to the uterus. The zygote is a solid ball of cells. Then it becomes a hollow ball of cells called a blastocyst. Inside the uterus, the blastocyst implants in the wall of the uterus, where it develops into an embryo attached to a placenta and surrounded by fluid-filled membranes.

Further development of the foetus

12th week of pregnancy

By the time you are 12 weeks pregnant, the uterus can be felt at the lowest part of your abdomen, just above the pelvic bone. The foetus is 6-7 cm long. All internal organs are formed, but are not fully developed. Fingers and toes can be seen and soft nails begin to form. The skin develops and is almost transparent. Some hair can be seen. Bones and muscles begin to grow. The hands are more developed than the feet. The arms are longer than the legs. The genitalia start showing the difference between male and female gender. The foetus has jerky, unstructured movements. Remember, you won't feel these movements. You will start feeling them much later but they can be seen clearly on an ulrasound scan.

The foetus is most vulnerable during the first 12 weeks of pregnancy, as all of the major organs and body systems are forming. The foetus can be damaged if exposed to certain drugs, German measles, radiation or chemical and toxic substances.

Even though the organs and body systems are fully formed by the end of 12 weeks, the foetus is a long way from surviving independently outside the mother's womb.

16th week

By the end of the 16th week, the foetus weighs about 110 grams. The length is 15-17 cm. Eyebrows, eyelashes, and fingernails have formed. The foetus can bend its arms and legs. The genitalia have formed. The skin is wrinkled and the body is covered with a waxy coating **(vernix)** and fine hair **(lanugo)**. The outer ear begins to develop. The foetus can swallow. The kidneys begin to produce urine.

20th week

You are now in the midpoint of your pregnancy, since a normal pregnancy lasts 40 weeks. The foetus weighs about 300 grams. and from this week on, the weight begins to increase rapidly. The foetus is about 25 cm long. The sucking reflex develops. If the hand happens to be near the mouth, the foetus may suck his or her thumb, and even develops a pattern of sleeping and waking. The nails grow to the tips of the fingers. He or she is more active. This is probably the first time that you might feel the baby move.

If the foetus is female, all the eggs that she will ever have are already formed in the ovaries. In a male foetus, the testicles begin to descend from the abdomen into the scrotum.

24th week

By the end of the 24th week, the foetus weighs about 630 grams and is about 30 cm long. The skin is wrinkled and fat deposition begins under the skin. The head is still comparatively large and hair begins to grow. The eyebrows and eyelashes are usually recognisable. The brain development is rapid. The eyes begin to open. Finger and toe prints can be seen. The lungs are fully formed, though not yet functioning. The foetus can hear. A foetus born at this time might make some attempts at breathing but the lungs will not function effectively.

28th week

The foetus is about 35 cm long and weighs about 1,100 grams. The eyes can open and close and changes in light can be sensed. The lanugo hair begins to disappear. The thin skin is red and is covered with a waxy white layer called **vernix**. The foetus can make grasping motions and responds to sound. It kicks and stretches, so much so you might feel as if the baby is playing football in there!

32nd week

The foetus is roughly around 45 cm long and weighs approximately 1,800 grams. With its major development completed, the foetus gains weight quickly. The bones harden, but the skull remains soft and flexible for delivery. The different regions of the brain form. Taste buds develop and the foetus can taste sweet and sour. Occasionally, you might feel a rhythmic movement that lasts for short periods of time – this is your baby hiccupping!

36th week

On an average, the foetus will be 50 cm long and weighs between 1,800-2,500 grams, and will gain about 400-500 grams per week this month. The skin is less wrinkled. Because of deposition of fat under the skin, the body becomes more rounded and the face appears less wrinkled. The lungs mature and are ready to function on their own. The foetus usually turns into a head-down position for birth.

40th week

The foetus is considered to be full term at 40 weeks. Though weight at term varies, the average Indian baby will weigh between 2,500 and 3,000 grams.

When is my baby due?

The average duration of a pregnancy is 280 days or 40 weeks, counting from the first day of your last menstrual period. It can be hard to predict the exact date of delivery. Only five per cent of babies are born on their due dates. A normal range, however, is from about 259 days to as many as 294 days (37-42 weeks).

Women with irregular periods may require an ultrasound scan in early pregnancy to establish the actual due date. Even women with very regular periods may be asked to have an ultrasound scan in early pregnancy to confirm the age of a foetus and thereby, the due date. The due date should be confirmed as early in pregnancy as possible. Later, it becomes harder to set the due date accurately.

> The day your baby is due is called the **estimated date of confinement or EDC.** (The estimated date of delivery or EDD is also used sometimes.) Calculating the due date helps the obstetrician know which month of pregnancy you are in and to monitor the growth of the baby.

> The 40 weeks of pregnancy are divided into **three trimesters.** These last about 12–13 weeks each (or about 3 months):
> 1st trimester: 0–13 weeks (months 1–3)
> 2nd trimester: 14–27 weeks (months 4–6)
> 3rd trimester: 28–40 weeks (months 7–9)

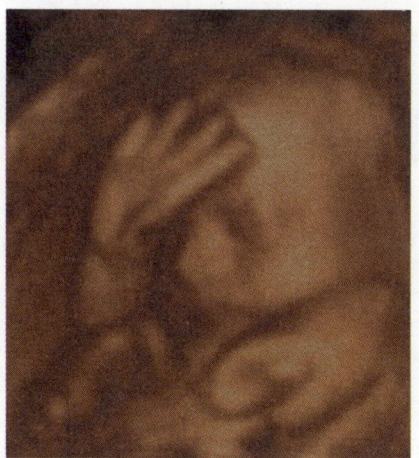

3D image of foetal face at 19 weeks

CHAPTER 2

Pre-pregnancy counselling

Smita has been married for a year and a half and had postponed a pregnancy because she and her husband are busy professionals. Now, they are ready for a baby, and have scheduled an appointment with an obstetrician for pre-pregnancy counselling (also called preconceptional care.)

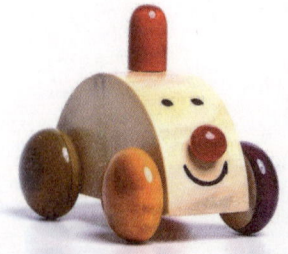

2 Pre-pregnancy counselling

What is pre-pregnancy counselling? Basically, it is a checklist for couples to make sure that they have a healthy pregnancy. Becoming a parent is a major decision. It brings with it its own uncertainty and apprehensions. Smita and her husband have made the right choice in seeking pre-pregnancy counselling.

Why is pre-pregnancy counselling important?

Planning your pregnancy can help you make sensible choices that will benefit both you and your baby. Most often, women do not realise they are pregnant until several weeks after they have conceived. The early weeks of foetal growth are crucial. During the early weeks, your health can affect your baby's growth.

During a preconceptional visit, your obstetrician will try to identify things that may pose risks to you or the baby you are planning to have. Keeping fit, eating healthy and avoiding certain things that could be harmful to the baby are the first steps to a healthy pregnancy.

Previous medical problems

Some women have medical problems such as diabetes, high blood pressure, anaemia, asthma, epilepsy or cardiovascular (heart and blood vessel) problems, which may increase risks for them or their foetus.

Diabetes

Women need to ensure tight control of their blood sugar levels during pregnancy. Women, who are on tablets for diabetes, may need to be switched to insulin. To avoid abnormalities in the baby, it is important that blood sugars at the time of conception are under strict control.

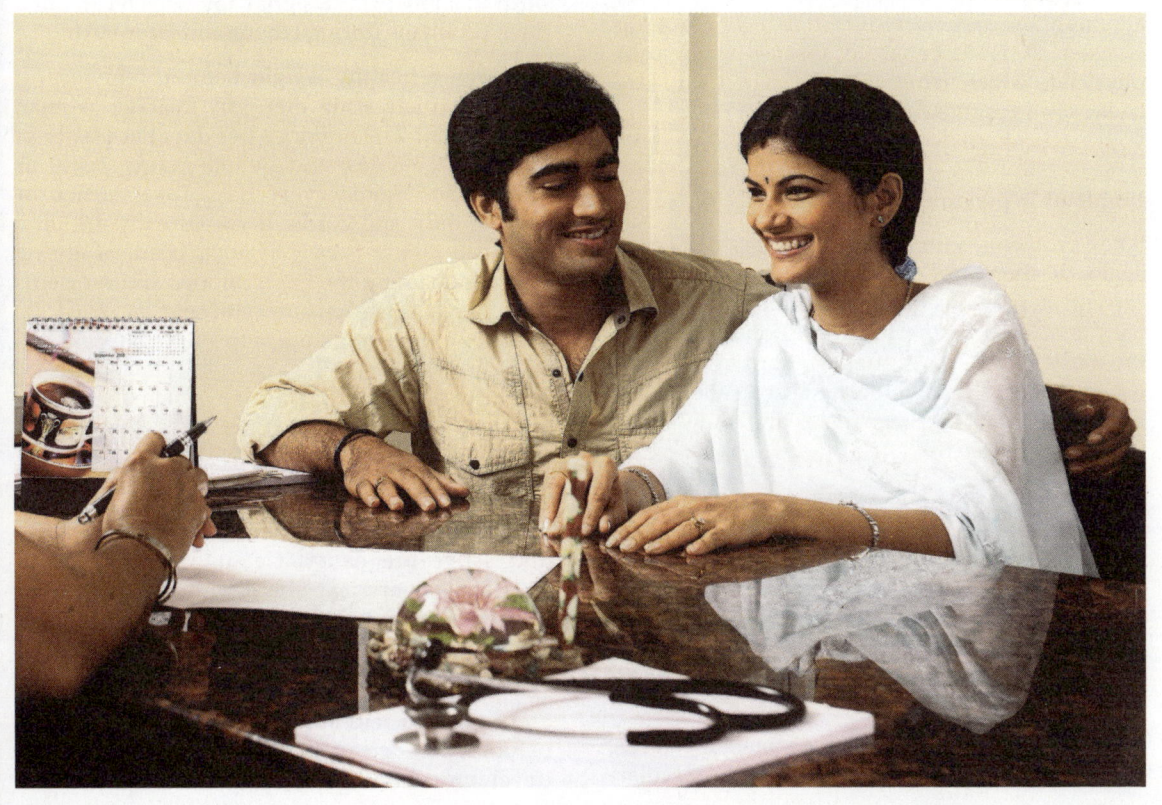

High blood pressure

If a woman has high blood pressure, it is important to make sure it is well under control before attempting pregnancy. Medications must be changed to those that are safe in pregnancy.

Anaemia

Anaemia due to iron deficiency is common in Indian women. Check your haemoglobin and if necessary start on iron supplementation.

Asthma

A high level of control is essential during pregnancy. Check with your doctor about which medications are safe when you are trying for a pregnancy. Inhalers, by and large, are safe because the medications do not get absorbed into the blood stream.

Epilepsy

It is safe for most epileptics on medications to try for a pregnancy. Most anti-epileptic drugs have the potential to cause foetal abnormalities although the risk is reduced if a single drug is used. It is essential to discuss with your physician which drug is safer when you are trying for a pregnancy. It is important not to stop your medication.

Problems in previous pregnancies

Some problems with past pregnancies can occur again. If there has been more than one miscarriage, a previous baby with a birth defect or a baby that died before birth or soon after birth, the obstetrician may suggest studies to find out the cause. It is important to keep all the records of previous pregnancies and show them to your obstetrician.

Family health history

Diabetes and high blood pressure are common conditions which may be present in the family. Even if the mother-to-be does not have these conditions, it is important to know if there is a family history because these conditions may show up in pregnancy.

Some genetic conditions such as mental retardation, cystic fibrosis, thalassaemia and muscular dystrophy, may run in the family. If there is a history of such a condition, then genetic counselling might be offered to help the couple find out the chances of having a child with a birth defect.

Optimising pre-pregnancy health

Being overweight or underweight before pregnancy may lead to problems in pregnancy. A healthy, balanced diet and regular exercise will ensure an optimal weight.

Being overweight can lead to high blood pressure or diabetes in pregnancy. It also puts a strain on the heart. Women who are obese have a greater chance of facing problems, posing risks for the baby as well as the mother. Remember that large women tend to have large babies and large babies may have trouble fitting through the birth canal, thus increasing the chances of having a caesarean.

Being underweight too can cause problems in pregnancy. It may increase the chances of giving birth to a low birth weight baby, which can often have problems during labour and after birth.

To reach a healthy weight before pregnancy, it helps to plan your diet. An average woman needs about 2,000 calories per day. Eat plenty of fruits, vegetables and whole-grains such as channa and rajma every day. Take fat-free or low-fat milk and curds. If you already are on a balanced diet, it is easy to make changes during pregnancy to get the extra calories and nutrients you need. Also ensure you get at least 30 minutes of brisk walking, 4 to 5 days a week.

Keeping fit

Good health depends on a balanced diet combined with exercise. Keeping fit and doing regular exercise even before you conceive, can improve your chances of having a comfortable and active pregnancy. Get into the habit of a brisk walk everyday. Check with your doctor on how active you can be after you get pregnant.

Vitamins and minerals

Starting **folic acid supplementation** 1-3 months before a planned pregnancy is important for the development of the baby's brain and spinal cord.

Calcium is important for both baby and mother. Milk and curds are a good natural source of calcium. **Iron** keeps the mother from developing anaemia during pregnancy. It is a good idea to have a blood test to rule out anaemia. If the haemoglobin levels are low, then an iron supplement should be taken for three months or more to ensure that the iron stores in the body are replenished and maintained.

Folic acid is present in
- Dark, leafy greens and vegetables
- Citrus fruits and juices (such as oranges)
- Organ meats (such as liver)
- Dried lentils (such as rajma, kabuli channa, black-eyed peas)
- Vitamin supplements

Preventing infections

Rubella or German measles is a viral infection which can cause severe abnormalities in the baby, especially if it occurs in the first three months of pregnancy. A woman planning to get pregnant should either be tested to see if she already has immunity or should directly be vaccinated against Rubella. It is important to avoid pregnancy for three months after the vaccination.

Viral hepatitis: It is useful to be vaccinated against Hepatitis B. If you already have Hepatitis B, inform your obstetrician so that she can take the appropriate steps to ensure your baby does not get affected.

Planning for insurance and maternity leave

Make sure your insurance covers pregnancy and complications which might arise from it. It is a good idea to find out how much maternity leave is allowed by your employer. This will help plan for family support after the delivery.

If you are going to your mother's house for delivery, do not postpone travelling till too late. If you are working or your first child is going to school and you want to travel as late as possible, remember that the optimum time to travel would be about six weeks before your due date i.e. 34 weeks. Check with your doctor if there is any condition which may require you to go to your new obstetrician earlier than that. It is in the last six weeks that the majority of complications can occur so it is safer to get to wherever you are going before that. This also gives you enough time to build a rapport with the obstetrician who is going to deliver you.

Pre-pregnancy check list

What to do before pregnancy to help you and your baby
- Take folic acid.
- Get a pre-pregnancy check-up, including a dental check-up.
- Eat right.
- Maintain a healthy weight and get fit.
- Avoid infections.
- Avoid hazardous substances and chemicals.
- Check for a family history of genetically transmitted problems.
- Avoid stress.
- If you smoke, stop smoking and avoid passive smoking.
- If you consume alcohol, stop drinking.

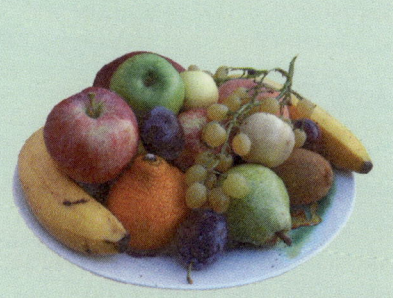

CHAPTER 3

Am I pregnant?

Stella is excited and overjoyed. She and her husband have been trying for a pregnancy for the past few months. She has just missed her period. Is she really pregnant?

Samhita has irregular periods. She has missed her periods by more than the usual time. She feels tired all the time and is plagued with nausea. Just yesterday, she almost threw up at the smell of fried potatoes, one of her favourite foods. Could she be pregnant?

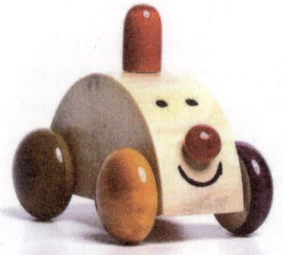

Am I pregnant?

One of the most commonly asked questions by women is, "Am I pregnant?" Even if they have never been pregnant before, most women are aware of the symptoms of early pregnancy. Women who have been pregnant before will recognise the symptoms which occurred in their previous pregnancy. Surprisingly though, some women may have severe symptoms during one pregnancy and hardly any in the next. The fact is that each pregnancy is different and a woman may not have the same symptoms or the same intensity of symptoms during each of her pregnancies.

When to suspect a pregnancy

Missing a period
This is one of the most common reasons for suspecting a pregnancy. Women who have regular periods will take this as the first sign of pregnancy. Only a urine or blood pregnancy test, followed by a pelvic exam, can confirm a pregnancy. Occasionally a period can be delayed due to hormonal problems, even in the absence of pregnancy. If you are trying for a pregnancy, keep track of your periods. Mark the first day of your period on a calendar, as that is what determines the due date of the pregnancy.

Why is a period missed?
Every month, signals from the brain cause the hormone **estrogen** to be released from the ovary. Estrogen acts on the lining of the uterus (endometrium). The endometrium responds by getting thicker and spongier in anticipation of a pregnancy. Most women produce an egg around the middle of the cycle, usually between the 11th and 16th day. Following this, the ovary produces the hormone **progesterone.** When the egg does not get fertilised in that cycle, the level of progesterone drops and the lining of the uterus is shed, leading to menstruation. In fact, the menstrual period has been described as 'the bloody tears of a disappointed uterus'! When fertilisation occurs, the levels of progesterone and estrogen rise dramatically and the lining of the uterus continues to get thicker to receive the embryo. In this case, the period is missed.

Calculating the due date
The due date is based on the assumption that the conception occurred exactly 2 weeks after the first day of the last period. The method used by

> Some women may have severe symptoms in one pregnancy and hardly any in the next.

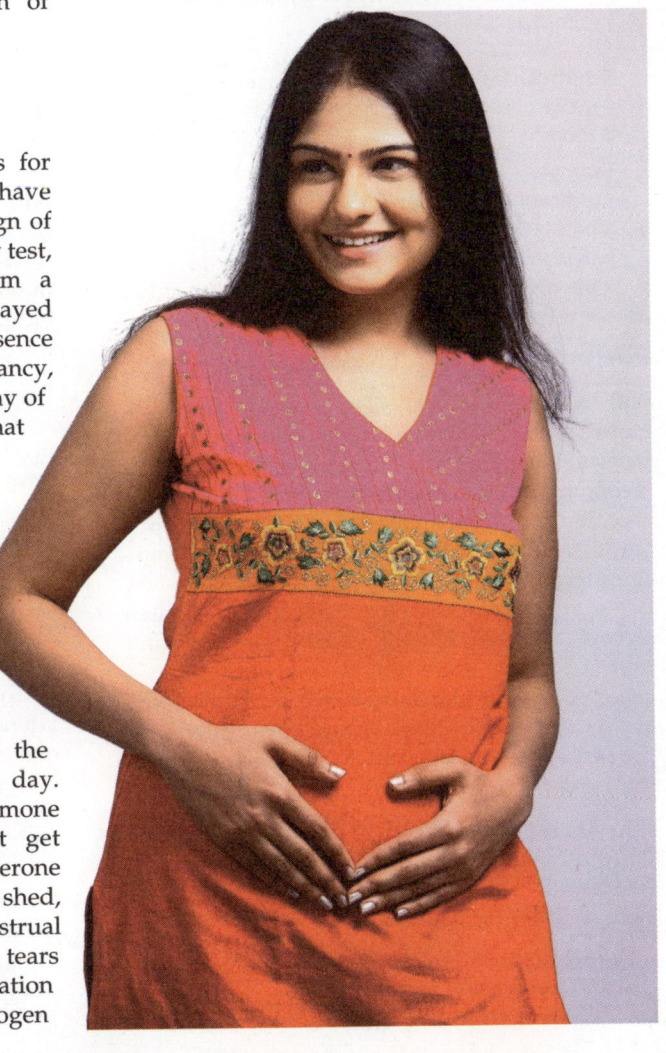

obstetricians around the world is to **add 7 days and subtract 3 months from the date of the first day of the last menstrual period.** For example, if the last menstrual period began on June 1, 2007, the due date is calculated as follows: June 1 + 7 days = June 8. June 8 minus 3 months = March 8. Therefore the estimated due date would be March 8, 2008.

> The **first day** of the last period is used to calculate the due date of delivery.

A normal pregnancy usually lasts 280 days (40 weeks). 37-40 weeks of pregnancy is called a 'term or full-term pregnancy'. If your periods are irregular, an early ultrasound scan may be done to fix the due date.

> **Formula for calculating due date:**
> 1st day of last period + 7 days minus 3 months
>
> Example:
> 1st day of last period: June 1
> June 1 + 7 days   =   June 8
> June 8 – 3 months   =   March 8
> **Therefore, your due date is March 8**

Swollen, tender or sore breasts and/or nipples

This is often the first sign of pregnancy. The breasts and/or nipples are often particularly painful during a first pregnancy. After the second month, the breasts start increasing in size and delicate veins may start being visible just beneath the skin. The nipples can become considerably larger, darker and can be very sore. Later on in pregnancy, the areola (the dark area around the nipple) will become broader and much darker. There are several tiny glands called sebaceous glands scattered throughout the areola. These become more prominent as pregnancy progresses and form tiny bumps on the areola.

Why are the breasts tender and sore?

The reason breasts and/or nipples are often sore, swollen or tender during early pregnancy is because there is an increased production of estrogen and progesterone. The breasts undergo changes to prepare for breastfeeding. The milk-producing glands within the breasts respond to the hormones and start enlarging.

Exhaustion or unusual tiredness

It is normal for a woman to feel extremely fatigued during the first 2-3 months of pregnancy. There is an intense desire to sleep and waking up seems to be a difficult proposition. This can become difficult and frustrating, especially for working women or for women who have to take care of another child. You will just not be able to find any energy to do your normal chores. It is not unusual to have a good night's sleep but still wake up groggy, lethargic and exhausted.

It is important to rest whenever possible. Learn to listen to your body and allow some periods of rest during the day. Don't overwhelm yourself with too many chores. Order out for food or have family and friends help out by sending food. Try to have early nights and get your full quota of sleep. Your husband can take your older child/ children out for a few hours so you have some respite and peace.

Relax! These symptoms only last for the first 12-14 weeks of pregnancy. Once your body gets used to the huge metabolic changes caused by hormones, these symptoms will subside. Soon you will feel energetic and some women actually say they "don't feel pregnant anymore"!

Why do you feel tired and exhausted?

These symptoms are caused by progesterone, which is produced in large amounts. This hormone can make a woman feel tired and intensely sleepy. In some cases, the tiredness may be compounded by the stress of daily living. If a woman has to go to work, she might also have to cook in the morning. If this is not your first pregnancy, you may feel constantly exhausted because your other child/children also need your attention.

> The breasts and/or nipples are often particularly painful during a first pregnancy.

> A husband who pitches in and allows his wife to sleep in a little longer, is worth his weight in gold!

Pregnancy tests

Urine pregnancy tests

These tests measure the levels of human chorionic gonadotropin (hCG), a hormone secreted during pregnancy, in your urine. The amount of urine each test can detect varies widely. The amount of hormone each woman produces may also vary, but not as widely. The home pregnancy kits commonly available in the market will measure 25-50 mIUs of hCG, which is usually the amount found in urine between the 4th and 5th weeks of pregnancy. First morning urine will always contain the highest concentration of hCG. However, most tests do not require that you use first morning urine. Wait four hours after you last urinated to take the test. This will allow hCG to build up in your urine. These tests are usually accurate but sometimes a false result can be obtained. A negative test which then turns out to be a pregnancy is usually the result of the test being performed too early. A false-positive test is a test where the test comes out positive even when you are not pregnant. Talk to your doctor if you have questions about your pregnancy test.

Blood pregnancy tests

Occasionally, your doctor might ask for a blood test to confirm your pregnancy or to determine if the pregnancy is growing normally. The weekly increase in the level of hCG in the blood usually follows a specific pattern. The level in the blood peaks between 60 and 80 days of pregnancy. The levels of hCG in your urine and blood will be different.

Levels of hCG in the blood

From conception	(mIU/ml or IU/L)
7 days	0 to 5
14 days	3 to 426
21 days	18 to 7,340
28 days	1,080 to 56,500
35 - 42 days	7,650 to 229,000
43 - 64 days	25,700 to 288,000
57 - 78 days	13,300 to 253,000
17 - 24 weeks	4,060 to 65,400
25 wks to term	3,640 to 117,000
4-6 weeks after delivery	nonpregnant levels (<5)

Nausea and vomiting

Nausea, with or without vomiting, is most common in the first three months of pregnancy. Unfortunately, some women experience this symptom almost throughout the pregnancy. Most women become oversensitive to smells and almost anything can trigger a bout of nausea and vomiting. The most common foods to trigger morning sickness are coffee, milk products, spicy and strong smelling foods and non-vegetarian dishes. Many women find that the nausea is precipitated on brushing their teeth.

Typically, the nausea starts around six weeks of pregnancy (or about two weeks after the period was due). Some women start experiencing nausea just a few days after missing the period. The symptoms may continue until about 12 to 14 weeks of pregnancy. However, morning sickness may start later than six weeks and may continue until 16 to 20 weeks of the pregnancy.

About 90 per cent of women will have relief by 22 weeks. Occasionally, some women may find a recurrence of the nausea in the last one or two months of pregnancy. This is usually due to increased acidity and the pressure of the growing baby on the stomach. Morning sickness may make you feel constantly nauseous or come as bouts of nausea at different times of the day. As for the vomiting, some women may vomit almost continuously whereas some may vomit without warning, usually in response to a particular smell.

> Though called morning sickness, it should really be called 'anytime sickness' because in 80 per cent of women, the nausea lasts throughout the day.

Increased salivation can occur by itself but it is usually associated with nausea and vomiting in early pregnancy. Some women also complain of bitter or metallic tasting saliva.

Most women will suffer partial or complete suppression of appetite because of the nausea, and will not gain weight initially and may even lose weight. This is quite normal though you and your husband might feel anxious that the baby is not getting enough nutrition. Actually, the foetus is not at all affected by your lack of appetite and poor intake of food. The pregnancy will only be affected if you have intractable vomiting and lose 4-5 kilos, which can happen with hyperemesis gravidarum.

What is hyperemesis gravidarum?

When the vomiting becomes uncontrollable, a woman might get dehydrated and require hospitalisation. Intractable vomiting is called **hyperemesis gravidarum.** There can be excessive loss of weight associated with hyperemesis gravidarum.

What causes nausea and vomiting?

The most common reason for this symptom is the rapid rise in estrogen and human chorionic gonadotropin (hCG), produced in large quantities in pregnancy. Since women carrying twins or triplets produce higher levels of these hormones, they can experience more severe morning sickness.

The nausea and vomiting can be aggravated by the increased acidity and low blood sugar which results from poor intake of food. Eating small quantities of food at frequent intervals can improve the symptoms. Dry, non-oily food is better than spicy, oily food. Salt biscuits, dry toast and bland food like idlis will be better tolerated.

Persistent emotional stress can often be accompanied by nausea and vomiting. This can make the situation even more difficult to deal with. The nausea may continue until after the pregnancy progresses beyond a certain point in time, or even until your baby is born. Sharing your fears with others you trust or seeking professional advice may be helpful.

Lower abdominal discomfort and cramping

Lower abdominal discomfort and cramping, similar to cramping during periods, occurs early in pregnancy. This happens because the uterus begins to expand as the baby grows. This discomfort can continue for the first few months and can get worse on getting up after sitting down for a while, or on turning from side to side while lying down. This pain is normal and does not need bed rest. If the pain occurs or worsens on walking briskly for a while, just rest for a few minutes and then continue walking.

> In early pregnancy, mild lower abdominal discomfort is common and does not signal an impending abortion.

Later on in pregnancy, some women experience pain on one or both sides of the lower abdomen. This is because of the stretching of the round ligaments which hold the uterus in position. Lying on the side of the pain relieves the stretching of the round ligament and therefore, will offer respite from the pain.

Frequent urination

In early pregnancy, there will be a frequent urge to pass urine. The bladder seems to fill up in no time at all and a woman will feel like using the bathroom very frequently. This usually eases off around 16 weeks but will recur in the last few weeks of pregnancy.

What causes frequent urination?

This problem is caused by the growing uterus pressing against the bladder. This symptom is worse in early and late pregnancy. Sometimes, women lose a few drops of urine on sneezing or coughing. This will usually disappear a few months after delivery.

Headaches

Headaches during pregnancy are often intense and occur usually in the early months of pregnancy. Though some of these headaches can be caused by eye strain or sinusitis, the vast majority have no known cause. Paracetamol can be taken for the headaches. Women who suffer from migraine may find the condition aggravated in pregnancy. This is because of the rise in the levels of estrogen.

Other symptoms

Mood swings are common in early pregnancy. Due to the sudden and huge increase of pregnancy hormones, women will face emotional ups and downs. It is common for a pregnant woman to burst into tears or get angry and upset for no apparent reason. This may leave her husband and family bewildered and a little concerned, but this phase is usually short lived. Once the body gets used to the surge of hormones, the emotional roller-coaster ride ends and stability usually returns.

Feeling weak, faint or dizzy is common in early and late pregnancy. In pregnancy, there is a great deal of dilatation of the blood vessels. This also leads to pooling of blood in the veins of the legs on standing for a long time. This can cause sudden dizziness or may even lead to fainting. When this happens, it is best to lie down for a few minutes with your feet raised on a pillow or cushion.

Feeling feverish and cold in the first few weeks of the pregnancy is something many women will complain about because the basal body temperature rises. This symptom will usually subside by the fourth month.

Constipation is a result of poor intake of food and fluids in the early weeks. Many women find that they cannot tolerate fluids, even water, due to the nausea. Therefore, even women who had normal bowel habits before pregnancy might find that they are having hard stools. This can lead to pain while passing stools and even bleeding. Increasing the intake of fluids and a reasonable amount of exercise will resolve the problem. If the nausea does not allow the increase in fluids, your obstetrician might prescribe a mild laxative. Later on, the intake of iron supplements can also aggravate constipation. Make sure you take enough fluids, fresh fruits and raw vegetables (as in salads) to relieve this problem.

Increased vaginal discharge results from increased mucus discharge from the cervix. It can be uncomfortable but is a normal and common symptom in early pregnancy. You need treatment only if the increased vaginal discharge is associated with itching or burning. When those symptoms are present, then you might have a vaginal infection. This will require treatment with specific antibiotics and local applications. **(See Chapter 39: Urinary tract infection and vaginal infection).**

Old wives' tales

- If the foetus has a lot of hair, vomiting will increase - **Not true!**
- If you don't eat well in the first three months of pregnancy, the baby will be affected - **Not true!**
- You should be under complete bed rest in the first three months of pregnancy - **Not true!**
- You should not climb stairs in the first three months of pregnancy - **Not true!**
- You should not eat papayas, mangoes or pineapples because they may cause an abortion - **Not true!**

CHAPTER 4

A visit to your obstetrician

Sabeeha is excited. She suspects she is pregnant. She and her husband have fixed an appointment with her obstetrician. She has apprehensions that she hopes her obstetrician will clear.

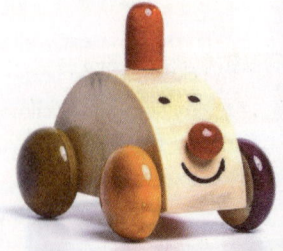

4 A visit to your obstetrician

The first visit

Your first visit to the obstetrician is an important milestone in your pregnancy. It is during this visit that your pregnancy will be confirmed. Usually this visit should be scheduled about six to eight weeks after your last period. You might need an earlier appointment if you have a medical condition, have had problems with a pregnancy in the past or are having symptoms such as vaginal bleeding, abdominal pain or severe nausea and vomiting. If you are taking any medication or think you may have been exposed to a hazardous substance, then schedule an early appointment.

In your apprehension and excitement, you may tend to forget your questions and doubts about the pregnancy. Make sure you jot down any queries you have so that you can have them answered. (You can use the pages provided in the **For You** section at the back of this book.)

The first visit is usually the longest. Your obstetrician will ask you several questions. From the date of your last period, she will calculate the expected date of delivery. She will find out if you have any symptoms such as nausea or vomiting, breast tenderness, frequent urination and excess sleepiness. This will help her in confirming your pregnancy. If you have some symptoms which might be alarming, for example spotting or bleeding from the birth passage, she might perform an ultrasound examination to confirm that the pregnancy is healthy.

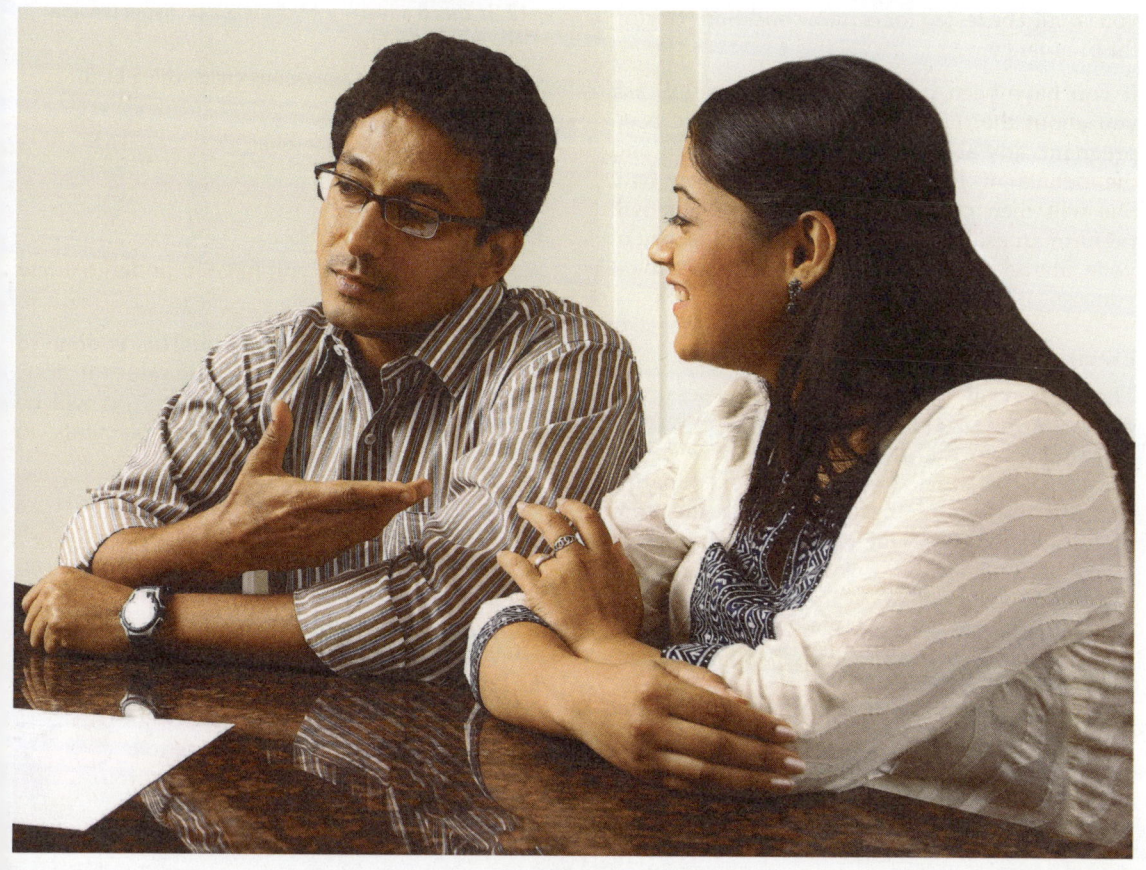

If this is your first pregnancy, you will be called a **primigravida**. A **multigravida** is one who has been pregnant more than once. A **primipara** is a woman who has delivered a child once.
A **multipara** is one who has delivered more than once.

If you have any medical conditions for which you are already on medications, let your obstetrician know at the first visit. Conditions such as asthma, epilepsy, hypothyroidism or hyperthyroidism, diabetes and hypertension might require modification of your medications. At the same time, make sure you do not abruptly stop your medications just because you are pregnant.

You will also be asked about your family's medical history. The emphasis will be on the presence of diabetes, hypertension and hereditary conditions. If you have any family history which worries you, this is the time to discuss it. Your family medical history will let your obstetrician know if you should be tested for certain conditions during the pregnancy.

If you have been pregnant before, she will ask you about the number of times you have been pregnant, any abortions you may have had and the details of the type of delivery you had. She will then confirm the pregnancy. She will perform an examination to determine the size of your uterus which will tell her how pregnant you are.

Examination of the uterine size

The first visit usually involves assessment of the uterine size to determine if the pregnancy corresponds to the dates that you have given. Your obstetrician will do an internal examination and feel the size of the uterus. After the third month of pregnancy, the examination is usually of the abdomen only. This is because, after the third month of pregnancy, the uterus can be felt abdominally. The doctor will examine the size of the uterus to know whether the baby is growing well or not.

Some questions you might be asked during your first visit:

1. What is the pattern of your periods?
2. When was your last menstrual period?
3. Do you take any medicines on a regular basis?
4. Do you have any allergies or health problems?
5. Have you been exposed to any infections?
6. What type of birth control have you used?
7. Have you been pregnant before?
8. Have you ever had a miscarriage?
9. Have you ever had an induced abortion?
10. If you have had a baby before:
    What did the baby weigh at birth?
    How long did labour last?
    Was it a caesarean delivery? Why was it done?
    Were there any problems?
11. Is there a history of birth defects in your family?
12. Is there a history of diabetes or hypertension in your family?
13. Have you had a previous child with a birth defect?
14. Do you drink or smoke?

Preliminary blood tests

At the first visit, you will have to undergo a few blood tests:

Haematocrit and haemoglobin: This is done to find out if you are anaemic. If these values are low, you are considered to be anaemic. You will be given iron and multivitamin supplements to improve your blood count.

Blood group and Rh typing: Your blood type can be A, B, AB or O. It can be Rh positive or Rh negative. If your blood lacks the Rh antigen, you are considered to be Rh negative. If it has the antigen, you are Rh positive. Problems can arise when the foetus is Rh positive and the mother is Rh negative. The mother's immune system

Write down any information you think is important for the obstetrician to know. Take along your records from a previous pregnancy, if you have had one. Do jot down any questions and doubts you have so that you can have them cleared.

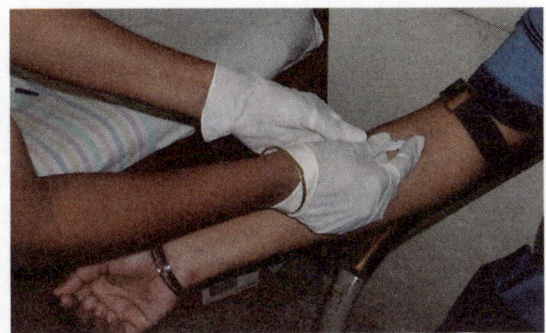

becomes sensitised to the Rh factor from the baby's blood and can create antibodies. These antibodies enter the baby's blood stream and destroy its blood cells leading to severe anaemia and water retention. The foetus can be severely affected. **(See Chapter 35: Rh factor: how it can affect pregnancy).**

Hepatitis B virus: This virus is present in the blood of infected individuals. If you have it, you can pass it to your baby. After the baby is born, you may be given a drug to help treat the virus. Your baby will be given an immunoglobulin and a vaccine against the virus after birth.

VDRL or RPR are tests for syphilis, a highly infectious disease caused by bacteria. Though rare, it can cause abnormalities in the baby.

Human immunodeficiency virus (HIV): HIV is a virus that attacks certain cells of the body's immune system and causes AIDS (Acquired Immunodeficiency Syndrome). If the mother has HIV, there is a chance that it can be passed to the baby. During pregnancy and delivery, the mother can be given medication to help reduce the risk of transmission to the baby.

Urine test

At each antenatal visit, you will be asked to give a sample of your urine for testing. Urine is tested for **sugar** and **protein (albumin).** Although the presence of sugar in the urine may be normal in pregnancy, high levels could be a sign of diabetes. Protein in the urine may be present if you have a urinary tract infection, kidney disease or high blood pressure that occurs in late pregnancy. The urine test is also used to check for infections of the bladder and kidneys. If these problems occur, they can be treated.

Testing for diabetes

Later in pregnancy, usually between 24 and 28 weeks of pregnancy, you may be tested for diabetes. This test is important for all women since diabetes is particularly common in Indians. If you have had a history of diabetes in your previous pregnancy, you might be tested during the first visit itself.

Testing for Down syndrome

Down syndrome is the commonest cause of mental retardation in humans. It is caused by the presence of an extra chromosome 21. Since it can occur at any age, all women should ideally undergo testing for it. The risk for Down syndrome increases with age. Therefore, women 35 years or older should definitely ask their obstetrician about this test. **(See Chapter 11: Tests in pregnancy: how do I know my baby is normal?).**

> **Down syndrome** is the commonest cause of mental retardation in humans. It is tested for with the first trimester screen or with the triple test.

During the first trimester, you may undergo a blood test that is done between 11 and 14 weeks. Combined with a **nuchal translucency screening** (the measurement of the foetal skin overlying the neck), the blood test and the ultrasound are known as the **first trimester screening for Down syndrome.**

In the second trimester, you may be offered the **triple screening or triple test,** done between 15 and 20 weeks of pregnancy.

If the screening test comes back as positive, you will have to undergo a test of the amniotic fluid surrounding the baby. This test is called an **amniocentesis. (See Chapter 13: Special tests in pregnancy).**

Listening to the foetal heartbeat

The foetal heartbeat can be heard from the third month using an electronic device called the Doppler device. If a regular stethoscope is used, then the heartbeat can be heard only from the fifth month onwards. Listening to the foetal heartbeat reassures us that the foetus is healthy and well.

Checking your blood pressure

During every visit, your blood pressure will be checked. The obstetrician looks for an abnormal rise in the pressure. There is truly no condition called 'low blood pressure'. The normal blood pressure for Indian women ranges between 90/60 mm of Hg and 120/80 mm of Hg. When the blood pressure is 140/90 mm of Hg and higher, high blood pressure is diagnosed.

Checking your weight

Your weight will be recorded at every check-up. It is normal to gain half to one kilo during each month of your pregnancy. A weight gain of about 10 to 12 kilos is considered normal for the entire pregnancy. If your weight gain is poor, the size of the baby may be small. If you gain too much weight, it increases the risk of developing diabetes in pregnancy, particularly if you are already prone to getting it. Also, if you have gain more weight than you should have, it will be difficult to lose the excess weight gained during the pregnancy.

Ultrasound examination

Your obstetrician may ask for an ultrasound examination in the first trimester to confirm the presence of a pregnancy, the size of the foetus and the number of foetuses present. An ultrasound scan is recommended at 11-14 weeks and 20-24 weeks of pregnancy. If necessary, an ultrasound examination might be repeated in the third trimester. **(See Chapter 12: Ultrasound scans in pregnancy).**

Repeat visits

Usually, you will be asked to come for a monthly check-up till the 28th to 32nd week of pregnancy. After that, you will have a check-up every two weeks. In the last month of pregnancy, you will be asked to come for weekly check-ups. Closer to your delivery date, your obstetrician may do an internal examination at each visit. This helps her determine whether the cervix (mouth of the uterus) is starting to thin out and dilate. She will also assess how far the baby's head has moved into the birth passage. If there is any complication in the pregnancy, you might be asked to come for more frequent visits.

The baby's head is engaged or fixed: what does that mean?

As the pregnancy crosses 37 weeks, the baby gets into the head-down position and starts entering the birth passage. Your obstetrician will assess how far the baby has dropped into the birth passage. When the baby reaches a certain point in the birth passage (the level of the ischial spines) the head is considered to be **engaged** or **fixed.** This is a good sign because it indicates that the baby's head fits well inside your pelvis and a vaginal delivery should be possible. However, just because the head is engaged does not mean that the baby is going to be born immediately. In women who have already had a baby earlier, the head may not get engaged till just immediately before labour. In some women the head might even get engaged after labour starts.

Tetanus toxoid immunisation:

The baby is born with no immunity to any infection. Tetanus is a dreaded, though extremely rare, infection which the baby can acquire at birth. During your pregnancy, you will be immunised with two doses of tetanus toxoid, six weeks apart, so that you can pass on your immunity to the baby. Some doctors will give the tetanus toxoid every month for three months. After the baby is born, he will receive immunisation against tetanus, along with other immunisations.

Optimise your visit to the obstetrician

- Note down any problems you have had between your last visit and now. In the short time you have with the obstetrician, you might forget to clear your doubts unless you have written down the problems. This is useful for both you and the obstetrician. It is no use going home and worrying about something: it is best to allay your fears while you are there.
- Listen carefully to instructions for any medicines which are being prescribed for you.
- Obstetricians are careful about any medicines which are prescribed to a pregnant woman but do not hesitate to check with her if you have any concerns.
- Don't forget to tell the doctor about known allergies you have to any medication.
- Take all reports of blood tests and ultrasound scans for each visit.
- Have only one person (preferably your husband) accompany you for the visit. When there are more people in the room (your parents, your in-laws), then they might be busy clearing their doubts and you will be left with no time to ask your own questions.

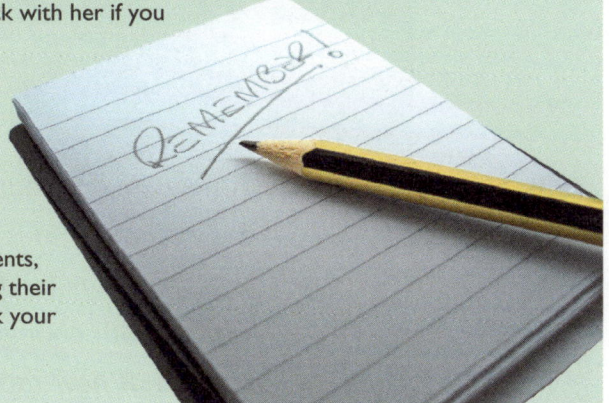

Checklist for tests and procedures in pregnancy

This is just a short checklist. Your obstetrician will guide you on everything else that is required especially for you.

First trimester
- Blood tests
- Ultrasound scan to look for age, growth and nuchal thickness.
- First trimester screening for Down syndrome (if available)

Second trimester
- Testing for diabetes in pregnancy
- Second trimester screening for Down syndrome (if not done in the first trimester)
- Ultrasound scan for foetal anomalies
- Immunisation for tetanus

Third trimester
- Ultrasound scan, if recommended by obstetrician
- Labour preparation class

CHAPTER 5

The first trimester (0-13 weeks)

A new life has found a home in your womb and is growing and developing day by day. It is a time filled with changes. You are amazed at how rapidly your body is adapting itself to provide a safe home for this new being. Your body is also preparing itself to nourish and nurture this baby after it is born.

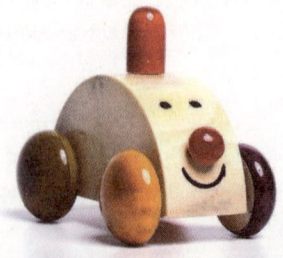

5 The first trimester (0-13 weeks)

To be equipped to take care of the growing baby inside you and yourself, you need to be aware of all the alterations and adaptations that your body is undergoing.

The most dramatic changes and development of the foetus occur during the first trimester. During the first 10 weeks, the growing baby is called an **embryo**. After 10 weeks, the **foetus** develops rapidly and by the end of the first trimester, it measures an average of 6-7 cm in length.

Week-by-week changes in mother and baby

Let us look at what happens to both you and the foetus. We will discuss the changes happening simultaneously in you and within you. We will count from the first day of the last period.

Week 1

Mother

You started your period on the first day of this week. This will be the last period you will have for at least the next nine or ten months. If you breastfeed, your periods might get postponed even more and you may not have a period for six to nine months after the delivery.

We start counting the weeks of the pregnancy from the first day of the last period because it is impossible to pinpoint the day ovulation and conception actually occur. Most women will remember the first day of their last period. If you are trying for a pregnancy, it is a good idea to note the first day of your periods on a calendar or a diary.

If you are planning to become pregnant, now is the time to improve your diet and add vitamin supplements such as folic acid and iron.

Week 2

Mother

Preparing for conception:

- Your last period is now over. Your uterus is lined with a new layer of cells to support and nourish your soon-to-be-conceived baby.
- An egg is growing in one of your ovaries. Soon it will ripen to the right size and you will ovulate.
- There is a surge in the estrogen levels accompanying ovulation. Many women find that they are at their peak level of energy and creativity during this week of their cycle.

Week 3

Mother

Congratulations! You are pregnant.

- Ovulation and conception will occur sometime during this week. One of your ovaries ripens and releases an egg (ovum). Pulled in by the finger-like projections of the fallopian tube, it begins its journey toward the uterus.
- During intercourse, your partner will ejaculate anywhere from 100 to 250 million sperm. If the conditions are just right with your cervical fluid, some of those sperm can live up to five days.

The first trimester :	0-13 weeks
The second trimester :	14-27 weeks
The third trimester :	28-40 weeks
Gestational age :	Weeks are counted from the first day of the last period
Conceptional age :	Weeks are counted from the age of conception, so conceptional age will be two weeks less than the gestational age.

In this book, we will use only gestational age i.e.
the weeks starting from the first day of the last period.

- Only about 200 sperm will actually make it through the uterus and into the correct Fallopian tube, eventually encountering the ovum.
- Sometime between 12 and 24 hours after you ovulate, a sperm (two in the case of twins) will break through the outer layers of the ovum and complete conception.
- Your progesterone levels will start increasing this week. High levels of progesterone keep the uterus quiescent, making it less likely to cramp. This helps the pregnancy continue. That is why progesterone is often called the **hormone of pregnancy.**
- Over the next seven days, the fertilised egg will move down the fallopian tube to the uterus. Once it reaches the uterine cavity, the embryo which is a ball of cells by now, will burrow into the lining of the uterus. You may experience a little bloody spotting at the time of this implantation. This is called **implantation bleed.** Some women may mistake this for a period.

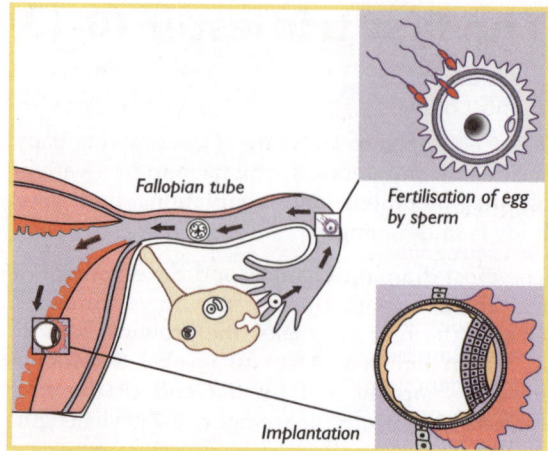

The process of fertilisation and implantation

Week 4
Mother
- If you have been trying for a pregnancy, you should avoid any medication at this point because some medications can be harmful to the developing embryo. If you need to take any medication, tell your doctor that you might be pregnant.
- Some women notice a metallic taste in their mouth, though no one knows the reason for this. It may probably be caused by the surge in hormonal levels.

Baby
- Although you are as yet unaware that you are pregnant, your baby is already undergoing great changes. The fertilised egg is now a quickly growing ball of cells called a **blastocyst.** It is embedded more deeply in the uterine wall and the amniotic cavity is being formed. The group of cells that will make up the placenta is being organised and circulatory networks containing maternal blood are being formed.
- Three layers of cells are forming within the blastocyst. The **ectoderm** will form the nervous system, hair and skin of your baby. The **endoderm** will become the lining of the gastrointestinal tract, and various organs such

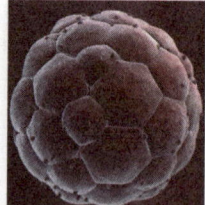

Blastocyst

The pregnancy test

Most chemical tests for pregnancy detect the presence of the **beta subunit of human chorionic gonadotropin (hCG).** A urine test can detect them as early as the 4-5th week from the first day of the last menstrual period. In most cases, the test is sensitive enough to detect pregnancy even on the day of the missed period. In some women though, the levels of hCG are not detectable so early. It is, in fact, advisable to wait a couple of days to a week after missing your period, before you perform the test. This will help avoid a falsely negative test.

Home pregnancy kits are easy to use and most require you to hold the strip in the urine stream. A specific change in colour in the line or dot will indicate a pregnancy.

Blood tests are more sensitive and may be ordered by your doctor if you have undergone treatment for infertility or if there is a doubt that the pregnancy may not be growing normally.

as thyroid, liver and pancreas. The **mesoderm** will develop into the skeleton, connective tissues, blood systems, urogenital system and most of the muscles.

Week 5
Mother
Am I pregnant?

- Your period is delayed and you are starting to wonder if you are pregnant. A pregnancy test can be positive at this point. A home pregnancy kit can be used. Don't be surprised if the pregnancy test comes negative. It will turn positive only when the hCG level reaches a certain threshold so you can repeat the test again after a few days.

- Your breasts become tender, particularly over the nipples. Due to congestion of blood in your pelvis, you may need to urinate more frequently than usual. Also, you may notice that you are more tired than usual. This is not surprising since your body is going through several physical and chemical changes.

- You may begin to experience nausea or vomiting. Many women feel this only in the morning, but some may have to deal with it all day long.

Baby

- Your baby is now an embryo with a little tail at the end of its developing spine and is only barely visible to the naked eye.

- The spinal column, brain and heart have begun to develop.

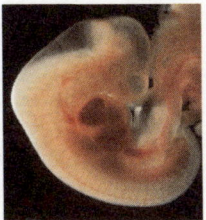

> **Travelling and transportation in the first three months**
> You can travel by any vehicle: two-wheeler, autos, buses or cars. The bumps on the roads cannot cause a miscarriage. You can travel by train or air. You will be asked to avoid travelling if you have had any bleeding in early pregnancy.

Week 6
Mother

- Your baby has been growing inside you for one month now though you may not find any physical changes. You might just find yourself sleepy and unusually tired.

- Occasionally, some women may feel dizzy or faint if they stand up for a long time. For many years, movies have used the fainting of a woman as a clue to the fact that she is pregnant!

- You may suddenly find an aversion to common smells. Cooking might become impossible as the smell of frying or for that matter, any smell in the kitchen may set off nausea. Many women develop an aversion to milk and milk products.

Baby

By week 6, the baby's heart has begun to beat. On an ultrasound, you can clearly make out the beating of the heart.

The baby is as big as your little fingernail. She has buds where her arms and legs will be and her head has the beginnings of eyes, ears and a mouth.

> **Relieving nausea and vomiting**
> Your obstetrician might recommend **meclizine** or **doxylamine succinate** tablets for nausea. These are safe and will relieve your nausea and vomiting without harming your baby.

Week 7
Mother

- You will stop looking tired and start getting the glow of pregnancy. Some women, however, may find themselves plagued with pimples on the face, chest and back. These are due to the changing hormone levels.

- Your appetite will be poor, though there are women who feel hungry all the time! Some women will find it difficult to take any liquids, including water. Constipation can be a problem because of the poor intake of food and fluids.

Acupressure point P6 has been scientifically proven to relieve nausea in pregnancy.

Location: On the inner forearm, about three fingers' width from the wrist crease.

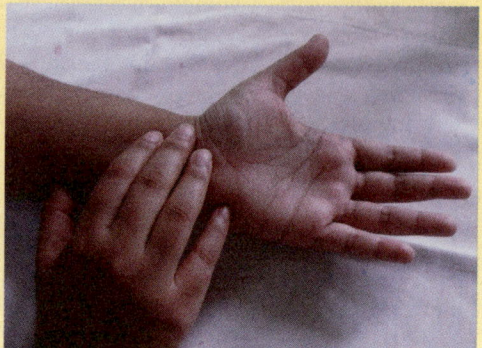

Finding the P6 pressure point for nausea

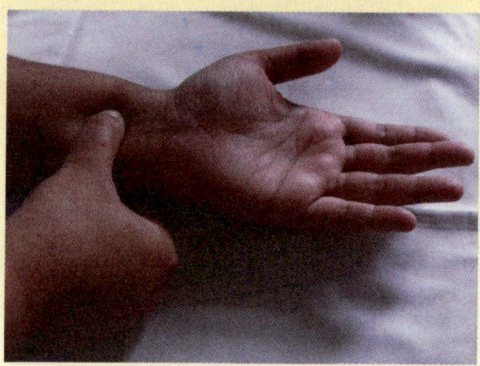

The P6 pressure point for nausea

Gently cradle your wrist on the palm of the other hand, and lightly press the point with your thumb. A light pressure is usually effective but you can experiment to see how much pressure is needed to relieve you of the nausea.

Be sure to relax both arms and shoulders; you can place your hands on a table or your lap to be comfortable. Hold for 30 seconds or so initially. Some women find immediate relief but for others it may take a little longer. Try for at least 5 minutes. The pressure should not be painful.

- You will definitely not be 'showing'- in fact, it is not unusual to lose weight at this point.

Baby

- The baby's heart is now beating regularly at 140-150 beats per minute.
- The arm buds have grown and the hands begin to develop.
- The whole baby is still only 5-7 mm long, about the size of your small fingernail, but the brain, intestines, pituitary gland and pancreas are growing.
- The baby's face is developing rapidly. The nasal pits form, the ears and lenses of the eyes are developing.

Week 8

Mother

- The uterus will feel enlarged on an internal examination by the obstetrician.
- The breasts get larger and heavier, and are probably still tender.
- The nipples may be darker and the little bumps around the edge of the areola more pronounced.
- You may feel the need to urinate more frequently as the growing uterus puts pressure on the bladder.
- Some women develop acidity which causes heartburn.
- Do not be surprised if you have recurrent headaches. It is quite safe to take paracetamol to relieve the ache.

Baby

- The baby is now about 10,000 times bigger than what it was at conception but is still only about 2.5 cm long.
- This week the gonads will either become testes or ovaries i.e. the baby will differentiate into a boy or girl.
- The eyes are formed and covered by a fold of skin, though the eyelid will not open as yet.
- The arms and legs are growing longer and the arms are bent at the elbow.

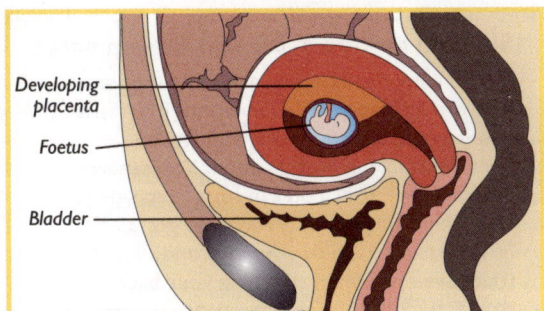

Foetus at 8 weeks

- The tip of the nose is visible and teeth are forming under the baby's gums.
- The foetus has started moving inside the uterus but the movements cannot be felt by you yet.

Week 9

Mother

- Your appetite might improve but do not be surprised if the nausea persists for another month or so.
- You might still lose weight but in most women, the weight will stabilise. Some may even gain a little weight.
- Due to hormonal changes, the gums become softer and thicker. You might bleed from your gums while brushing your teeth. Be sure to use a soft toothbrush.

Baby

- Bones and cartilage are beginning to form.
- The umbilical cord and placenta are forming and growing.
- The fingers have formed but are webbed.

Week 10

Mother

- You will have mood swings because of the surge in hormone levels. You might swing from happiness to crying to anger in minutes. Your husband and family have to be prepared for this!
- If you are feeling a little more energetic, start going for walks. This will make you feel healthy and fit and is a good practice to follow throughout pregnancy.
- You may feel breathless. This may cause you to take deep breaths and sigh a lot. This is an effect of the increased levels of progesterone in your blood. The breathlessness will reduce at the end of the first trimester but will come back in the third trimester.

Baby

- This week, your baby graduates from being an embryo to a foetus!
- Most of the joints are formed - shoulders, elbows, wrists, hands and fingers, knees, ankles, feet and toes.
- All of the organs are there, but not fully formed or functional.

Week 11

Mother

- Your uterus just about fills your pelvis. If you press your fingers into your lower abdomen, just above the pubic bone, you may be able to feel it. Your obstetrician may be able to feel the uterus abdominally. A Doppler device may be used to hear the baby's heartbeat. The first time you hear the baby's heartbeat is an amazing milestone!

> **Intercourse in the first three months**
>
> Though some women may feel less interested in sex because of the nausea and tiredness, there is no need to avoid intercourse, if you feel like it. If you have had any bleeding in early pregnancy, your doctor might advise you to avoid intercourse for two weeks.

> **Hormone tablets and injections in the first three months**
>
> There is no need for hormonal tablets or injections in the first three months. Research over many years has proven that they are of no benefit. If the pregnancy is normal, it will continue without any external hormonal 'support'. If it is an abnormal pregnancy, it will miscarry in spite of tablets and injections.

- You may still suffer the effects of morning sickness, but it will soon disappear.
- You might be advised to have your first ultrasound scan to assess the growth of the baby. The thickness of the skin over the neck (**nuchal thickness**) is also measured. This provides information about the health of the baby.

Baby
- Nails are just starting to develop on the baby's little fingers.
- The length of the baby will probably double this week.
- The irises of the eyes are developing now.

Week 12

Mother
- Your uterus will shift upwards a bit so that it does not press on your bladder as much as before.
- This is the turnaround week - your tiredness and exhaustion will be replaced with a sense of well-being and you will feel energetic again.
- You may notice more changes in your skin. Some women will have irregular brown patches, called the 'mask of pregnancy' (chloasma) on their face or neck.
- Look for the linea nigra, a dark line of pigmentation running from the top to the bottom, in the midline of your abdomen. This may develop even later in pregnancy.
- The placenta will take over the production of hormones.

Sleeping posture in the first three months

Sleep in any position you are comfortable in. You can still sleep on your stomach because soon, as the uterus grows, you will be uncomfortable in that position. You can sleep on your back too. You can turn from side to side while lying down. When you get up from a lying posture, turn to your side and then get up (this saves you from spraining your back and stomach muscles as the pregnancy progresses).

Baby
- The baby is about 6 cm long, fully formed and looks like a human being. She would fit in the palm of your hand!
- The beginnings of hair are seen on the scalp.
- Skin and nails have developed.
- The webbed hands and feet develop into fingers and toes.
- The baby's chest rises and falls as it practises breathing movements.
- With kidneys fully functioning, the baby can swallow amniotic fluid and excrete it as urine.
- The amniotic fluid is completely replaced every three hours, so the baby's environment stays fresh.

Week 13

Mother
- You will start to feel some heaviness and a mild ache in your lower abdomen, as the uterus grows and stretches. You might find it uncomfortable when you get up after sitting down or when you turn from side to side

---

Activity in the first three months
- Keep up your usual level of activity. Lie down or sleep when you feel very tired but don't spend the day in bed!
- You can carry on all normal housework but avoid lifting anything very heavy. You can carry your older child, if you have one, but see if you can pick her up from a chair or have somebody hand her to you.
- If you have a job, there is no need to take leave of absence from work.
- You can climb up and down stairs any number of times.
- If you have had any spotting or bleeding, your obstetrician might advise you to restrict your activities for a few days or weeks.

when you are lying down. This feeling increases over the following few weeks.
- The veins on your breasts are probably much more noticeable and your nipples will become darker in colour.

Eating in the first three months
Your appetite may be very poor. Eat small quantities and frequently. Avoid oily and spiced food. Salt biscuits / crackers help in suppressing the nausea. Bland foods such as dry toast and idlis are well tolerated. Drink plenty of fluids. Remember, this too shall pass!

Baby
- Your baby is almost 8 cm long.
- The vocal cords begin to develop.
- All the twenty baby teeth are formed and waiting beneath the gums until well after birth. However, every once in a while a baby is born with a tooth already showing.
- The baby's bone marrow, liver and spleen have taken over the production of red blood cells.
- Initially, the eyes on the foetus are on the sides, but this week, they move to the front and appear closer together (to begin the makings of the face). The ears also move to the proper position on either side of the head.

The role of the father-to-be
The first trimester can be a roller coaster ride for the father-to-be. You may feel helpless as you see your wife tired and exhausted, nauseous and unable to eat. If she does not eat, will the baby's development be affected? Do not worry; the baby does not require more than what your wife is able to eat. Once her appetite is back to normal, she can start eating nutritious food.

You may also be filled with anxiety about your ability to handle the pregnancy and its demands on your feelings. Your wife might be emotionally labile, with mood swings which leave you bewildered and sometimes, upset.

How can you help?
Just being there for her is an enormous mood elevator for a new mother-to-be. With words and deeds, let her know you are delighted that she is pregnant. Help her out with housework because she may find it hard to do all the household chores, especially during the first trimester when she seems tired all the time.

Make sure you go to all her antenatal check-ups. This will allow you to clear your doubts too. Knowing what is happening with her pregnancy will enable you to be a supportive and comforting husband.

First trimester screening for Down syndrome
This screening test is done between 11 and 14 weeks of pregnancy. It combines the results of a special ultrasound test called nuchal translucency screening and certain blood tests (PAPP-A and hCG) to look for signs of Down syndrome, trisomy 18, and heart defects. If this test is available, it might be a good idea to have it done.

Old wives' tales
- Having intercourse in the first trimester will cause an abortion- **not true!** If you have had any spotting or bleeding in the first trimester, your obstetrician might ask you to avoid intercourse for a period of time.
- Avoid bumpy rides – it might lead to an abortion. **Not true!**
- Do not climb stairs in the first few months because it can lead to an abortion. **Not true!**
- Do not eat papayas, pineapples or mangoes in the first few months- they may cause an abortion. **Not true!**
- The computer screen can cause radiation and harm the baby. **Not true!**

CHAPTER 6

The second trimester (14 - 27 weeks)

The first trimester has come to an end! You are feeling great, the nausea has subsided or almost subsided and you and your husband may have heard the baby's heartbeat at your obstetrician's clinic. Let us now move on to the second trimester.

Most women consider this stage of pregnancy the easiest to deal with. The nausea has disappeared or almost subsided. Energy levels are rising and the intense sleepiness of the first three months is letting up.

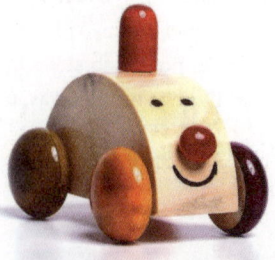

6 The second trimester

Week 14

Mother

- Having made it through the first three months, your risk of miscarriage is very low.
- You might just be able to feel a little bump at the lowest part of your abdomen. This is the growing uterus.
- You might start developing acidity, leading to heartburn. Your doctor will prescribe antacids to relieve it. Try to finish your last meal for the day early, so that you have at least an hour and a half or two hours between your meal and lying down.
- Your breasts are heavy but the tenderness should have subsided by now. Some women find that they may have to change their bra size to one size larger.
- Constipation can still be a problem. Start adding more fibre to your diet e.g. leafy greens. Make sure you drink plenty of fluids.
- You may just about start 'showing'. Many first-time mothers are concerned that they do not show yet. Remember that in the first pregnancy, you may not start showing till another month or so, especially with loose Indian clothing.
- If your interest in sex had decreased in the first three months, you might find it easier to have sex now.

Baby

- Your baby is about 7.5 cm long and the weight has tripled to about 45 grams.
- The facial features become more defined. The facial muscles become active and the baby is able to smile, frown and wrinkle its forehead.
- The baby's neck becomes well defined.
- Reflexes begin to operate. She will start opening and closing her fists.
- The external genitalia have clearly differentiated into that of a boy or a girl.
- Whorls start developing on the finger tips and will become the future fingerprints.

Week 15

Mother

- The heaviness in the lower abdomen is likely to increase. The top of your uterus (the fundus) is now half way between your pubic bone and umbilicus. It can be easily felt and your obstetrician will be able to assess if the uterus is growing normally.
- Have the palms of your hands started looking red and feeling warm? This is because of the increased blood circulation in pregnancy.
- From the 15th week onwards, you can undergo the triple screen test for Down syndrome.

> **Screening for Down syndrome:**
> The triple screening test for Down syndrome is done between 15 and 20 weeks of pregnancy. It combines an ultrasound with blood tests of estriol, hCG and alphafoetoprotein. If this test is available, it is a good idea to have it done.

Baby

- Your baby is more than 10 cm long.
- Colourless eyebrows and eyelashes have now appeared.
- The baby's heart is beating well and the blood circulation is fine.
- The hair on the top of the head is starting to show up more.
- Skin formation is progressing, but is thin (you can even see small blood vessels forming underneath).
- At this point, the baby is exploring everything and sometimes, on ultrasound, can even be seen sucking his thumb!

Week 16

Mother

- If you have had a baby before, you might start feeling the slightest of flutters as your baby

starts moving. First-time mothers have to be patient for at least another two to four weeks to start feeling the baby's early movements.
- Sleeping on your stomach might start becoming uncomfortable. You can sleep on your back but you can start learning to sleep on your sides so that later on in pregnancy, you will be more comfortable in that position.
- The placenta is now fully formed and functional.

Baby
- Your baby is about 11 cm long and the average weight is about 100 grams.
- The head is erect.
- The lower limbs are well developed.
- The baby's eyes are moving though the eyelids are still not open.
- The skin is getting thicker and is less transparent.

Week 17
Mother
- You slowly start gaining weight. Make sure you start a regular antenatal exercise programme and stick to it.
- If you have not started your iron supplementation, this is a good time to do it.

Baby
- Loud noises outside the uterus may cause the baby to startle and move jerkily.
- The baby will make purposeful movements.
- Fat starts getting deposited under the baby's skin.

Week 18
Mother
- You still feel good. Your energy levels are high.
- Many women get worried because they do not seem to have symptoms of pregnancy anymore: the nausea is gone, the appetite is healthy and you have become used to the weight of the uterus so there is no abdominal discomfort. Don't worry; this is the good time of pregnancy, so enjoy it!

- The uterus is not big enough yet to cause any discomfort though you may continue to feel the weight in the lower abdomen, especially when you sit down and get up.
- Have you started thinking of a name for the baby? Pick a boy's name and a girl's name so that you will be ready when the baby is born.

Baby
- Your baby weighs 200 grams.
- The ears stand out from the head.
- The baby's bones are growing harder and stronger.
- The kidneys are producing 7-14 ml of urine every day.
- Meconium, a greenish substance, is beginning to accumulate in the bowel. It is made up of undigested debris from the amniotic fluid and various secretions of the digestive tract. This will come out in the early days after birth as the baby's first few bowel movements.
- The placenta transfers nutrients and oxygen from your blood to the baby via the umbilical cord.
- The baby is beginning to be covered in a white, waxy substance called **vernix**. This protects the baby's delicate skin from getting wrinkled due to constantly being in the amniotic fluid.

Week 19
Mother
- Your lower abdomen starts to get fuller. If this is your first pregnancy, this is when all your friends can easily notice that you are pregnant!
- The skin over your abdomen may start developing 'stretch marks' in the coming months. Though you cannot always avoid them, this is a good time to start applying moisturisers over the abdominal skin to minimise the stretch marks.

Baby
- If your baby is a little girl, millions of undeveloped eggs will start forming in the ovaries. By the time she is born, she will

have about a million undeveloped eggs in her ovaries.

- Buds for permanent teeth start forming behind the buds for the baby (milk) teeth.
- The toenails grow but not as rapidly as the fingernails.
- Don't be surprised if the baby does not seem to be moving all the time - she will be sleeping a lot.

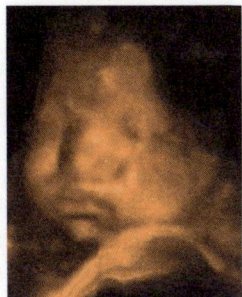

3D ultrasound of face at 19 weeks

Week 20

Mother

- You have reached the midpoint of your pregnancy.
- The top of the uterus reaches the level of your umbilicus.
- Your umbilicus might start looking a little protuberant and as the pregnancy progresses, may protrude quite a bit.
- Right from the beginning of pregnancy, you might have noticed increased vaginal discharge. It might get more pronounced now. If it is accompanied by itching or burning, contact your obstetrician.

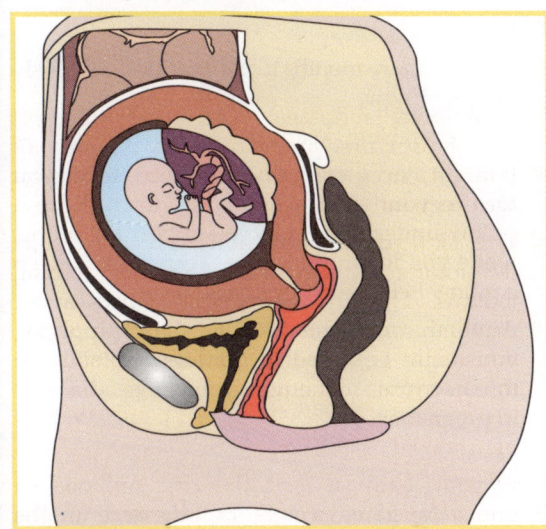

Foetus at 20 weeks

- If your feet start to get a little puffy, there is nothing to be concerned about. As the pregnancy progresses, you will retain more and more water in your body and the feet will get more swollen. Putting up your feet will help reduce the oedema.

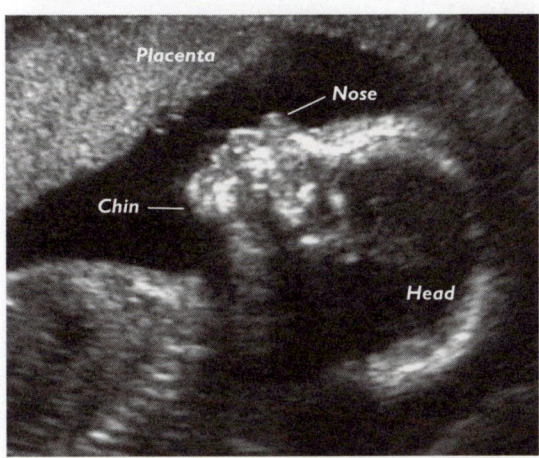

Ultrasound at 20 weeks showing profile

Baby

- Your baby weighs approximately 320 grams.
- If the baby is a girl, the uterus has started developing.
- Your baby's heart is beating at a rate of 120 to 160 beats per minute.

Week 21

Mother

- For the past few weeks, you might have asked your husband to feel the baby's movements by placing his hands on your abdomen. Now, he will be able to feel the baby move really well, without having to pretend he does!
- Be as active as you can. Keep up the daily walking and don't forget to do your prenatal exercises.
- You may notice some swelling in your legs. Try to avoid standing for long periods of time and put your feet up when you sit down.

Baby

- Your baby will be moving well now but don't worry if she sleeps for a while. Her

movements will be felt vigorously one day and may be mild another day.
- The baby's bone marrow starts making blood cells. This was done by the liver and spleen till now.

Week 22
Mother
- You may feel the effects of the change in your centre of gravity. Your gait will change when you walk.
- Avoid wearing high heels. You may be more comfortable with a slight heel on your footwear, rather than completely flat footwear.
- You might develop haemorrhoids ('piles'). In pregnancy, it is common to develop haemorrhoids. If they are painful or cause a small amount of bleeding, you can ask your doctor for a stool softener and an ointment to reduce the pain. Make sure you avoid constipation.

Baby
- Your baby weighs about 460 grams and is about 25 cm long.
- There is a downy layer of hair on the skin, called **lanugo**. This will disappear before the baby is born or soon after birth.
- Taste buds are starting to form on your baby's tongue.
- The brain and nerve endings can process the sensation of touch. Your baby may experiment by feeling his or her face or anything else within reach.
- For boys, the testes begin to descend from the abdomen into the scrotum this week.

Week 23
Mother
- The baby's movements are quite obvious now. Is he playing football in there?
- Your sides may ache, in the lower abdomen. This is due to the stretching of the round ligaments which hold the uterus up. Lying down and resting on the same side as the pain will help relieve it.

- When you sit for a long time, your lower ribs may ache as the uterus pushes against them. Try to lean back when you sit, so that the uterus does not push directly into the ribs.

Baby
- Your baby weighs about 500 grams.
- The pancreas is developing well and even begins to produce insulin.
- The bones in the little one's middle ear are hardening now and the baby can hear muffled sounds. In fact, she can hear the rhythmic beat of your heart!

> **Stretch marks**
> Between 75% and 90% of women develop stretch marks to some degree during pregnancy. Stretch marks are the result of the rapid stretching of the skin associated with rapid growth. They first appear as reddish lines, but tend to gradually fade to a lighter colour. The affected areas feel empty and soft to the touch. Stretch marks may start appearing from the fifth month. Applying moisturisers on the skin may help reduce the amount of stretch marks but **do not waste money on creams and ointments which promise to prevent stretch marks.**

Week 24
Mother
- Just four more months to go! You look obviously pregnant now.
- Keep exercising, keep fit.
- It might start getting uncomfortable when you turn to your sides while lying down. Keep a pillow under your belly to support the uterus while you lie on your side. You can also keep a pillow between your knees.
- Anytime from the 24th to the 28th week, you might be asked to undergo a blood test to determine whether you have diabetes in pregnancy.

Baby
- The baby gains weight rapidly and weighs about 630 grams.

- The lungs are developing blood vessels now, preparing them to take over the task of getting oxygen into the blood stream.
- The lungs begin to produce **surfactant**. This substance allows the air sacs in the lungs to inflate and prevents them from collapsing. This substance is the reason why newborn babies can breathe air as soon as they are born.
- Remember: babies have just the opposite of our sleep rhythms. That is why you will find her jumping around at night and sleeping more during the day.
- Your baby is developing the ability to suck.
- Remember that the baby can hear muffled sounds. Play some music. She can't hear the words but she can definitely listen to the intonation and the rhythm.

Week 25

Mother

- Your face looks rounder. The nose may start changing shape and may get a little plumper.
- Your skin may darken in various places: neck, abdomen, and around the mouth. Don't worry, this will fade after the baby is born and your skin colour will return to its normal tone.

Baby

- The hands are fully developed. With her sense of touch well developed, she spends her time trying to touch everything!
- The spine has developed completely.

Week 26

Mother

- Have you had your tetanus toxoid injection? If not, make sure you start your immunisation schedule now.
- Do you feel your abdomen tighten and relax at irregular intervals? These painless contractions are called Braxton-Hicks contractions. They help the uterus prepare for the birth.

Baby

- The baby may weigh about 800 grams.
- The skin is becoming less transparent.

> **Back pain**
> Your back will ache a little more as the curve gets exaggerated due to the growing uterus. Try this simple exercise to relax your back muscles: Stand with your back against the wall, knees slightly bent. As you inhale, press the small of your back against the wall. Exhale and relax your back.

- The baby's brain is now registering brain wave activity for sight and hearing.
- Your baby's body still appears lean.

Week 27

Mother

- You will gain weight more rapidly now. Make sure you do not put on more than one to two kilos per month.
- You may find yourself short of breath at times. That's because the baby pushes against your ribs, giving less space for the lungs to expand.
- Your baby has plenty of amniotic fluid to swim in - this fluid cushions him well. You will be able to see parts of your baby move around in your abdomen, as he pushes against your body!

Baby

- This week marks the end of the second trimester. The baby's lungs, liver and immune system are continuing to mature. At 27 weeks, your baby's length would have tripled or even quadrupled from the length she was when you were 12 weeks pregnant.
- The baby's skin is still wrinkled and red. The fat deposited under the skin will start to slowly even out the skin texture.
- Your baby's eyelashes are developing. The hair on the head is getting thicker.

The role of the father-to-be

The second trimester is the good part of pregnancy. Your wife feels energetic and is able to carry on all her work. The size of her pregnancy has still not made her very uncomfortable. Her appetite is back to normal.

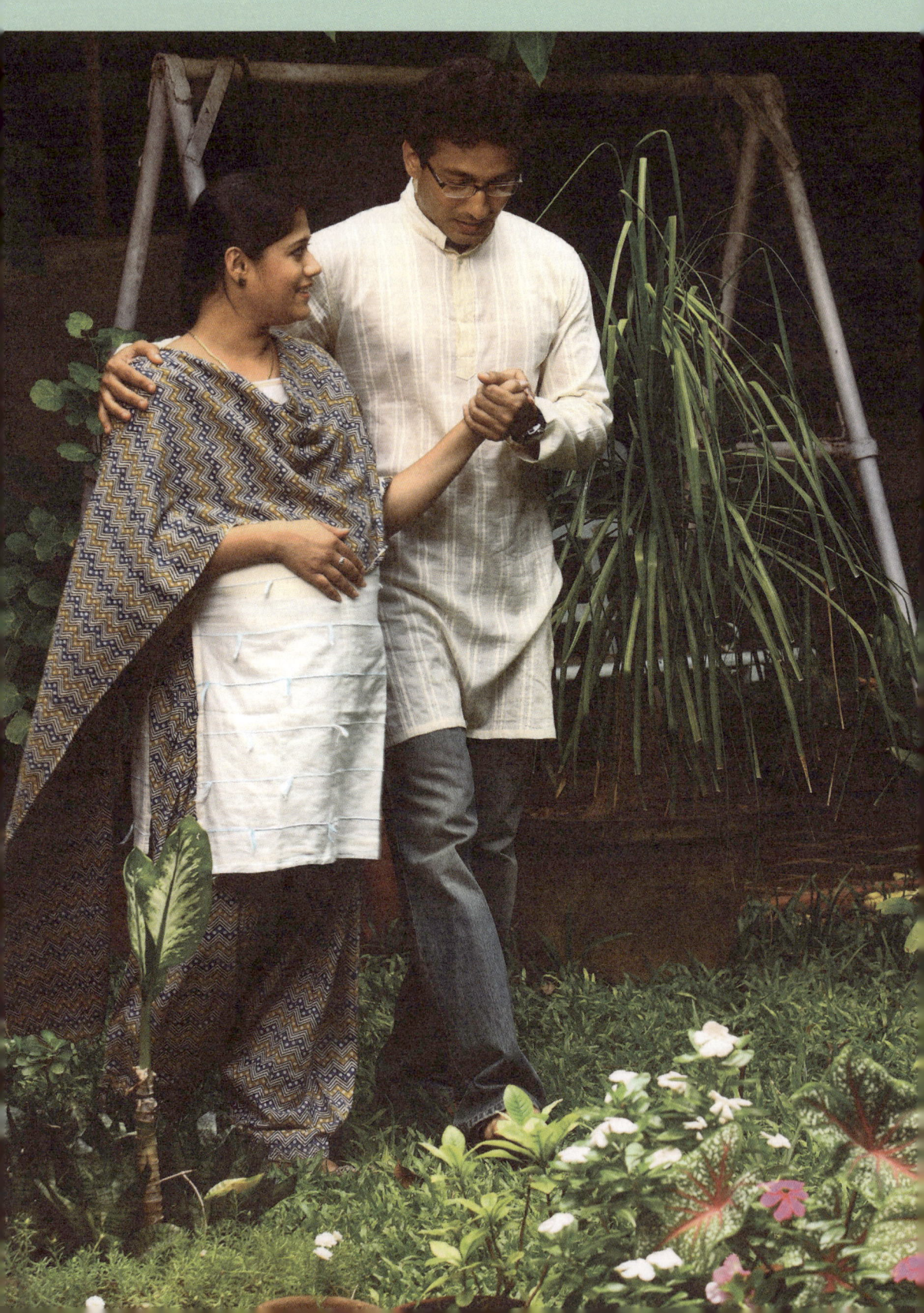

How can you help?

Make sure your wife gets a healthy, nutritious diet. At the same time, do not get carried away and force her to eat so much that she puts on unnecessary weight. If you insist on overfeeding her, the excess weight gain may leave you, at the end of the pregnancy, with more wife than you bargained for! Remember that the redundant weight put on during a pregnancy is difficult to get rid off and can be the beginning of lifelong obesity.

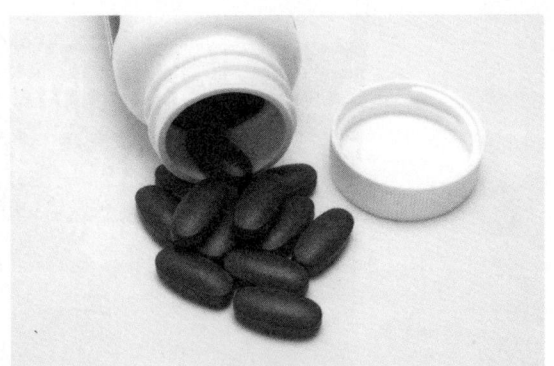

She may have leg aches and back pains. Help her exercise by taking time to walk with her. You can also help by massaging her legs and lower back.

Those dark skin patches

During pregnancy, many women notice darkening of the skin. This might happen on the face, breasts, nipples, neck or inner thighs. This darkening is due to an increase in **melanin,** which is the pigment which gives our skin the brown colour. More than 90 per cent of pregnant women will get these dark patches.

Brownish marks that appear around the eyes, nose, and cheeks are called **chloasma** or "mask of pregnancy." Some women also notice a faint, dark line that runs from their belly button to their pubic hair. This is called **linea nigra.** These dark areas are harmless and usually fade a few months after delivery. However, they are unlikely to go away completely. There are no creams which will prevent this darkening and applying turmeric powder will not make them go away.

CHAPTER 7

The third trimester (28 - 40 weeks)

You have officially entered your third trimester now. In a few short months, you will become a mother! You will be getting impatient.

The baby moves more now. This is the time to make sure you are fit and healthy enough to face labour. It is also time for you to prepare yourself by learning more about the process of labour and delivery.

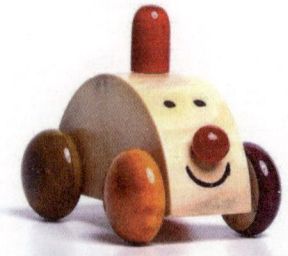

7 The third trimester

Week 28

Mother

- You may lose a few drops of urine when you cough or sneeze. This is quite normal in pregnancy. Make sure you learn Kegel's exercises to make your pelvic muscles supple and strong. **(See Chapter 24: After delivery care).**

- Have you been tested for diabetes in pregnancy? If not, you should be getting the test done now.

- If you are Rh negative and your husband is Rh positive, your obstetrician may suggest that you take an injection now to prevent any problems for the baby. The injection at this stage is optional but if your baby is born as Rh positive, you definitely need to take the injection after birth. **(See Chapter 35: The Rh factor: how can it affect pregnancy)**

Baby

- Your baby reaches the 1 kilo (1000 grams) mark!
- The hair is growing thicker and is getting darker.

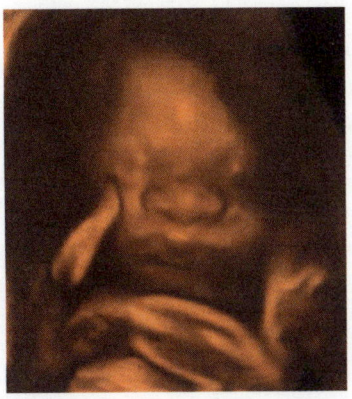

3D ultrasound of face at 28 weeks

- The lungs are more mature and if the baby is born now, the lungs are capable of breathing air.
- The baby's eyes are partially open and sensitive to light.
- The surface of the brain, smooth till now, will start developing wrinkles called sulci and gyri. This is part of the normal development of the brain.

Water retention

You will retain a large amount of water as your pregnancy progresses. By the time you are ready to deliver, there will be 3.5 litres of water in the baby, placenta and the amniotic fluid around the baby. You will accumulate another 2.5-3 litres in your uterus, breasts and blood. So by the end of a pregnancy, you would have about 6.5 litres of extra water in your body!

Your feet will swell up by the end of the day because there is about one litre of water in your legs.

Week 29

Mother

- Your breasts may feel heavy. The nipples and the area around them (areolae) become larger and are deeply pigmented. You might feel small bumps on the areolae. This is normal. Some women will notice a clear discharge

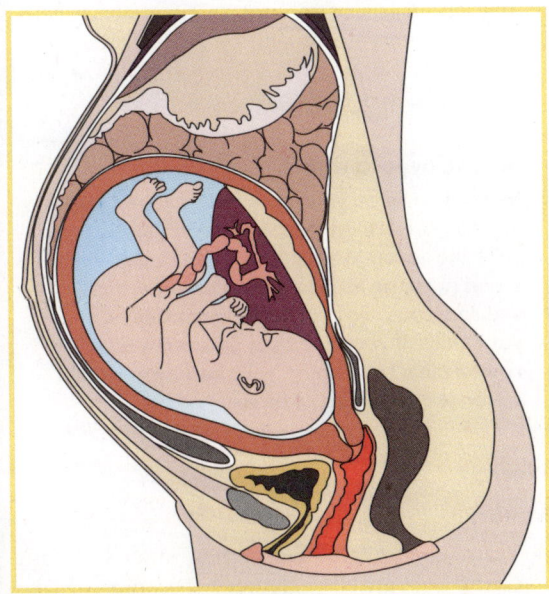

Foetus at 28 weeks

from the breast. This is common and just a sign that the breasts are getting ready for breastfeeding.
- The amount of circulating blood in your body almost doubles.
- Acidity and heartburn become more common now. Take an antacid if you need it.
- Are you regular with your iron supplement? Remember that the iron you get from your diet is insufficient to prevent anaemia.
- You may be unable to sleep too well. This is common - your body is preparing itself for the sleepless nights after the baby is born! Make sure you have enough magazines and books to take to bed so that you have something to do when you are unable to sleep at night.

Braxton-Hicks contractions
You might start feeling tightening of your uterus on and off. These painless contractions are called 'Braxton-Hicks contractions' and are just preparing your uterus for childbirth.

Baby
- You will find the baby tucking itself under your ribs. Sometimes, you might experience pain under the ribs on the right side - this is because the baby is pushing against your liver. Just push her away gently.
- She will now be in the classic 'foetal position' with her arms and legs curled over the body.
- The bone marrow takes over production of red blood cells.
- You will find plenty of movements and kicks - he is building his muscles by moving around.

Week 30
Mother
- Your antenatal check-ups will become more frequent now. You will be seen every two weeks from now on.
- You might have pain in the lower sides of the abdomen. This is because the ligaments which hold the uterus in place (called the 'round ligaments') get stretched. Lying down on your side on the same side as the pain helps.

- The nagging low back pain gets worse. This is because of the exaggeration of the normal curve of the lower back. Prenatal exercises will relieve the pain so don't stop your exercises.

Itching in pregnancy
You might itch all over the body. This is usually mild but some women have severe, incessant itching. You might find rashes all over the body. This is called **PUPPP** (pruritic urticarial plaques and patches of pregnancy). It is treated with moisturisers, local steroid creams or oral steroid tablets. It does not harm the baby in any way.
The most important thing to remember is that scratching makes the condition worse. The good thing is the rashes and itching disappear after the birth of the baby.

Baby
- Your baby now weighs about 1,250 grams.
- Your baby's skin is getting smooth though some wrinkles still remain.
- The downy hair over the body (lanugo) is starting to disappear.
- The baby's brain is growing rapidly, developing hundreds of billions of new nerve cells. No new nerve cells will be added after birth, though the brain will not reach full size until your child is 5 years old.

Supine hypotension
When you lie on your back, the enlarged uterus causes pressure on the large blood vessels (vena cava and aorta) in your body. This causes your blood pressure to fall and you may feel dizzy and nauseous. To avoid this, try to sleep on your sides. If you have back pain and it feels comfortable to sleep on your back, you can do so for short periods of time.

Week 31
Mother
- Your gait might be getting altered. Your centre of gravity changes because of the protuberant stomach.

- The hormones produced in pregnancy cause relaxation of the joints between the bones in your pelvic area. This relaxation will cause you to waddle. The back pain can get worse as the pregnancy progresses.
- Finding a comfortable position to sleep in can be difficult. Try lying on your side with pillows to support the uterus and a pillow between your knees. If you want to sleep on your back, bend one knee. This will relieve the pressure on your low back.

> **Back pain**
> If you have to stand for a long time, place one foot on a low stool. Sit on chairs with good back support. Apply a hot water bottle or ice pack to the painful area. Ask your husband to massage your back. Ask your obstetrician whether you can take a paracetamol or ibuprofen tablet for pain relief.

Baby
- As the baby gets more padded with fat, her skin goes from deep red to pink.
- The eyes are open now.
- She has plenty of hair on her head.
- Do you feel your baby jump when there is a loud noise near you? Some babies even respond and move a great deal when they hear music!

Week 32
Mother
- Getting nervous and anxious? Remember that every mother-to-be, specially a first time one, worries about the baby and the coming labour. Prepare yourself by reading about labour and delivery and by attending labour preparation classes.
- The baby will still be tumbling around in your uterus. It may not get into a head down position for another week or two.
- If you are carrying twins, your uterus is already as large as if you were full term with a single baby.

Baby
- Your baby is starting to fill out and probably weighs around 1,700 grams.
- From this point on, your baby's weight will increase faster than the length.
- As your baby continues to grow, her movements will become more frequent and vigorous. Some of your baby's kicks may actually be painful!

Week 33
Mother
- You might feel breathless most of the time as the uterus pushes your diaphragm up and that in turn compresses the lungs.
- You will be urinating more often. As the baby pushes against your bladder, you might get up more often in the night to go to the toilet.
- Pressure on the bowels may cause you to have frequent or irregular bowel movements.
- Start planning for what you will need to do when you go into labour. Start buying the things that you need for the newborn baby to avoid a last minute rush. **(See Chapter 15: Preparing for labour).**

Baby
- Do you feel taps or thumps in one particular point in your abdomen, lasting for a few minutes? That's your baby having hiccups! This is common and she will continue to have them even after she is born.
- Iron is being stored in the baby's liver.
- If it is a boy, his testicles are descending into the scrotum.
- Your baby may practise breathing by moving his or her diaphragm in a repetitive rhythm.
- The waxy layer of vernix covering the skin gets thicker now.

Week 34
Mother
- Do you know how to recognise when labour has started? Read about it or attend labour preparation classes.

- Make sure you keep up with your walking and exercise regimen. Keeping fit is particularly important at this point.

Baby
- Your baby weighs about 2 kilos by now.
- Your baby's nails are long enough to reach to the tip of the fingers or beyond. When she is born, the nails might be long and she might even scratch herself. She may require the first nail trimming soon after birth!
- If you are carrying twins, they will probably be in the position now that they will stay in until birth. A single baby may still change its position, though not so frequently.
- If for any reason your baby is born now, she has a good chance of survival.

Week 35

Mother
- You may find a lot of pressure in your pelvic area. When you walk, you might feel the weight in your vagina. There may be pain and discomfort when you get up after sitting for a while.
- There might be numbness over the front of the thighs because the enlarged uterus is pressing on some nerves.
- The cramps in your calf muscles might become more frequent. Remember to stretch your calf muscles.

Baby
- Your baby is getting into the head down position.
- The movements are changing- instead of kicks, the baby will roll and wriggle. This is because the space is getting less in the uterus as she continues to grow.
- The fat deposition all over the body continues and the baby is starting to look plump now.

Week 36

Mother
- You will start your weekly check ups now.
- The baby should have got into its final position by now. Most babies will be in the

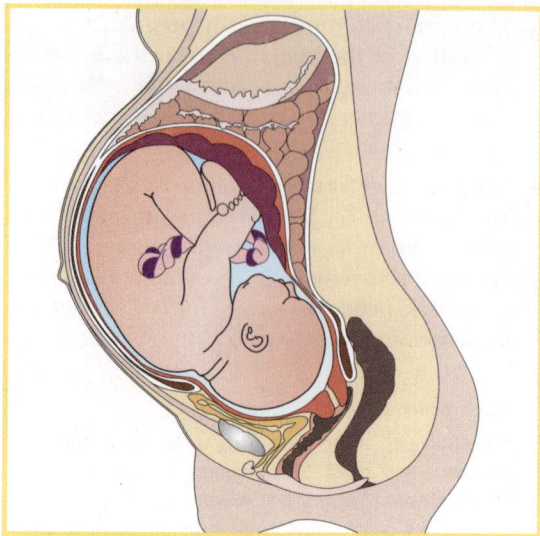

Foetus at 36 weeks

head down position but about 4 out of 100 will be in a breech (buttocks down) position.
- Besides examining your abdomen, your obstetrician may start doing a vaginal examination this week or the next week. This is to assess the condition of your cervix and the position of the baby's head.
- Your uterus has grown to 1,000 times its non-pregnant volume.
- It is important to keep checking to see if the baby is moving well. Though the force of the movements will get less, the baby should move for a minimum of 20 times during the day.

Baby
- Your baby's face is getting rounder now. There is fat being deposited on its cheeks. This 'buccal pad' of fat helps the baby suckle at the mother's breast.
- The baby's head is finding its way into the birth canal.
- The movements are not so vigorous now.

Week 37

Mother
- Once you have completed 37 weeks of pregnancy, you are considered to be 'full term'.

If the baby is born any time after this, she is considered mature. If she is born before 37 weeks, the baby is considered 'premature'.

- The pressure on your ribs may have eased off considerably now. This is called 'lightening' because the baby's head has dropped into the birth canal. The older women in your house might point out that the abdomen has 'dropped'!
- The mucus or watery discharge from your vagina will increase since the cervix has started to open up a little.
- Learn what the signs of labour are and check with your obstetrician when you are supposed to go to the hospital. Have you attended a labour preparation class yet?
- If you are keen on having epidural analgesia, now is a good time to discuss it with your obstetrician. **(See Chapter 20: Pain relief in labour and delivery).**

Baby

- The waxy white coating over the baby's skin lessens. If the baby is born now, you will find vernix over the scalp and in the creases of the joints.
- As the baby occupies more and more space, the movements become less. Keep counting the movements to ensure the baby is healthy.
- Your baby can survive comfortably if born now.

Week 38

Mother

- You might have frequent false pains. False pains are irregular, more over the low back and do not progress in frequency and intensity. These pains are there because the cervix is thinning out (effacing) and starting to open slightly (dilating) in preparation for labour.
- You can be as active as you want to be.
- Your obstetrician will do an internal examination to find out how your cervix is preparing for labour and also if the baby's head has dropped into the birth canal. If this is your first baby, the head will usually be in the birth canal by now. If it has not dropped in, do not worry, some babies drop in once labour has started. If you have already had a baby or babies before, the head might not drop in till labour starts.

Baby

- The baby weighs between 2,500-2,900 grams on an average.
- The downy hair over the body (lanugo) is almost gone.
- The baby is plump because of a good deposition of fat under the skin.

Week 39

Mother

- The last weeks are the toughest to get through. Everybody will call to find out if you have delivered the baby yet!
- You might not want to do much since the uterus is so stretched out and you are really uncomfortable.
- Be sure to have all your stuff ready to take to the hospital. Make all the arrangements at home for you to go to the hospital.

Counting your baby's kicks:

It is a good idea to keep an eye on your baby's movements. A healthy baby will move well, whereas a baby which is experiencing trouble inside the uterus will move very little.

From the time you wake up in the morning till 12 noon, you should be able to count at least 10 movements. From 12 noon to 6 in the evening you should be able to count at least another 10 movements. Most babies are active from the evening through the night. If you feel the movements are decreasing, lie on your side for an hour. If you feel at least three movements in that hour, then your baby is healthy. If it has not, then it is important for you to go and see your obstetrician immediately.

Baby

- Your baby is preparing for life outside the uterus. He will have plenty of breathing movements - pushing his little chest in and out.
- He might weigh between 2,700-3,000 grams on an average. An Indian baby is considered large if he weighs 3,500 grams or more.

Week 40
Mother

- The days are dragging! Though you may be a little apprehensive about the labour, you wish it would be over with.
- Remember that most babies are born a week before or after the due date. Only four per cent of babies are born on the exact due date.
- Your obstetrician will make sure the baby is doing well inside. She might want to wait till 41 weeks to induce labour **(See Chapter 30: Postdated pregnancy).**

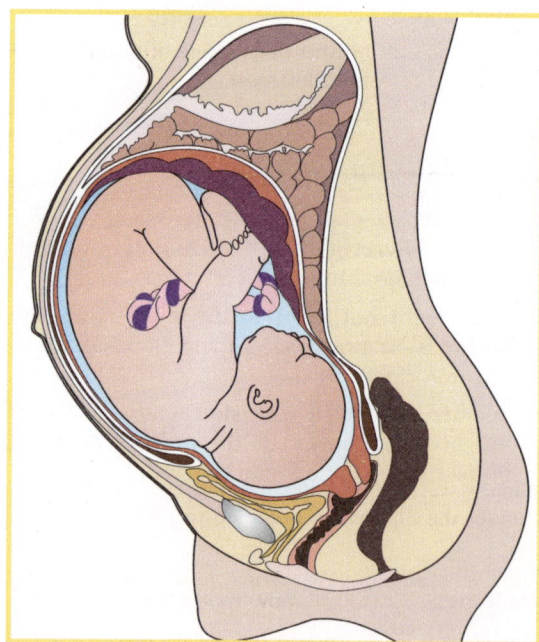

Foetus at 40 weeks

Baby

- Your baby is now mature enough to face life outside your womb and the vital organs are ready to function.
- The baby's bowels are filled with meconium, a greenish black stool which is the first motion that the baby passes.
- Though most of the lanugo is gone, the baby may still be born with downy hair over the forehead, on top of the ears and over the shoulders.

The role of the father-to-be

The third trimester can be as stressful for you as it is for your wife. You might be worried about how she is going to handle labour. Also, the reality of having a new person in your life is just about sinking in.

How can you help?

Be prepared for labour by reading about it and also by attending labour preparation classes with your wife. Talk to the obstetrician and find out if you will be allowed into the labour room to provide comfort and support to your wife during labour. Seeing your baby born before your eyes can be one of the most miraculous experiences in your life.

Be prepared for the eventuality of a caesarean. Nearly 20 to 25 per cent of pregnant women may end up having a caesarean section. Make sure you have already discussed with your obstetrician what your wife will face if she needs a caesarean section. If an elective caesarean section has been planned and blood is being reserved as is usually done, you can make arrangements for blood donors from your circle of friends or relatives.

As a husband, you may have eagerly waited to play a part in the birth of your baby. When you learn that your wife will be undergoing a caesarean section, you may at first feel a little cheated that you are not able to be in the labour room participating in the birth of the baby. Don't worry. You can provide emotional support for your wife after the baby is born, for there will be plenty of opportunities to participate in the bringing up of your baby.

Bond with your baby

Make sure that you are allowed to hold the baby as soon as possible after the birth. This strengthens the bond between you and your newborn. It is important to cuddle your baby so that she can recognise and become familiar with your feel and touch.

Never forget: all babies need their dad as much as they need their mother!

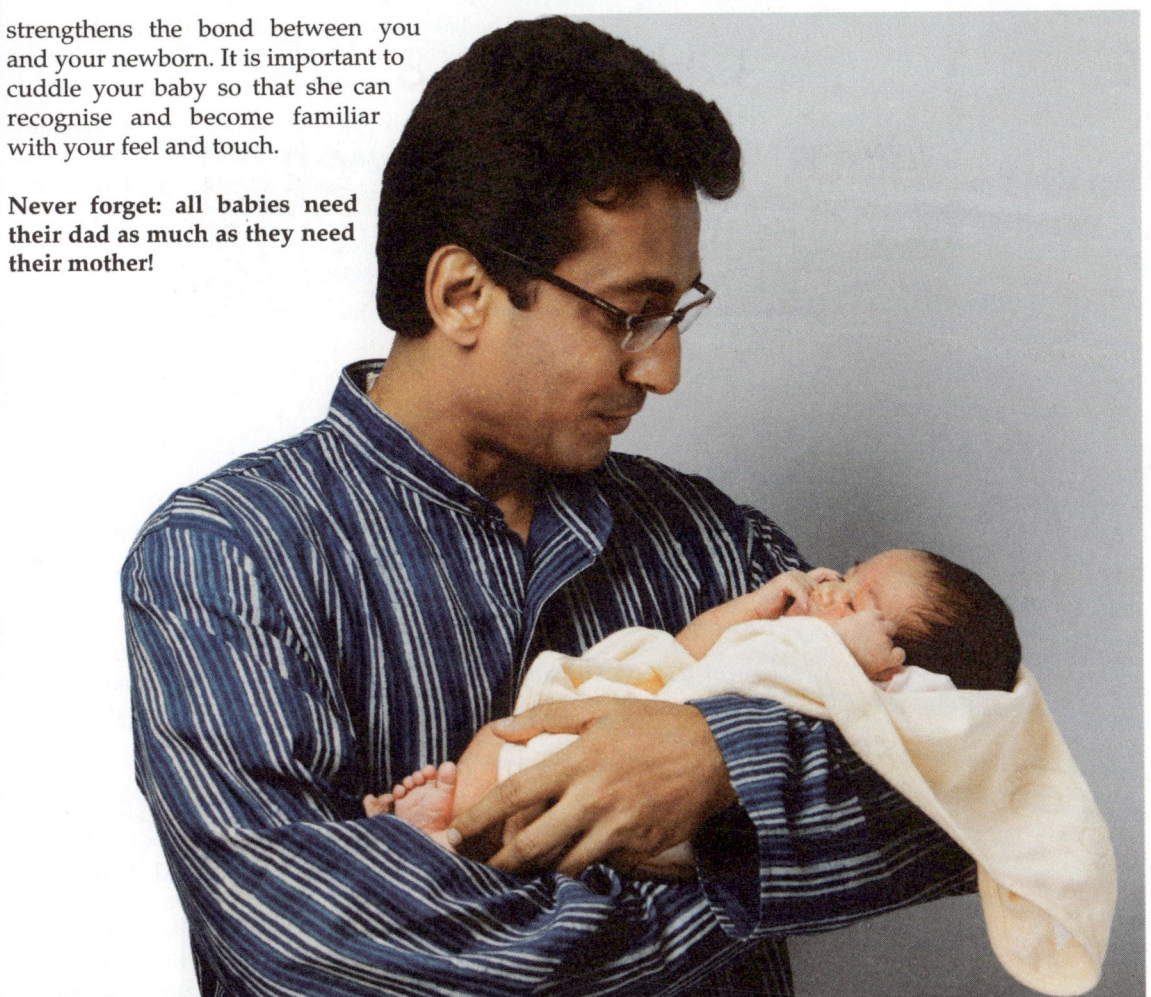

Old wives' tales
- You should not travel in the 'even' months of pregnancy i.e. 6th month or 8th month. Actually it does not matter which month you travel in. If you are going elsewhere for your delivery, then make sure you travel before 34 weeks of pregnancy. Medically, we know that some complications of pregnancy are more common after 34 weeks, so it is better to be under the supervision of the obstetrician who is going to deliver you.
- Avoid sleeping on your back or, always sleep on your left side. **Not true.** For normal, healthy women in an uncomplicated pregnancy, the best position for sleeping is the one that's most comfortable.
- You must have intercourse to have a normal vaginal delivery. **Not true!** Though there is no reason to avoid intercourse, you may feel uncomfortable closer to term so you may not want to have sex. This will not prevent you from having a normal vaginal delivery.
- You should eat well when labour starts because you will not be given food for another few hours. **Not true.** It is very important that you do not eat or drink anything once the water breaks or pains start. (See Chapter 17: **Labour and delivery**).

CHAPTER 8

Eating healthy in pregnancy

Seetha is pregnant! She is excited and happy as she tells her family the wonderful news. There are smiles and an occasional tear of happiness as the news sinks in. The first reaction to the news is, "Now you must take good care of yourself. You must eat for two, sleep well and be happy!" But does she really need to eat for two?

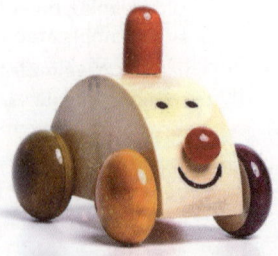

8 Eating healthy in pregnancy

Eating healthy

Good nutrition helps a woman's body prepare for motherhood. The complex processes that occur during pregnancy require a rich supply of protein, vitamins and minerals for both mother and child.

> Eating a balanced diet, rich in nutrients, during your pregnancy is one of the best things you can do for yourself and your baby.

Getting an early start

When is the best time to start eating a healthy diet? Obviously, before you become pregnant. This will ensure that both you and your baby start out with the right balance of nutrients required.

If you are planning a pregnancy, it would be a good idea to start taking **folic acid.** This vitamin prevents you from having a baby with certain spinal defects. Folic acid occurs naturally in green leafy vegetables, citrus fruits or dried lentils. In addition, your doctor will prescribe a folic acid supplement. It is recommended to start this at least 1-3 months before you get pregnant and to continue it for the first three months of the pregnancy.

Do I need to eat for two?

This is a time which is exciting and yet a bit scary. Having a baby means so much more than just carrying around some extra weight for the next nine months. That new life growing inside you will depend on you for everything it needs, to be healthy and strong, before and after he or she is born.

Do you really need to eat for two? Not really. The growing foetus doesn't 'eat' food! It only absorbs the essential nutrients it requires from the blood circulating through the placenta. In the las six months of a normal pregnancy, you require 300 calories more per day. These 300 calories are really not much in terms of food quantity (see box). There is no need to overeat to achieve this.

I don't want to gain too much weight during pregnancy!

Many women today are conscious about their weight. They dread getting out of shape during

The extra 300 calories per day: how can you get them?	
2 cups of cow's milk	200 calories
2 medium chapathis with small cup of vegetables	300 calories
100 gm of cooked rice	325 calories
3 idlis with ½ cup of sambhar	300 calories
2 small vegetable sandwiches	300 calories
Egg (whole)	75 calories
White of egg	15 calories

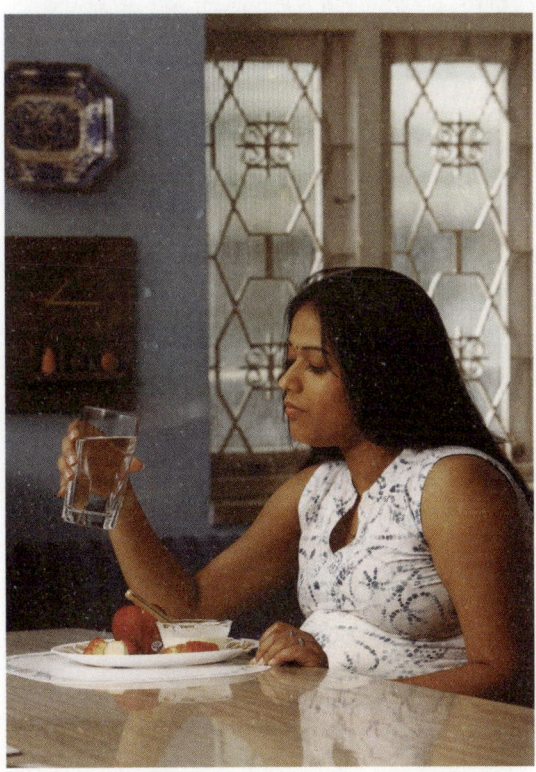

pregnancy. It is difficult to expend too much energy while being pregnant. Therefore, there's no need to increase your intake drastically. A healthy weight gain is between 8 and 10 kilos for the entire pregnancy. After the first three months, a healthy weight gain is usually between 1-1.5 kilos per month.

It is not all baby

During her monthly check-up, Shantha was found to have put on 4 kilos in one month. Her husband was happy because he had visions of a cute, chubby baby. He believed if the mother put on a lot of weight, the baby would be 'healthy'. He had to be gently reminded that the weight gain could not be all baby. In fact, if she continued to put on too much weight, at the end of the pregnancy he would have more wife than he had bargained for!

Ideal weight gain in pregnancy

A healthy weight gain for a pregnancy would be between 8-10 kilos. If you are obese at the start of the pregnancy, it is important to restrict the weight gain to 6-8 kilos. If you are underweight to begin with, it might be advisable to put on 10-12 kilos.

Where does the weight gain come from?

Average sized baby	2.8-3.5 kg
Uterus, placenta and amniotic fluid	1.5 kg
Blood and retained water	2.5 kg
Body stores (mostly fat)	4.0-4.5 kg

The extra fat stores are difficult to get rid of after a pregnancy. If there has been too much weight gain due to fat accumulation, then a strict diet regimen needs to be followed after the delivery. **Remember, future obesity starts with excessive weight gain during pregnancy.**

The first three months

Sahana is two months pregnant. "I hate the sight of food," she bursts out. Her husband is frustrated because he has the mistaken belief that if she does not eat well, the baby will not be healthy. This is not true. In the first three months, pregnant women may not like the smell and taste of many foods and at the same time, may develop strange cravings.

At this time, it is easier to eat bland, dry food like salt biscuits, dry toast, dry chapathis or idlis. Identify healthy snacks that you can eat during the day. This is a good way to get the nutrients and extra calories you need. You may find it easier to eat small meals at frequent intervals rather than three big meals a day. This also may help avoid nausea. It is enough to avoid getting dehydrated and feeling rundown. Avoid long periods of starvation because this will increase acidity and increase nausea.

Getting through those first three months

In the first three months, eat small, healthy snacks or meals at frequent intervals to avoid nausea. Try to avoid long periods of starvation.

Eat low fat foods that are rich in carbohydrates such as toast, idlis or chapathis. Bland foods will keep your nausea under control. Avoid strong smelling, oily, spicy foods. If you can tolerate milk, have a bowl of cereal with cold milk.

A mid-morning and mid-afternoon snack keeps the acidity down and can decrease nausea. It can be a fruit juice, salt or sweet biscuits or fruits (fresh or dried fruits like raisins, dates, apricots).

If you are vomiting a lot, you may tend to get dehydrated. This will make you feel exhausted and can cause constipation. Try and consume at least two litres of fluid every day. You may not even like the taste of water, so you can drink other fluids: dilute buttermilk, tender coconut water, thin soups and juices like sweet lime or lemon.

Your obstetrician will prescribe medication to control the nausea and the vomiting. This will definitely help you get through the first few weeks of pregnancy.

A balanced diet

A healthy diet in pregnancy should include proteins, carbohydrates, fats, vitamins and minerals too.

Dairy products

Pregnant women should try to drink two glasses of milk and eat two cups of curds (yogurt) a day. Dairy products are an excellent source of protein and calcium. If you are trying to control your weight, then low-fat milk and curds will give you the protein and calcium you require, without the fat. Cheese and paneer are also good sources of milk protein. Restrict ice-creams because though they are dairy products, they are high in calories derived from fat and sugar.

Protein

Proteins are the building blocks for the baby. Make sure your diet includes dairy products, grains, nuts and pulses, meat, fish or poultry.

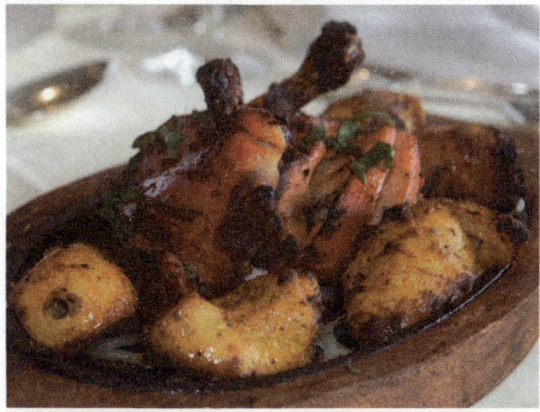

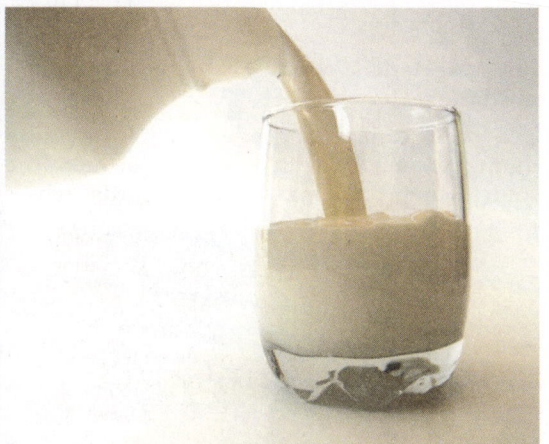

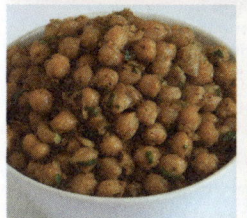

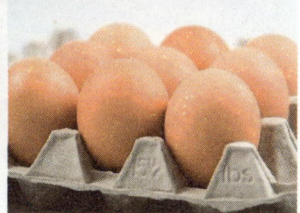

To be sure your diet provides you with the right amount of nutrients, you should know which foods are good sources of each.

Nutrient	How does it help?	Best sources
Iron	Helps in producing red blood cells which carry oxygen to your baby	Green leafy vegetables, dates, iron supplements
Calcium	Helps build strong bones and teeth	Milk, curds, paneer, cheese
Vitamin A	Healthy skin and good eyesight.	Carrots, dark-green leafy vegetables
Vitamin C	Helps in absorption of iron; promotes healthy gums, prevents colds	Citrus fruits, tomatoes, amla
Vitamin B_6	Helps body utilise protein, fat, carbohydrates and helps in formation of red blood cells	Whole grains, bananas
Vitamin B_{12}	Important in the formation of red blood cells, maintains nervous system	Found only in animal foods- vegetarians need to take a supplement
Folic acid	Prevents spinal abnormalities in the foetus. Needed to produce blood and protein	Green leafy vegetables, dark yellow fruits and vegetables, legumes and nuts, vitamin supplements.

Carbohydrates

Carbohydrates provide you with energy. When taken in larger quantities, you will only get empty calories. You need not increase the quantity of rice you normally take. Substitute chapathis for rice at one meal, if you are gaining too much weight.

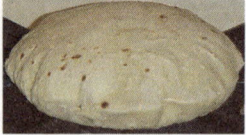

Vegetables and fruits

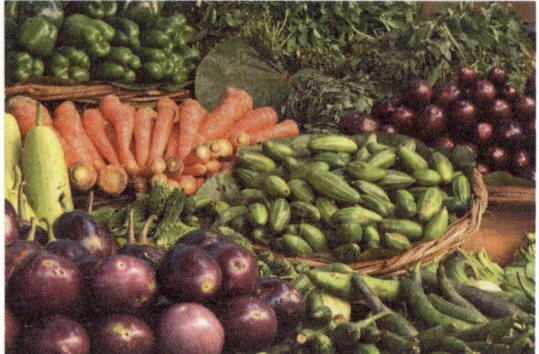

Vegetables provide vitamins, minerals and roughage. Try to include 3-4 servings per day. A salad with fresh, raw vegetables is highly recommended. This will provide the fibre and roughage that will prevent constipation. About 2-3 servings of fruit should be included daily. The old wives' tale of not eating papaya, pineapple and mangoes in pregnancy has no basis in science.

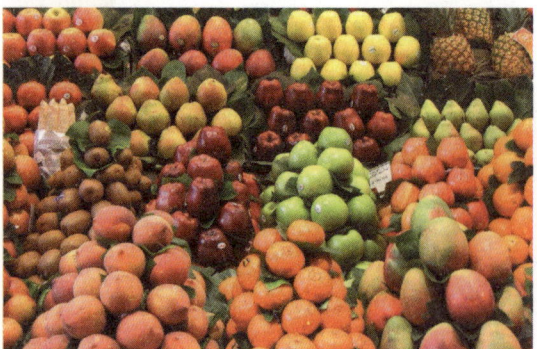

Vitamins and minerals

Many women of childbearing age have low iron stores. It is important to be on a combination supplement of iron, B-complex and folic acid. Calcium requirements double during pregnancy.

A mother's body adapts to absorb more calcium from the foods eaten and so keep up your intake of dairy products.

Pregnant women need extra iron and folic acid, and these are usually prescribed in tablets or capsules. A prenatal supplement that contains these two nutrients plus vitamins and minerals is recommended.

Special concerns

I'm a vegetarian. Will my baby receive enough nutrition?

Yes, you can still get adequate nutrition during pregnancy with a vegetarian diet. The sources of protein will be milk, curds, whole

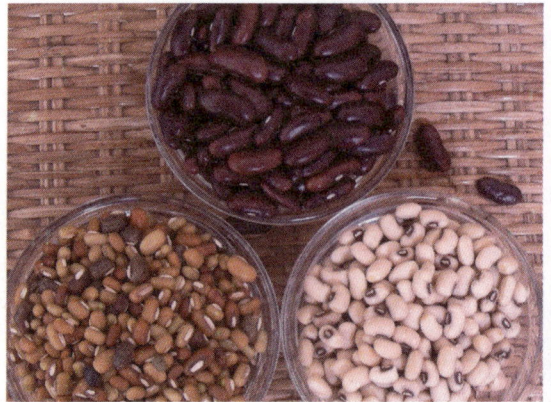

Folic acid

Women should take 400 micrograms of folic acid daily, in addition to a well balanced diet, for at least 1-3 months before pregnancy and during the first 3 months of pregnancy. This can help prevent neural tube defects, which affect the spine and skull of the foetus.

Women who have had a child with a neural tube defect are more likely to have another child with this problem. These women need much higher doses of folic acid—4 milligrams daily. It should be taken for 1-3 months before pregnancy and during the first 3 months of pregnancy. Women who need 4 milligrams should take folic acid as a separate supplement, not as part of a multivitamin.

grains and pulses. You will need to take supplements, especially iron, vitamins B12 and folic acid. There is no need for commercial food preparations like "health drinks" or "protein supplements".

I am unable to tolerate dairy products. Will that harm my baby?

Some women cannot stand the taste of milk, and even have symptoms such as bloating, diarrhoea, gas and indigestion after drinking milk or eating dairy products. This is known as **lactose intolerance.** Milk and other dairy products are the best sources of calcium in your diet. If you are absolutely unable to tolerate dairy products, you need **calcium supplements** during pregnancy.

I have the urge to eat the strangest things!

It is commonly known that women have a craving for some foods which they may not even like when they are not pregnant. Most women feel like eating sour or spicy food, especially in the early months of pregnancy. Occasionally, some may take a violent dislike to what used to be their favourite food.

A strange phenomenon called **pica** occurs sometimes in pregnancy, where women feel strong urges to eat non-food items such as clay, ice, mud or chalk. Pica can be harmful to your pregnancy. It can affect your intake of nutrients and can lead to constipation and anaemia. Luckily, pica lasts for only short periods of time.

> Healthy eating also means avoiding things that may be harmful. This includes alcohol (beer, wine, or mixed drinks) which may cause birth defects and other problems for the baby. Smoking cigarettes is especially harmful to a pregnant woman and her baby.

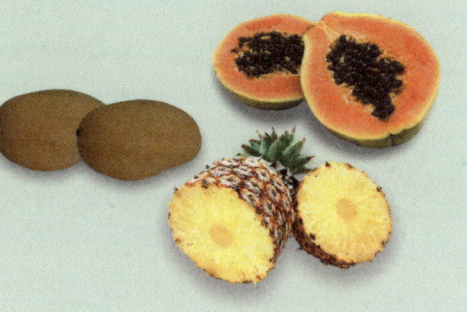

Old wives' tales
- Saffron makes your baby fair skinned. **Not true!** No food that you eat can have any effect on the colour of your baby's skin. That is determined by genetics.
- Mangoes, pineapples and papayas can cause an abortion. **Not true!**
- Sesame seed (*til* seeds) can cause an abortion. **Not true!**

CHAPTER 9

Exercising in pregnancy

Santoshini is pregnant for the second time. She was active throughout her first pregnancy, keeping up a regular exercise programme. Her friends were amazed at how fit she was through her pregnancy and how quickly she lost the pregnancy weight after delivery.

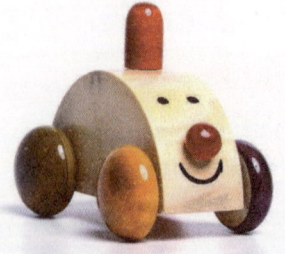

9 Exercising in pregnancy

There is no doubt about it: exercising throughout pregnancy has great benefits. The level of exercise you do depends on how fit you were before your pregnancy. Discuss with your obstetrician what adjustments you need to make to your normal exercise routine. Even if you did not have a regular exercise routine earlier, you can keep yourself fit with a sensible fitness regimen. Walking is an excellent form of exercise and should be part of your fitness programme.

Why exercise?

It is common knowledge that exercise has immense benefits at any stage of life. In pregnancy, exercise can

- **Make you feel better:** As the pregnancy progresses, your sense of balance will be challenged because of your changing posture. Exercise improves your balance. It also boosts energy levels.
- **Relieve backaches and improve your posture** by strengthening and toning muscles in your back, buttocks and thighs. As your body undergoes changes, you will develop aches and pains caused by the growing uterus. There is additional strain on the muscles of your back, abdomen and legs. Exercise will help relieve these pains.
- **Reduce constipation** by improving intestinal movement.
- **Help you sleep better** by releasing muscle tension and relieving stress.
- **Prepare you and your body for birth** by strengthening your muscles and gently stretching your pelvic muscles.
- **Return to your pre-pregnancy shape faster** because you will not gain unnecessary weight.

What is the best exercise plan?

Nothing beats the benefits of brisk walking. You should build up your stamina till you are walking at least 30-45 minutes a day, at least five times a week. If you are just starting, begin with a moderately brisk pace for a kilometre, five days a week. Add five minutes every few days till you are walking the optimal time. As the

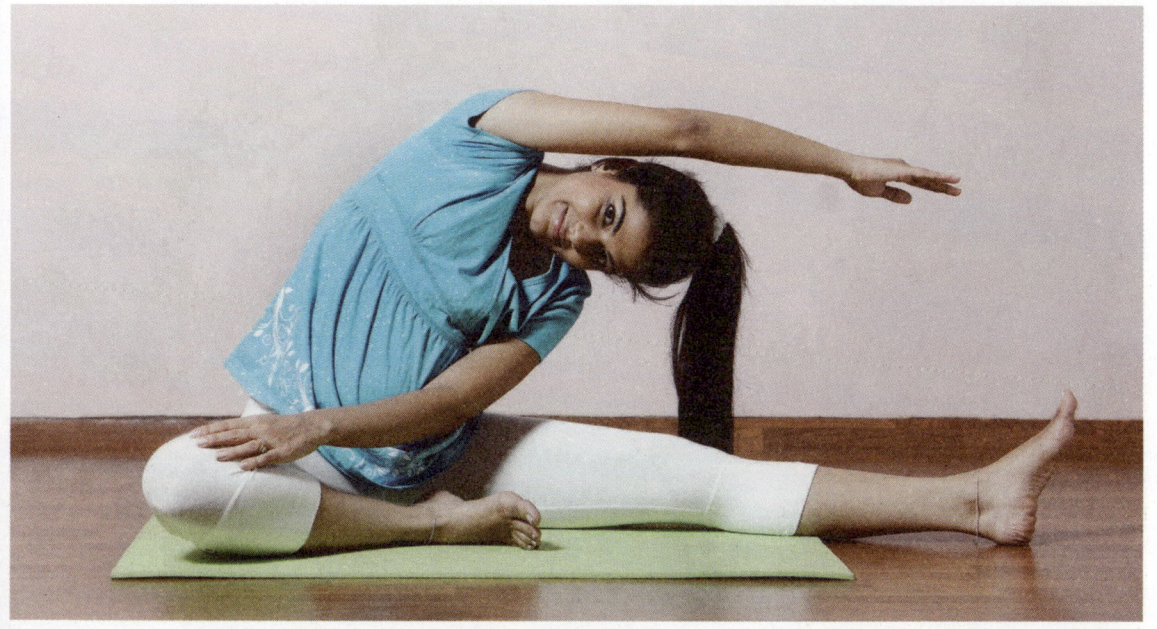

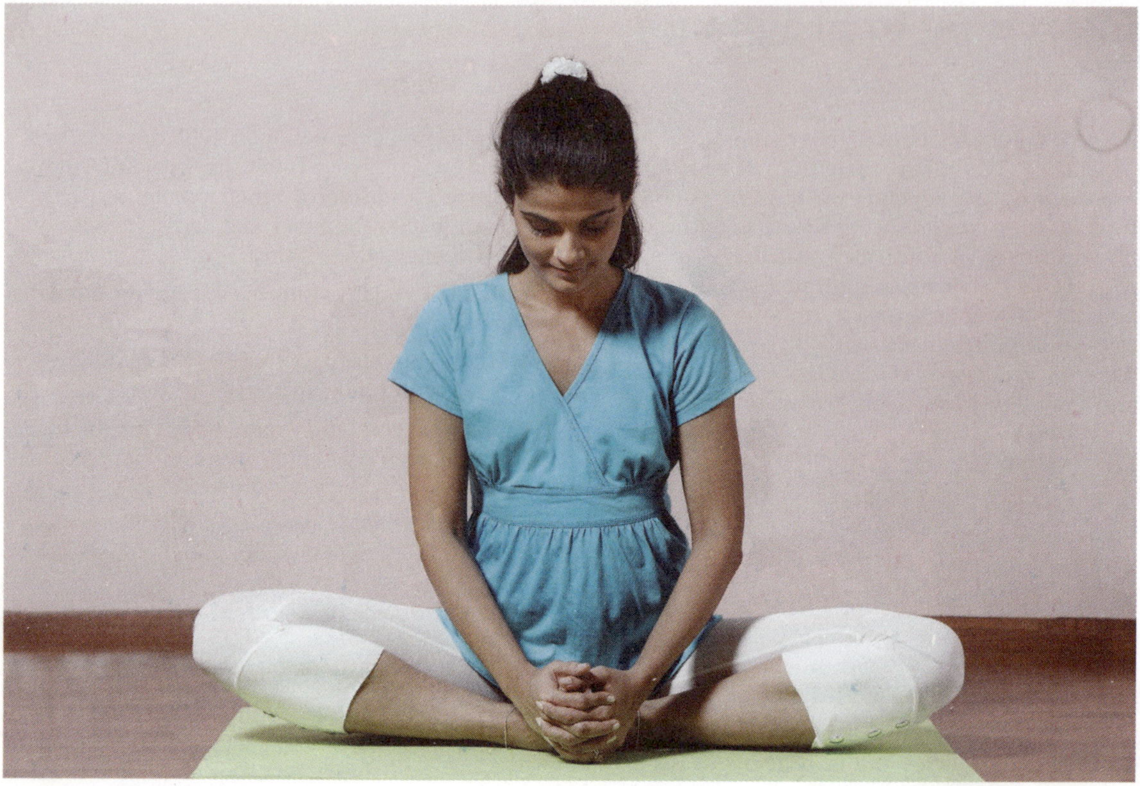

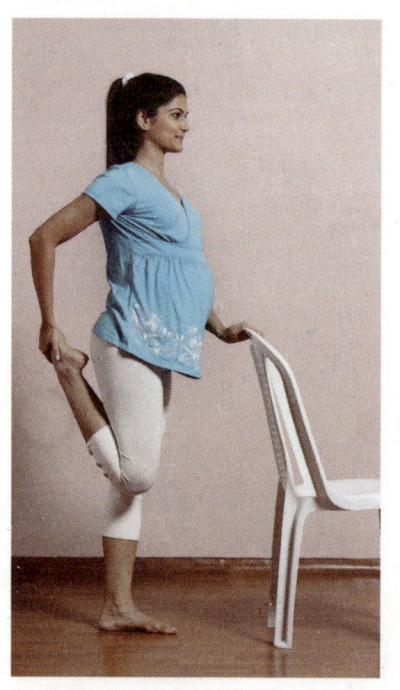
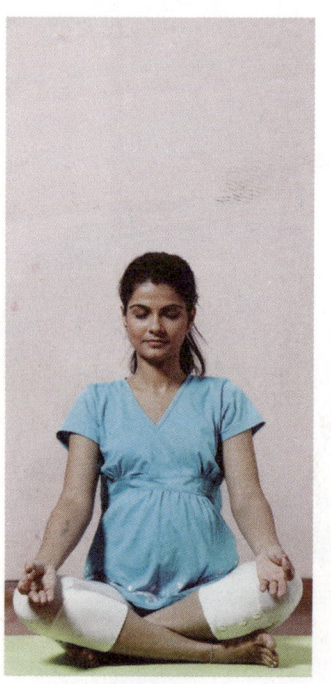
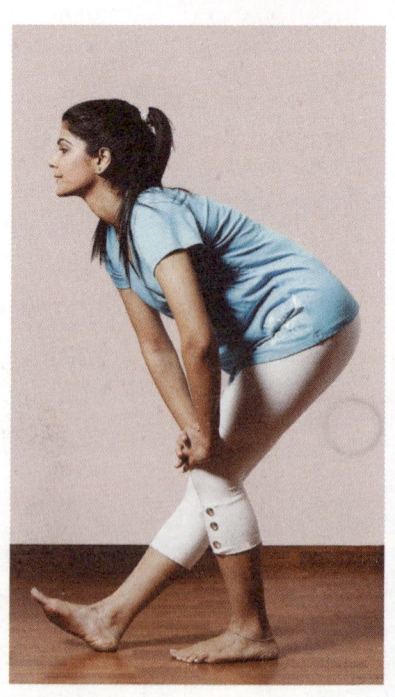

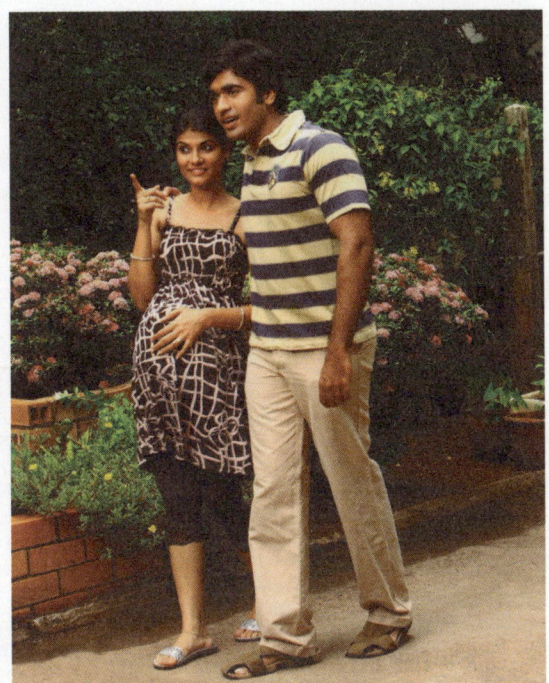

pregnancy progresses, especially in the last few weeks, you might find yourself tiring easily and getting breathless. Pace yourself and modify your regimen but do not give up completely. Remember – walk slowly for the first five minutes as a warm up. Similarly, slow down in the last five minutes to cool down.

Stretches and yoga

During pregnancy, it is important to gently stretch the major muscle groups and ligaments of the body. **Yoga** is one option to stretch different muscle groups. **Pranayama** (rhythmic deep breathing) improves oxygenation to all parts of the body and also to the uterus.

A combination of cardio (aerobic), strength and flexibility exercises is the best for you. Find out if there are any antenatal exercise classes near you and enrol into one of them.

Discuss any concerns you have with your obstetrician.

When should exercise be avoided?

Your obstetrician may ask you to limit your exercise if you have:

- pregnancy-induced high blood pressure
- early contractions
- vaginal bleeding
- premature rupture of your membranes (leaking of the amniotic fluid)

Tips for healthy exercising

When you exercise, make sure that you warm up and cool down. Wear loose fitting, comfortable clothing, non-skid shoes that are supportive, and a well-fitting bra.

Watch your centre of gravity and always keep your balance. Bouncing or jerky exercises are best avoided. Your joints loosen up in pregnancy and care must be taken not to sprain them. Make sure that you don't get overheated. Always drink water before, during and after exercising. Listen to your body when something hurts or doesn't feel right. Your heart rate should stay below 130 beats per minute. When you are walking or exercising, you have reached the right target if you are mildly breathless but still able to carry on a conversation.

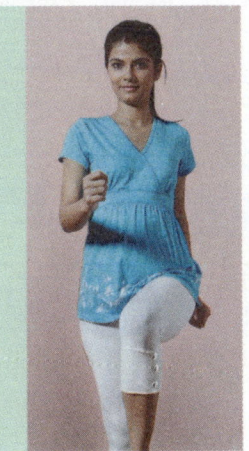

CHAPTER 10

The role of the father-to-be

A few years ago, it was uncommon to see a husband accompany his wife for an antenatal check-up. With encouragement, and the prospect of being allowed into the labour room, more and more husbands have started accompanying their wives. The support that a woman gets from her husband during pregnancy is invaluable.

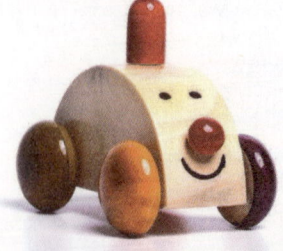

10 The role of the father-to-be

The days when women came for their obstetric consultation with only their mother or another female relative, are long past. A few years ago, it was uncommon to see a husband accompany his wife for an antenatal check-up. Nowadays, with encouragement, and the prospect of being allowed into the labour room, more and more husbands have started accompanying their wives. Today, the majority of women come for their consultation with their husbands and this is how it should be.

Pregnancy is replete with changes. The physical and emotional changes that occur in the pregnant woman can leave her partner bewildered and sometimes a little worried. To truly enjoy the pregnancy, it is important for the husband to have a complete understanding of the process and the innumerable adjustments needed.

Many men get involved right from the time the pregnancy test comes back as positive. They go for antenatal appointments with their wives, and attend classes for labour preparation. At the same time, they may be filled with anxiety about their ability to handle the pregnancy and its demands on their feelings and emotions.

The father is important too

Children need their fathers as much as their mothers. A man's role as a father can begin long before the baby is born. A supportive husband can make his wife's pregnancy easier and healthier. There is no doubt that labour and delivery are easier and shorter for women whose husbands actively participate in the process.

A husband's role during labour and birth is to provide emotional support and comfort to his wife. Being part of the child's birth is a significant and incomparable experience.

The birth of a child is such an intense and emotional experience that the significance doubles when it is shared by the couple.

Support in early pregnancy

Early in pregnancy (up to the first 14 weeks), your wife may feel tired, may need more sleep, urinate frequently and have sore breasts. Nausea and vomiting are quite common. Although these symptoms are known as "morning sickness," they can happen at any time of the day or night. Your support is important at this time. Try to spend as much time as you can with her. Take over some household chores so that she can sleep a little longer.

> A husband who pitches in and lets his wife sleep a little longer, is worth his weight in gold!

You may be concerned that she is not eating properly. If she does not eat, will the baby's development be affected? Don't worry. The baby will not be affected. In a few weeks, her appetite will be back to normal and she can start eating nutritious food again.

What may catch you by surprise are her mood swings! Early pregnancy can be an emotional roller-coaster for a woman. Sudden changes in mood are common. You may feel hurt and upset by her labile moods. At the same time, you may feel left out as she focusses on her changing body and emotions. Knowing that these changes are a natural part of early pregnancy will help you support your wife and deal with her feelings.

Working together for a healthy lifestyle will benefit you, your wife and your baby. You both can adapt your lifestyle to include a balanced

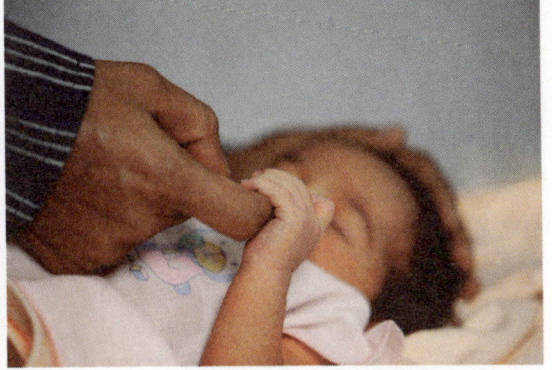

diet and plenty of rest. Since she must stop any use of alcohol and tobacco, this is a good time for you to stop as well. Remember, if your wife inhales tobacco smoke from your smoking, this affects the baby.

How can you help?

Just being there for her is an enormous mood elevator for the new mother-to-be. With words and deeds, let her know that you are delighted that she is pregnant. Help her out with housework because she may find it hard to do all the household chores due to the tiredness of early pregnancy. Plan short weekend trips to nearby destinations. Spend time together as much as possible. For, once the baby is born, it can be quite a while before you take a holiday.

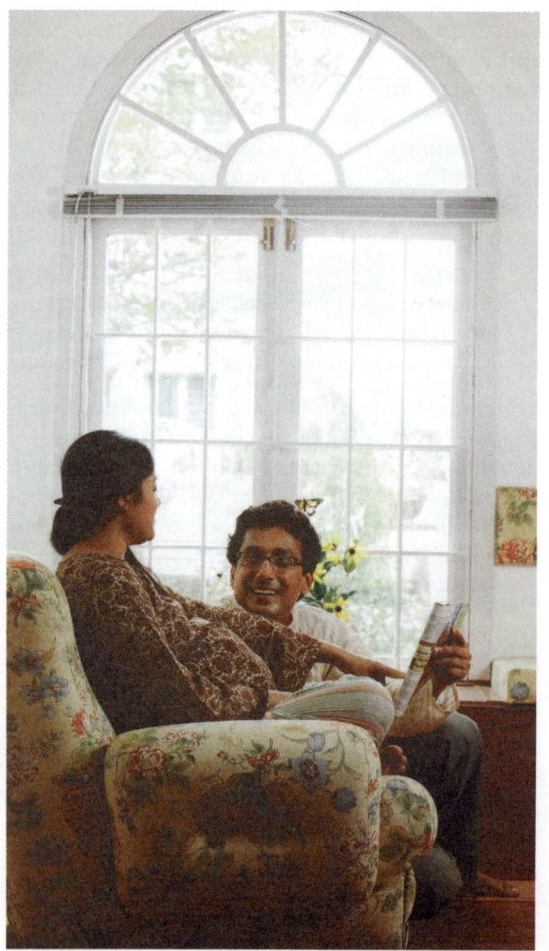

Make sure that you go to all her antenatal check-ups with her. This will allow you to clear your doubts too. Knowing what is happening with her pregnancy will enable you to be a supportive and comforting husband.

The second trimester (14-28 weeks)

The second trimester is the good part of pregnancy. Your wife is energetic and will be able to carry on with all her work. She is still not very uncomfortable because of the size of the pregnancy. Her appetite is back to normal.

How can you help?

Make sure your wife gets a nutritious diet. At the same time, do not get carried away and force her to eat so much that she puts on unnecessary weight. If you insist on overfeeding her, the excess weight gain may leave you, at the end of the pregnancy, with more wife than you bargained for! Remember that the redundant weight put on during a pregnancy is difficult to get rid off and can be the beginning of life-long obesity.

She may have leg aches and back pains. Help her exercise by taking time to walk with her. You can also help by massaging her legs and lower back.

Make sure that she takes her iron and vitamin supplement everyday.

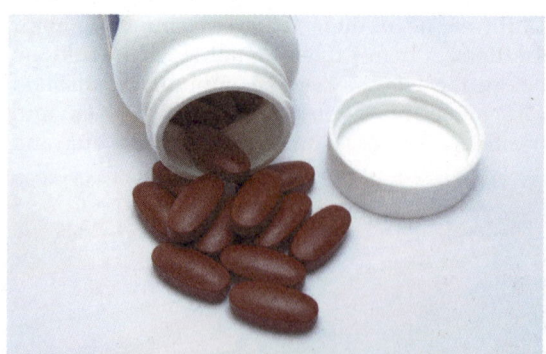

The third trimester (29 weeks to delivery)

The third trimester can be as stressful for you as it is for her. You might be worried about how she will handle labour. The reality of having a new baby is also sinking in.

Many couples wonder if it is safe to have sex during pregnancy and if intercourse will harm the baby. In most pregnancies, sex is considered safe and healthy. The woman's comfort should be the most important guide during sex. As pregnancy advances, have intercourse in positions that do not put pressure on her abdomen, such as with her on top or lying side by side. If you have any concerns about having intercourse during pregnancy, talk to your doctor. If your wife is having bleeding in pregnancy, you might be asked to avoid intercourse for some time.

How can you help?

Be prepared for labour by reading about it and by attending labour preparation classes with your wife. Have a checklist and make sure you are prepared when she goes into labour.

- Know the phone numbers of the hospital and the doctor and keep them handy.
- Keep a packed suitcase to take to hospital.
- Make sure there is somebody who can take her to the hospital if she goes into labour when you are not around.
- Do trial runs to see how long it takes to get to the hospital.
- Make sure you always have petrol in the car!
- If you are going to use a call taxi, keep that number handy.

Being in the labour room

Talk to the obstetrician and ask her if you will be allowed into the labour room. Seeing your baby born before your eyes can be one of the most miraculous experiences of your life.

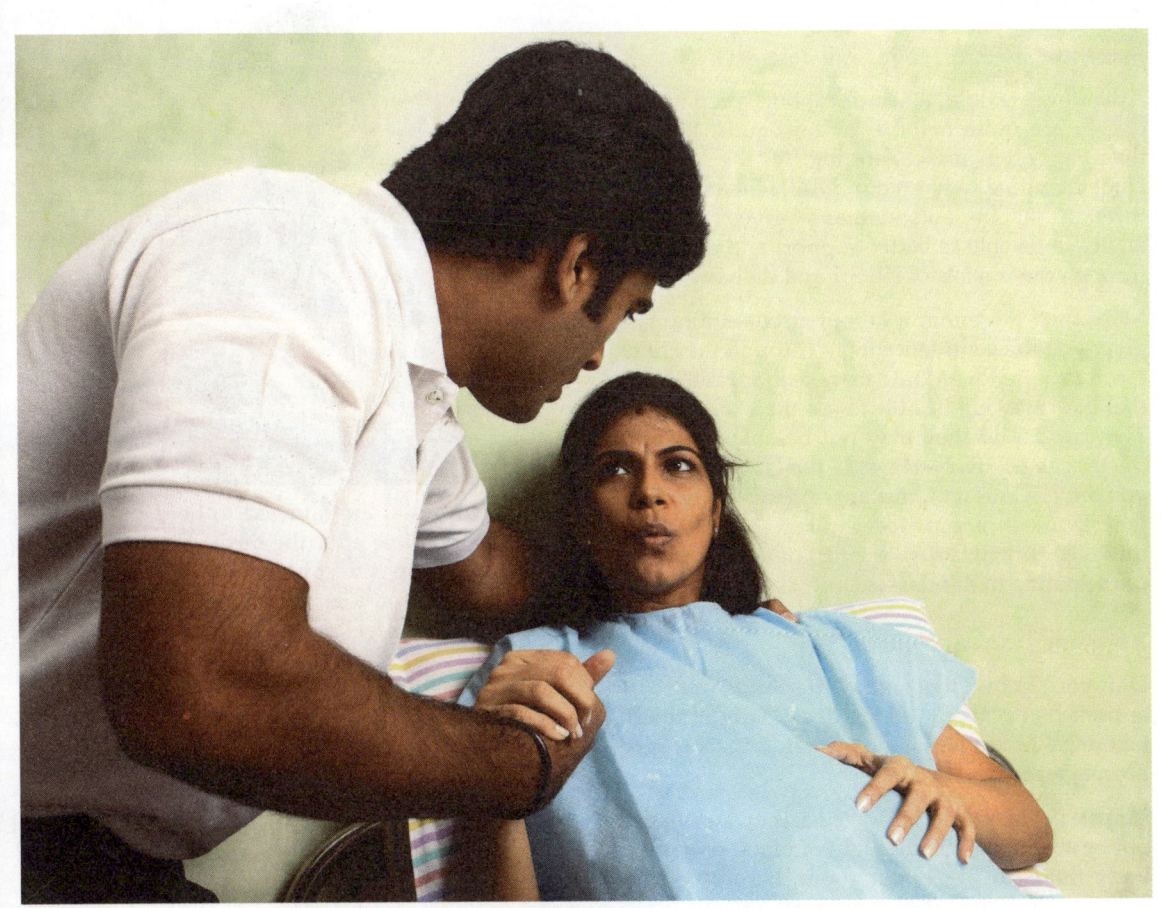

Be prepared for the eventuality of a caesarean. Nearly 20-25 per cent of pregnant women may end up having a caesarean section. Make sure you have already discussed with your obstetrician what your wife will face if she needs a caesarean section. If an elective caesarean section has been planned and blood is being reserved as is usually done, you can make arrangements for blood donors from your circle of friends or relatives.

As a husband, you may have eagerly waited to play a part in the birth of your baby. When you learn that your wife will be undergoing a caesarean section, you may at first feel a little cheated that you are not able to be in the labour room participating in the birth of the baby. Don't worry. You can provide emotional support for your wife after the baby is born, for there will be plenty of opportunities to participate in the bringing up of your baby.

Being prepared for labour and delivery

Attending childbirth and labour preparation classes are quite helpful for husbands. It gives them a better understanding of the process. Understanding what your wife will be facing through labour and delivery gives you the ability to be able to better support and assist her through the travails of labour and delivery.

More than anything, a labour preparation class gives you the confidence to go through the childbirth experience. Many men are apprehensive that they may not be able to see their wife suffer. They are afraid they may not be able to handle the processes involved inside the labour room. If you are anxious and hesitant, attending the class will lay most of your fears to rest. You will feel more confident after seeing other men also participating in the classes.

It is normal to be nervous!

Did you know that most husbands may be apprehensive about taking their wife through labour? You are not alone in that. This is a very normal reaction.

Your wife may also be worried that you might not be able to handle the sight of blood and other body fluids in the labour room. Do not worry.

When your wife is in labour and when she is going to deliver, you will be so involved with encouraging her and giving her moral support that you will forget about everything else.

Remember that most of the times, you will be sitting or standing near your wife's head. You can turn your eyes away from anything else that is going on and only concentrate on talking your wife through her pains. Usually a chair or stool will be provided for you to be comfortably seated while you talk to your wife.

If a problem arises, you may be asked to leave the delivery room. In the best interest of the mother and baby, you should leave right away if asked.

Bond with your baby

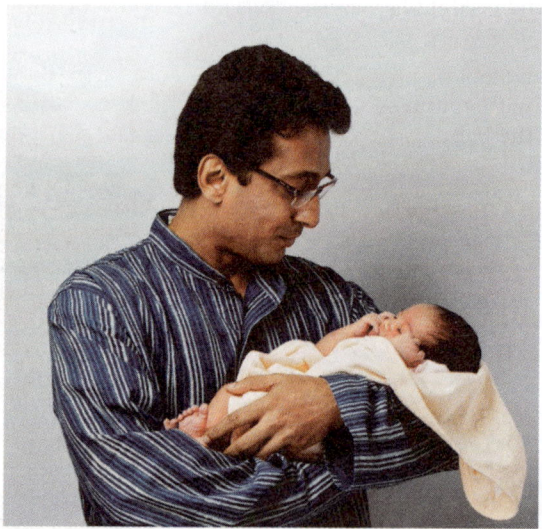

Make sure you are allowed to hold the baby as soon as possible after the birth. This strengthens the bond between you and your newborn. It is important to cuddle your baby so that she can recognise your feel and touch.

Never forget: all babies need their father as much as they need their mother.

After the baby's birth

The first six weeks after birth are considered the postpartum period. During this time, your wife's body again goes through dramatic changes as it recovers from the physical stress of pregnancy and birth. She will have some bleeding for 4-6 weeks. If she has had an episiotomy, she may have pain and discomfort from the stitches. Her breasts may be sore. She may be anxious about breastfeeding and may worry whether the baby is getting enough milk.

If the baby was born by caesarean birth, the incision on the abdomen may be uncomfortable. It will take time for her to regain her usual strength.

How can you help?

If you do not have other family members to help out, the postpartum period can sometimes be overwhelming. New parents are often nervous about taking care of the newborn. It is important to maintain a sense of humour at this time to help both of you cope with the demands of your new baby.

Do not be afraid to take care of your baby. Bond with your newborn by changing diapers, bathing the baby and rocking your baby to sleep. If you have older children at home, spend extra time with them to help them get used to being big brother or sister. By sharing the care of the baby with your wife, you will provide the support she needs and at the same time, gain confidence in your own parenting skills.

Resuming intercourse after delivery

After a vaginal delivery or a caesarean section, it is usually safe to resume intercourse six weeks after birth. By that time, your wife would have had her postnatal check-up and her obstetrician would have made sure she has healed well. Your wife may be a little apprehensive about pain the first few times and it is important to make sure she is comfortable.

Remember that even if a woman is not having a period or is breastfeeding, she can become pregnant. Birth control should be used when you resume intercourse. Talk to your obstetrician about the safest and most suitable birth control option **(see Chapter 43: Methods of birth control).**

'**Postpartum blues**' is a term used when new mothers feel sad, afraid or anxious after childbirth. Most new mothers experience these feelings in a mild form. When these feelings are extreme and last longer, however, they signal a more serious condition called **postpartum depression.** Postpartum depression may require counselling and treatment

---

To-do list for dad

Pack a bag
Discuss with your wife what she needs to take to the hospital. Keep a suitcase handy in which you can pack all the essentials. As you buy things for the baby or for the delivery, keep putting them in the bag. Keep this bag in a convenient and prominent place so that you won't forget to take it when the time comes to go to the hospital.

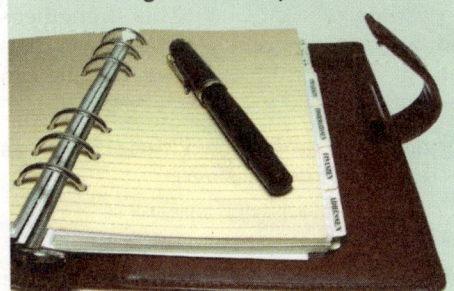

Insurance and hospital payments
Do you have medical insurance? Find out if they will pay for pregnancy and pregnancy-related procedures. Check with the hospital whether they will accept payment by cash only, cheques or credit card.

Names for the baby
Shortlist names for the baby. You have several months to decide. Do not delay this important task. Choose names for both a boy and a girl. (See the **For You** section in this book).

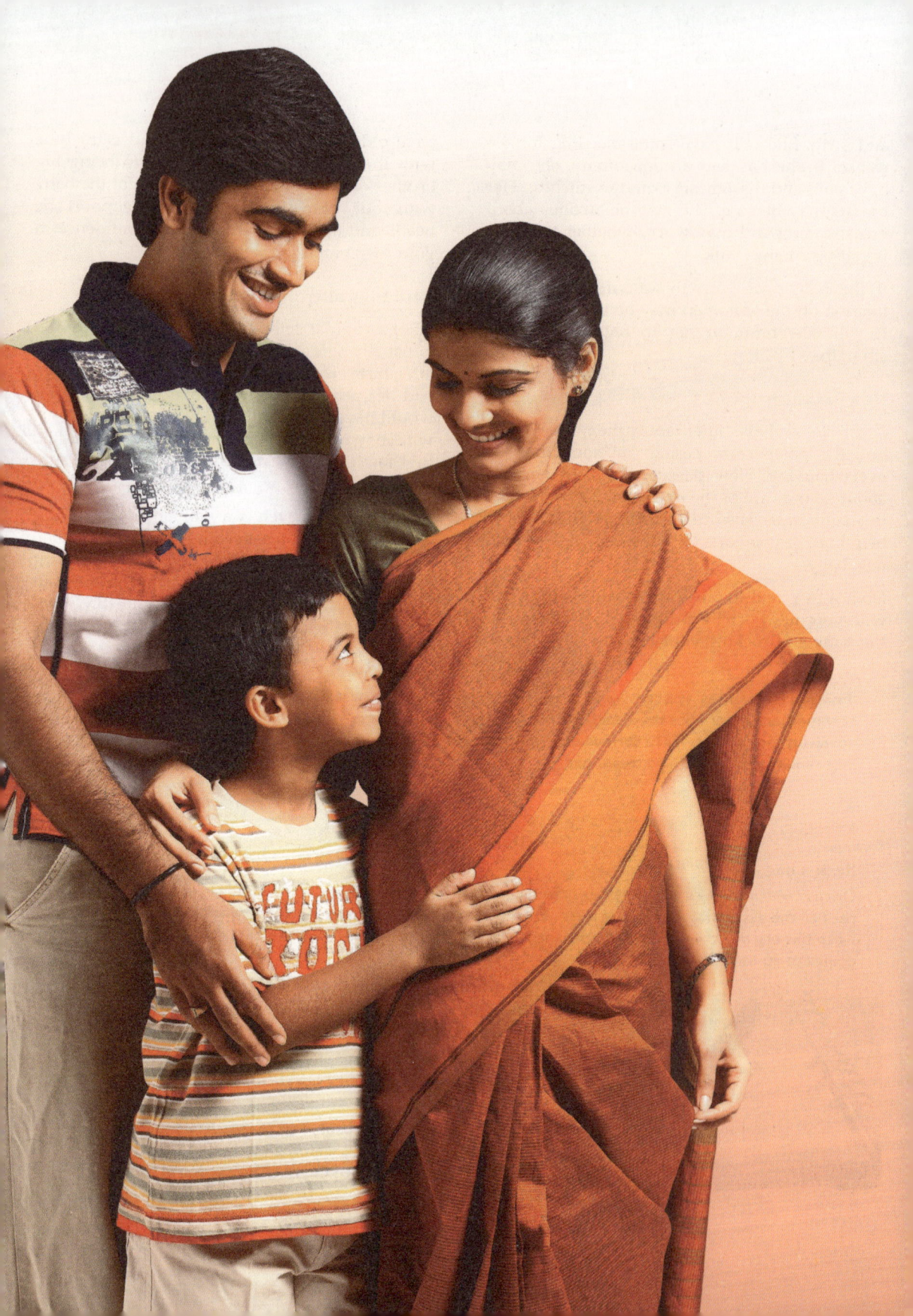

How is the baby doing?

CHAPTER 11

Tests during pregnancy:
how do I know my baby is normal?

Sheri is pregnant for the first time. She heard from her cousin about a friend who had a baby with a birth defect. Like all mothers-to-be, Sheri is concerned. Will her baby be perfect in every way? Is there any way she can find out if her baby has a birth defect? What tests should she undergo in pregnancy to ensure that the baby is normal?

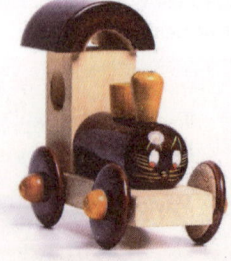

11 Tests during pregnancy:
how do I know my baby is normal?

It is important to know that out of every 100 babies born, only two or three will have major birth defects. For several centuries after the science of obstetrics came into being, all that an obstetrician could monitor were the external manifestations of pregnancy: the size of the mother's abdomen and the baby's heart beat. It was only in the 1970s, with the advent of ultrasound scanning, that we could actually unravel the physical mysteries of the unborn baby. Ultrasound scanning allows us to observe the baby from the early stages of pregnancy and look for various signs which can reassure us of the health of the baby or warn us of impending problems. The late 20th century, therefore, saw the emergence of a window to the womb, giving us a glimpse into the hitherto hidden world of the foetus.

What is a birth defect?

A birth defect (also called a **congenital abnormality, anomaly or malformation)** is a physical problem present at birth. The cause for a congenital abnormality is not known in about 70 per cent of babies. In other cases, birth defects are inherited through genes or chromosomes. Occasionally, the defect can be caused by the mother being exposed to an infection or a harmful drug in early pregnancy.

Birth defects are caused by a mishap in the way the baby develops. A birth defect may affect the structure of a body part or its function. The baby's organs develop in the first three months of pregnancy and this is when most birth defects occur. Most birth defects are mild, but some can be severe enough to jeopardise the baby's life. Babies with birth defects may need surgery or medical treatment.

Some congenital anomalies can be identified before birth with special screening tests. Others may be recognised only at birth or later in a person's life.

What is the risk of your baby having a birth defect?

Every couple worries about their baby being born with a birth defect. In the majority of cases, this worry is unnecessary. Across the world, only two or three babies out of a 100 newborns will have a major birth defect.

What causes birth defects?

If you consider the fact that just two cells (the egg and the sperm) combine to form a complex being made of billions of cells and with intricate functions, it is astounding that only 2 to 3 per cent end up with a major abnormality!

Birth defects are caused by an error in the way complex organs such as the heart, kidney, bone, muscles, brain or skin develop. A birth defect may affect how the body looks, functions or both. Rarely, the birth defect can be so complex that the baby may not survive.

What are the commonly detected birth defects?

Some of the most common birth defects found through prenatal testing include:

- **Neural tube defects:** There is incomplete closure of the foetal spine that can result in **spina bifida** or the skull does not form (**anencephaly**).
- **Abdominal wall defects:** One type of defect occurs when the muscle and skin that cover the wall of the abdomen are missing and the bowel protrudes through a defect in the abdominal

---

Two cells - the egg and the sperm - get fertilised and develop into a complex organism composed of billions of cells with intricate organs which can see, hear and taste, among other things, and perform complicated tasks. It is not surprising that sometimes the process can go awry and some part of the body may be deformed or there is a chromosomal abnormality. What is amazing is that this so uncommon!

wall (**gastroschisis**). Another type is when the tissue around the umbilical cord is weak and allows organs to protrude into this area (**omphalocoele**).

- **Heart defect:** The chambers or blood vessels of the heart are not properly developed.
- **Down syndrome:** Mental retardation, abnormal features of the face and medical problems such as heart defects occur because of an extra chromosome 21.

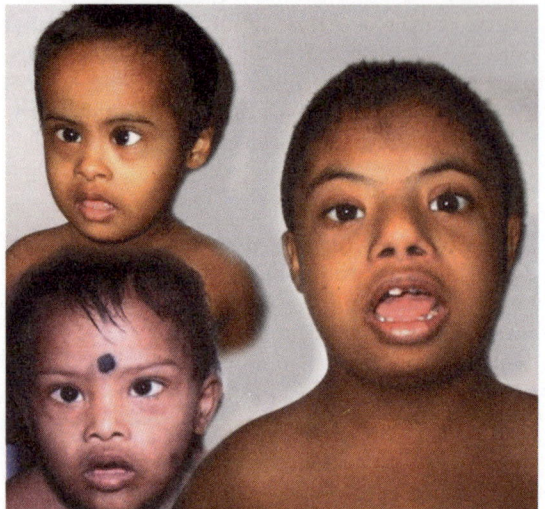

Children with Down syndrome

- **Trisomy 18:** There is an extra chromosome 18, which causes severe problems with growth and development.

What is your risk of having a baby with a birth defect?

Though many babies with birth defects are born to couples with no risk factors, the risk of birth defects increases in the following situations:

- Family or personal history of birth defects
- Previous child with a birth defect
- Diabetes before pregnancy
- Woman aged 35 years or older at the time of delivery
- Certain medicines used around the time of conception

Couples with these risk factors should have counselling and testing. Some genetic disorders occur more often in certain communities, and testing may be offered to detect them. However, most birth defects occur when there is no history of problems. There are many genetic disorders which cannot be detected by testing.

Some women or their husbands may be carriers for a genetic disorder e.g. thalassemia or cystic fibrosis. Carrier testing can be done before, during and after pregnancy to see if a woman is at risk for these genetic disorders. If the test results show that both parents are carriers, genetic counselling is needed to identify the risk of having a baby with the disorder. Diagnostic testing of the baby can show if the defect is present.

If a woman is at risk for a specific disorder such as haemophilia, the cells of the foetus can be tested by a special prenatal procedure,to see if the baby is likely to have this condition.

Screening tests for abnormalities

Screening tests are done during pregnancy to assess the risk of certain birth defects. These tests do not diagnose birth defects. A number of tests are available to screen mothers for a variety of possible foetal abnormalities which can indicate the risk of having a certain abnormality:

- Ultrasound scans
- Maternal serum screening
- Carrier screening for genetic disorders

> If the test comes back as **screen negative,** the chance of the baby having the abnormality is low. If the test comes back as **screen positive,** other diagnostic tests need to be done to make sure the baby does not have the problem. **(See Chapter 13: Special tests in pregnancy).**

What types of tests are available?

There are two kinds of tests: screening tests and diagnostic tests.

Screening tests

Screening tests are done during pregnancy to assess the risk of certain birth defects. These tests do not diagnose birth defects. A number of tests are available to screen mothers for a variety of possible foetal abnormalities. These tests can indicate the risk of having a certain abnormality. If the test comes back as **screen negative,** the chance of the baby having the abnormality is low. If the test comes back as **screen positive,** other diagnostic tests need to be done to make sure the baby does not have the problem. For example, screening for Down Syndrome can be reported as screen negative or screen positive.

Ultrasound scanning

Ultrasound scanning is a test in which sound waves are changed to images which enable us to examine internal structures.

The two most important times that an ultrasound should be done to screen for birth defects are at 11-14 weeks and at 20-22 weeks.

Ultrasound scan at 11-14 weeks

An ultrasound scan done at this time is important because it:

- Confirms the age of the foetus
- Confirms the presence of one or more foetuses
- Confirms the presence of a heart beat
- Checks the **nuchal translucency** which measures the thickness of the skin at the back of the neck of the foetus. This is an important indicator of chromosomal abnormalities and possible heart defects.

Ultrasound scan at 20-22 weeks

An ultrasound scan done at this time is important because it:

- Checks the organs of the foetus and detects birth defects
- Confirms that the foetus is growing well

Even in the best of hands, some birth defects may not be detected by ultrasound and may be found only at the time of birth or even some time later.

Maternal serum screening

Maternal serum screening tests are done to find out if there is a higher-than-normal risk of having a baby with Down syndrome, trisomy 18 (both chromosomal disorders) or neural tube defects. Down syndrome is a genetic disorder in which mental retardation, abnormal features of the face, and medical problems such as heart defects occur. Though the risk of Down syndrome increases with increasing age of the mother, it is difficult to predict who will have a baby with Down syndrome. It is therefore important for all women to undergo this test.

If the screening test is positive, it only means that there is a risk of having a baby with a problem; it does not mean that the baby actually has the problem. A further test like a **chorionic villus sampling** or an **amniocentesis** will be required to confirm the diagnosis. **(See Chapter 13: Special tests in pregnancy).** If the screening test comes back negative, it means that the chances are low that the baby will have the problem.

If someone is already at an increased risk of having a baby with one of these problems, for example, someone who already has had a baby with Down syndrome, she may directly be offered a chorionic villus sampling or an amniocentesis.

First trimester screening

This screening test is done between 11 and 14 weeks of pregnancy. This screening can be done as a single combined test or as part of a step-by-step process. Some women may not need further testing.

First trimester screening is a combination of an ultrasound scan and blood tests done on the mother.

An ultrasound exam called **nuchal translucency screening,** is used to measure the thickness of the skin at the back of the neck of the foetus An increase in nuchal translucency may be a sign of Down syndrome, trisomy 18 or other chromosomal problems.

The blood tests measure the level of two substances in the mother's blood:

- Pregnancy-associated plasma protein-A (PAPP-A)
- Human chorionic gonadotropin (hCG)

Nuchal translucency (NT)

The risk of having a baby with Down syndrome or other defect can be assessed around 11-14 weeks using a special ultrasound scan called a nuchal translucency scan. The ultrasound measures the thickness of the skin lying over the back of the neck of the foetus. This skin is thicker in babies with Down syndrome or heart defects.

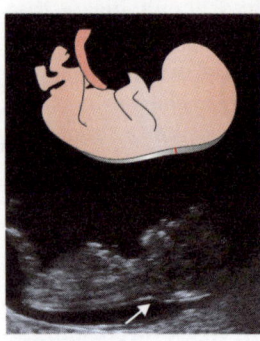 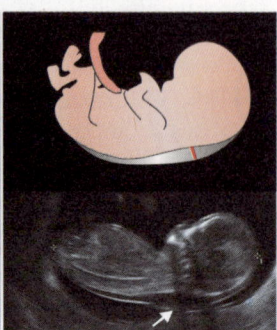

The foetus on the left has a normal nuchal translucency measurement (red line). The foetus on the right has an increased nuchal translucency measurement (red line)

The results of the nuchal translucency screening are then combined with those of the blood tests and the mother's age, to assess the risk for the foetus. **In the first trimester, this combined test detects Down syndrome in 85 per cent of cases.**

When the nuchal translucency is increased but the blood tests are normal, the foetus may still have a heart defect or other genetic condition. In this case, a more detailed ultrasound exam around 20 to 22 weeks of pregnancy is essential to detect any abnormality.

Triple screening test

This screening is done between 15 and 21 weeks of pregnancy. The week of pregnancy at the time of the test is important because levels of the substances measured change during pregnancy. Blood levels of estriol, human chorionic gonadotropin and alpha-foetoprotein (AFP) are tested. The blood levels of these hormones are put through computerised testing which calculates the risk of having a baby with Down syndrome, trisomy 18 or neural tube defects. The triple screen test detects Down syndrome in about 70 per cent of cases. The AFP test detects neural tube defects in 80 per cent of cases.

The triple test measures the level of the following substances in your blood:

- **Estriol** is a hormone produced by the placenta and the liver of the foetus.
- **Human chorionic gonadotropin (hCG)** is a hormone secreted by the placenta.
- **Alpha-foetoprotein (AFP)** is a substance produced by the foetus, which is found in amniotic fluid, foetal blood, and, in smaller amounts, in the mother's blood.

What is a genetic or chromosomal disorder?

The nucleus of each cell in the body contains chromosomes. Each chromosome has many genes. Traits like height, colour of the skin, hair texture, and shape of the nose are passed from parent to child through genes and chromosomes. A baby gets an equal number of chromosomes from the mother and the father. Similarly, half of the genes are from the mother and the other half come from the father.

A gene or a genetic disorder can be **dominant** or **recessive.** If one gene in a pair is dominant, the trait it carries cancels out the trait carried by the recessive gene. For a recessive trait to appear, the gene that carries it must be inherited from both parents. This is one of the reasons that a marriage between close relatives carries an increased risk of a chromosomal or genetic disorder.

Carrier screening for genetic disorders

Some birth defects are inherited, just as a baby can inherit the shape of the nose or the colour of the skin from one of the parents. A carrier is a person who has no manifestation of a particular disorder but carries the defective gene and can pass the gene on to his or her children. Carrier screening is done to see if the husband, wife or both carry a defective gene for certain inherited disorders. A carrier screening test can be done if there is a strong history of a particular genetic disorder in a family e.g. **thalassaemia, cystic fibrosis, sickle cell anaemia, fragile X syndrome, Duchenne muscular dystrophy, haemophilia** and **Huntington's disease.**

For this test, a sample of parental blood is processed in a specialised genetic lab. If you already have a child with the genetic disorder, the blood sample of that child will also be tested to pinpoint the exact genetic defect. If the test result shows that both parents are carriers, a genetic counsellor can provide more information about the risk of having a baby with the disorder.

Some genetic disorders are more common in certain ethnic groups in India. Carrier testing can be done before, during or after pregnancy to assess the risk of some of these disorders. This type of testing is available only for a limited number of genetic disorders.

Do you need to be tested?

Are you at an increased risk of having a baby with a birth defect? If you are, then a direct diagnostic test may be offered instead of a screening test.

You are at high risk for having a birth defect if you have:

- A family or personal history of birth defects
- A previous child with a birth defect or genetic condition
- Used certain medicines around the time of conception
- Diabetes before getting pregnant

Screening tests are offered to all pregnant women to assess their risk of having a baby with a birth defect or genetic disorder. If a screening test shows an increased risk of having an affected baby, further tests may be used to diagnose the problem. An abnormal screening test result, while alarming, only signals a possible problem. In most cases, the baby is healthy even if there is an abnormal screening test result. In a small number of women, a birth defect can occur even if the test result does not show a problem.

Is it safe to marry a close relative?

Traditionally in India, some women are married to a close family member i.e. a cousin or an uncle. Sometimes this is carried out generation after generation. When close relatives marry, it increases their chance of having a child which has inherited a genetic disease.

This is how it happens: the mother may have a defective gene but it may not cause the disease in her because she may also have a corresponding normal gene. Similarly, the father may be normal appearing but may also be carrying the defective gene. When the baby gets the mother's defective gene as well as the father's defective gene, the baby will have the genetic disorder. It is therefore safer to avoid marrying close relatives.

CHAPTER 12

Ultrasound scans in pregnancy

Sumithra is excited. She is three months pregnant and has been scheduled for an ultrasound examination. She and her husband will actually be able to see the baby! At the same time she is a bit nervous. Will the baby be normal? Will the doctor be able to tell her that the baby is growing normally? Does she have twins?

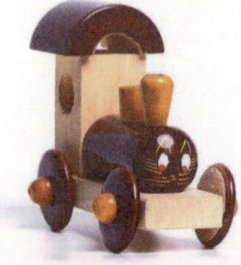

12 Ultrasound scans in pregnancy

What is an obstetric ultrasound scan?

In the 1970's, ultrasound scanning was introduced to image the foetus growing inside the uterus. Prior to the introduction of ultrasound scans, the obstetrician could only depend on hearing the baby's heart beat to predict if the baby was doing well or not. Ultrasound scans literally threw a new light on the growing foetus. We are now able to get a peek into the hitherto hidden world of the foetus. We can now measure its growth, and watch and make sure that most of its organs are functioning well. We can see it moving, blinking its eyes, breathing, swallowing, waving its fingers, sucking its thumb and even urinating inside!

Ultrasound scan is a safe, non-invasive, accurate and cost-effective investigation in a pregnancy. It has increasingly become an indispensable obstetric tool and plays an important part in the care of every pregnant woman.

How does ultrasound scanning work?

Very high frequency sound waves are generally used for scanning the uterus and the foetus. These sound waves are generated from a **transducer** (or probe) which is placed in contact with the mother's abdomen. Ultrasound beams scan the foetus in thin slices and are bounced back on to the same transducer.

The information obtained is recomposed back into a **picture** on the monitor. Using these images, measurements of the different parts of the foetus can be made accurately. Abnormalities in the foetus can be assessed. The movement of the foetal heart can be seen. Other movements and functions of the baby can be monitored.

A **full bladder** is often required for the procedure when **abdominal scanning** is done in early pregnancy. The bladder acts as a window for the sound waves and allows the foetus to be seen clearly. An internal scanning may also be

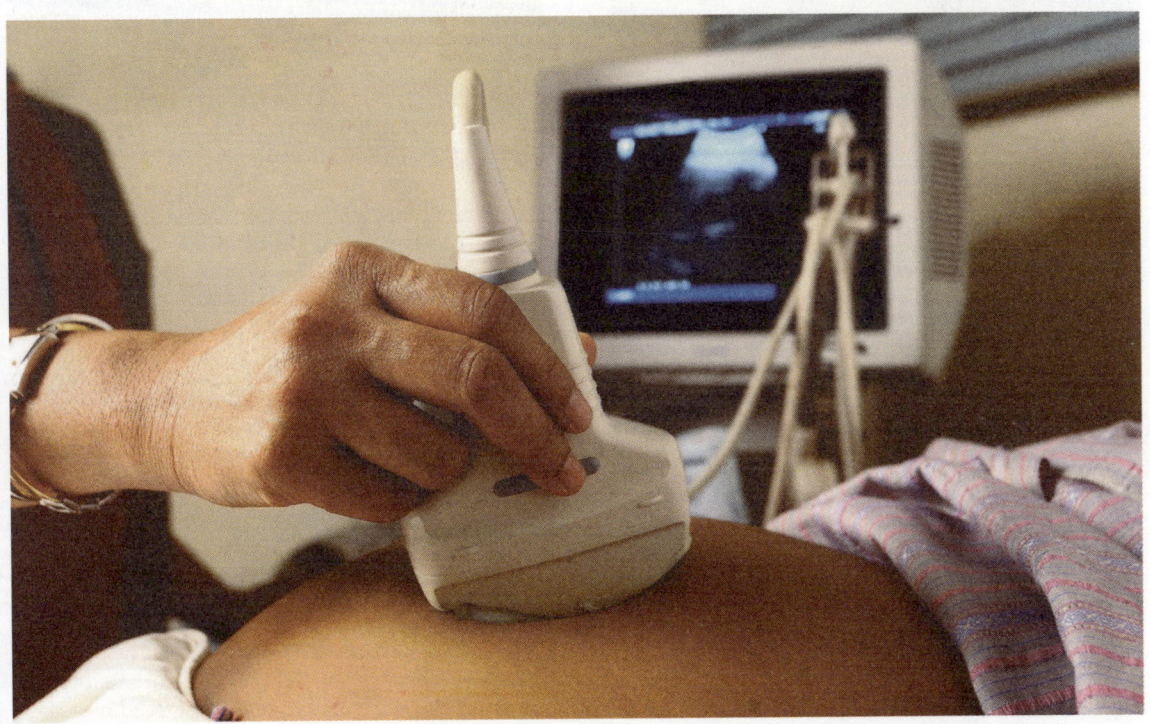

done using a probe which is inserted into the vagina. This is known as **transvaginal scanning.**

Can ultrasound scanning harm the baby?

Since ultrasound scanning only uses sound waves, it does not harm the growing foetus in any way. This method has been used for many decades, and on millions of babies, and to date no harmful effects have been documented.

The role of ultrasound scanning in pregnancy

Am I pregnant?

The gestational sac can be recognised as early as four and a half weeks of gestation and the yolk sac at about five weeks. The embryo can be observed and measured by about five and a half weeks. One of the important uses of ultrasound in early pregnancy is to confirm that the pregnancy is growing inside the cavity of the uterus and not in the Fallopian tube.

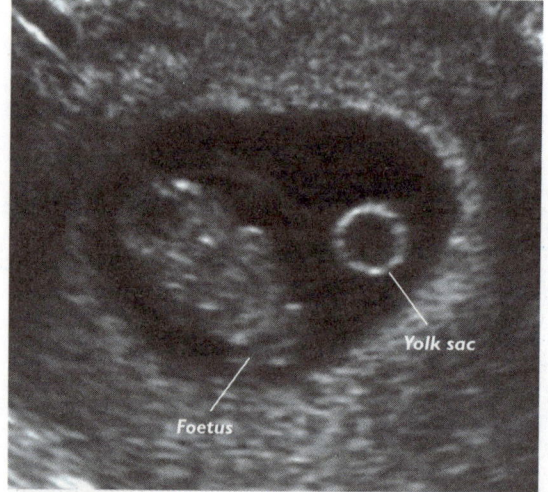

Foetus and yolk sac at 8 weeks

Am I having a miscarriage?

When there is **vaginal bleeding in early pregnancy,** ultrasound examination is important for confirming the viability of the foetus. In a normally growing pregnancy, the heartbeat can definitely be identified by six weeks of pregnancy. If the heartbeat is identified, the chance that the baby will go to term is almost 95 per cent. In case the pregnancy is not growing well, the gestational sac may be irregular and the foetus may not be identified. This is called a **blighted ovum.** If the foetus is seen but there is no heart beat, a diagnosis of **missed abortion** will be made.

Since some women do not have regular periods, the findings after a single scan may be interpreted with caution. You may be asked to repeat the ultrasound scan in 7-10 days to confirm a missed abortion.

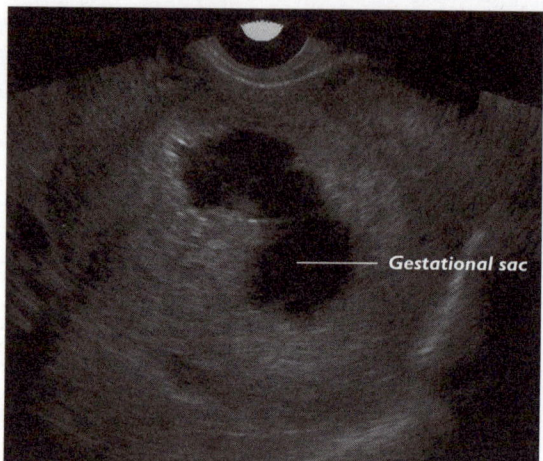

Empty gestational sac - blighted ovum

Occasionally, the pregnancy may not be growing inside the uterus but may actually have formed inside the Fallopian tube. This is called an **ectopic pregnancy.** In the presence of first trimester bleeding, an ultrasound scan along with a blood test for pregnancy, can help in the early diagnosis of an ectopic pregnancy.

How many weeks pregnant am I?

Foetal body measurements give us the gestational age of the foetus. A scan done between 7-13 weeks of gestation will give us the most accurate age of the foetus. In women who have irregular periods or who do not remember the first day of the last period, such measurements must be made as early as possible in pregnancy to arrive at a correct **dating** of the pregnancy.

In the second half of pregnancy, measuring body parameters will allow assessment of the size and growth of the foetus. The measurements help in determining if the baby is growing well or not.

Foetal measurements by ultrasound

Crown-rump length (CRL) is a measurement of the foetus from the tip of the head to the buttocks. This measurement can be made between 7 to 13 weeks and gives an accurate gestational age. When the due date has been set by an accurately measured CRL, it should not be changed by a subsequent scan.

Biparietal diameter (BPD) is the diameter between the 2 sides of the head. This is measured after 12 weeks.

Femur length (FL) measures the thigh bone.

Abdominal circumference (AC) is the single most important measurement to assess foetal growth and weight.

Is my baby normal?

Many physical abnormalities in the foetus can be reliably diagnosed by an ultrasound scan. A few abnormalities can be seen even in the early weeks of pregnancy but the best time to look for most defects is between 20-24 weeks of pregnancy. It is important to remember that even with the most advanced ultrasound technology, nearly 15-20 per cent of foetal defects may be missed.

Am I having twins?

Ultrasound scanning is invaluable in the diagnosis of twins, and is used to monitor the growth of the babies.

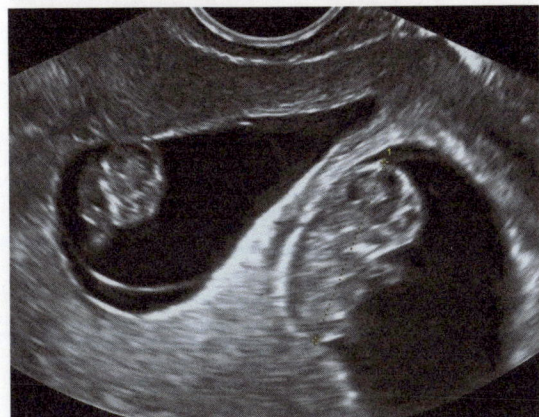
Twin pregnancy at 8 weeks

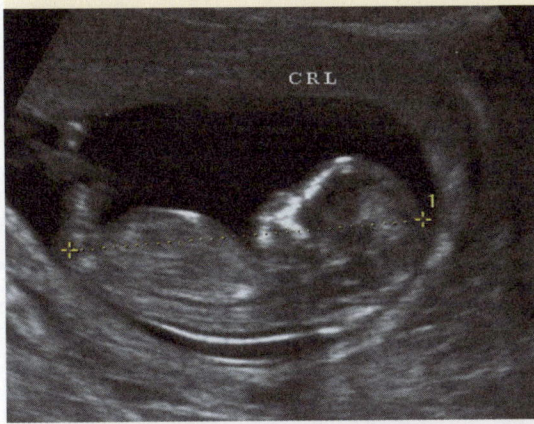
Crown-rump length (CRL)

Screening and diagnostic procedures

Ultrasound scanning is an important part of screening for chromosomal abnormalities such as Down syndrome. **(See Chapter 11: Tests in pregnancy: how do I know my baby is normal).**

Ultrasound can also assist in procedures for prenatal diagnosis such as amniocentesis, chorionic villus sampling and foetal blood sampling. **(See Chapter 13: Special tests in pregnancy).**

Assessment of amniotic fluid

The amniotic fluid around the foetus is a good indicator of the health of the baby. Ultrasound helps in assessing and measuring the amount of amniotic fluid. Too little fluid **(oligohydramnios)** and too much fluid **(polyhydramnios)** may both be indicators of foetal problems.

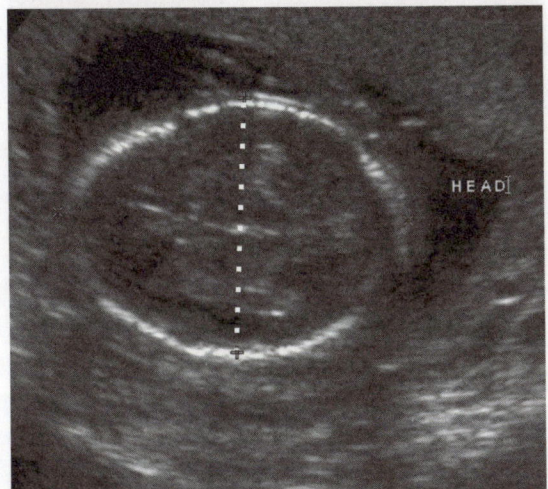
Biparietal diameter (BPD)

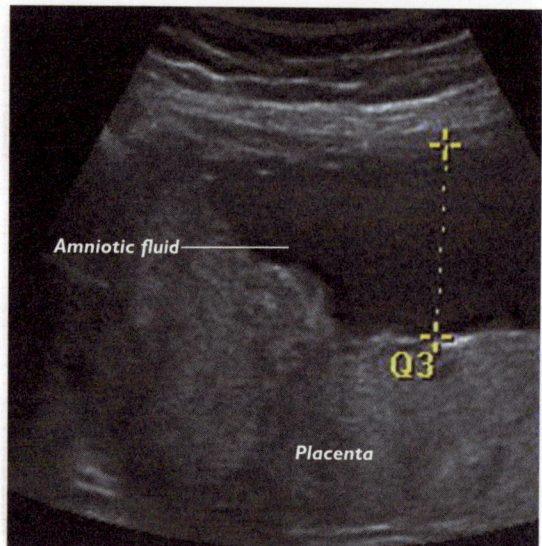

Measuring amniotic fluid volume

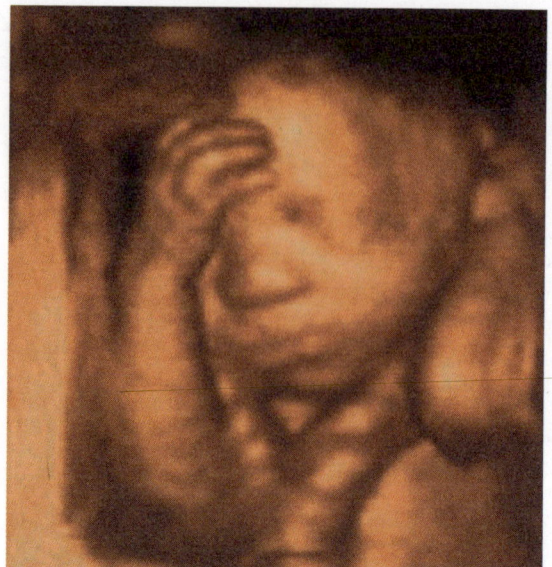

3-D image of foetal face

Other uses for ultrasound in pregnancy:

In situations where your obstetrician is not sure which part of the baby is coming down into the birth canal, ultrasound is used to confirm the position of the baby. It is also used to assess foetal health by evaluating movements, tone and breathing movements of the baby. In some cases, where foetal movements have stopped and the heart beat is not heard, ultrasound is used for confirmation of intrauterine death. Ultrasound can correctly identify the position of the placenta. Ultrasound scanning also helps in diagnosing the presence of fibroids and ovarian cysts in pregnancy.

Special ultrasound scans

Doppler ultrasound: This imaging technique is used to measure the flow of blood in the blood vessels of the placenta and the foetal blood vessels.

3-D ultrasound: This technology uses specially designed probes and software to generate 3-D images of the developing foetus. It helps in clearly defining certain foetal abnormalities, for example, cleft lip.

4-D or dynamic 3-D ultrasound: This uses specially designed scanners to combine 3-D images with imaging of the movements of the baby.

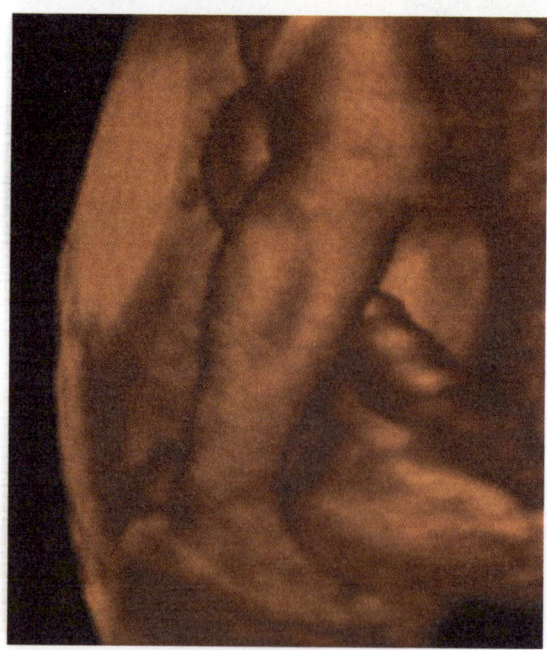

3-D image of foetal legs and feet

Foetal echocardiography: This technology is extremely useful to assess the baby's heart structure and function. This is particularly helpful in assessing suspected congenital heart defects.

How often will I have a scan?

There is no hard and fast rule as to the number of scans a woman should have during her pregnancy but certainly there is no need for an ultrasound scan at every checkup.

An early scan may be done at **7-8 weeks** to confirm pregnancy, exclude ectopic or molar pregnancies, confirm the presence of a heart beat, confirm the number of foetuses and measure the crown-rump length for dating.

A scan between **11-14 weeks** of pregnancy is useful to check nuchal translucency and can be combined with blood tests to rule out Down syndrome.

An ultrasound scan at **20-22 weeks** is important to rule out foetal abnormalities. Growth can also be assessed. Placental position is also determined. Further scans may be necessary if abnormalities are suspected.

Your obstetrician may ask for a scan in the **third trimester** to assess foetal growth and also to evaluate foetal size and weight. The scan might also be done to follow up on possible abnormalities seen at an earlier scan. Placental position is further verified. The most common reason for having more scans in the later part of pregnancy is foetal growth restriction. Doppler scans may also be necessary in that situation.

Ultrasound cannot diagnose all malformations and problems in the unborn baby. A 'normal scan' report is not a guarantee that the baby will be completely normal. Some abnormalities are difficult to find or to be absolutely certain about.

Some conditions, like hydrocephalus (where the baby is born with fluid collected in the brain), may not be obvious at the time of an earlier scan and may develop late in pregnancy. The position of the baby in the uterus may also make it difficult to visualise certain organs such as the heart, face and spine. Sometimes a repeat examination has to be scheduled the following day, in the hope that the baby has moved and made it easier to visualise certain parts.

It is also easier to see the baby more clearly in a thin patient with plenty of amniotic fluid. Increased abdominal fat in a woman can make it difficult for the sound waves to penetrate and may make it difficult to diagnose abnormalities.

CHAPTER 13

Special tests in pregnancy

Sathya has just confirmed her pregnancy. Instead of being happy, she is consumed with worry. Sathya's brother has Down syndrome. Will her baby also have Down syndrome?

Santhoshi is 37 years old. This is her second pregnancy. Her first child suffered from cystic fibrosis, which is a lung condition which can prove fatal. She wants to know if this baby is normal.

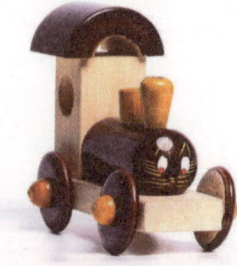

13 Special tests in pregnancy

During your regular antenatal check-ups, several tests may be offered to screen for and rule out abnormalities in the baby. The commonest test done is an ultrasound scan **(See Chapter 11: Ultrasound scans in pregnancy).** In addition to this, there are a number of special screening and diagnostic tests to check for various complications or defects affecting the baby. These tests serve two purposes. If the doctor suspects a problem in the baby, or if you or your husband has a family history of a genetic problem, these tests can reassure you that the baby is normal. On the other hand, the tests may also reveal a problem that may require some serious thought on whether to continue with the pregnancy or not.

It is important to understand why these tests are done. You must also discuss with your obstetrician the implications of an abnormal result and the choices that you will have. Most birth defects occur even when there is no history of problems. There are many genetic disorders which cannot be detected by testing.

A woman or her husband or both may be carriers for a genetic disorder e.g. thalassaemia or cystic fibrosis. Carrier testing can be done before, during and after pregnancy to see if a woman is at risk for these genetic disorders. If the test results show that both parents are carriers, genetic counselling is needed to identify the risk of having a baby with the disorder. Diagnostic testing of the baby can show if the defect is present.

If the foetus is at risk for a specific disorder such as haemophilia or thalassaemia, the cells of the foetus can be tested by a special prenatal procedure, to see if the baby has this condition.

Diagnostic tests

These tests are used to confirm abnormalities in the foetus. These are only used after screening tests or ultrasound scans have shown that you may be at high risk for having a baby with an abnormality.

The three diagnostic tests commonly offered are **amniocentesis, chorionic villus sampling (CVS)** and **foetal blood sampling.** Amniocentesis is the most common diagnostic test offered. CVS is used when an early diagnosis is required because it can be done around 11-12 weeks of pregnancy.

It is important that you and your husband have counselling about the implications and suitability of these tests before you go ahead with the testing.

Amniocentesis

The foetus is constantly shedding cells into the amniotic fluid from its skin and other organs. These cells can be used for tests. Amniocentesis is the procedure where amniotic fluid is withdrawn from the surrounding of the foetus.

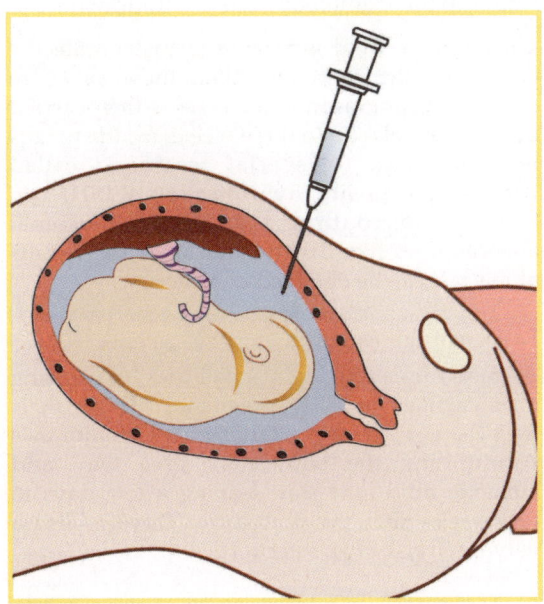

Amniocentesis

When is amniocentesis advised?

Amniocentesis is offered as an option if a screening test has come back positive, if you are 35 years or older or if an ultrasound scan reveals an abnormality which may be caused by a chromosomal aberration or an infection.

Analysis of amniotic fluid

- The cells from the amniotic fluid can be cultured and tested for chromosomal abnormalities. This is known as **karyotyping**.
- The amniotic fluid can be tested for the presence of certain intrauterine infections such as rubella, cytomegalovirus or toxoplasmosis. These infections can cause major problems in the baby. These tests are done when the mother is suspected of having had the infection and there is a chance that it may have crossed over to the foetus.

How is an amniocentesis done?

Amniocentesis is usually done between 16-18 weeks. At this time, there is enough amniotic fluid around the baby so that withdrawing a small amount will not harm the baby. Using ultrasound guidance, a needle is inserted into the amniotic sac through the abdominal wall. About 20 ml of amniotic fluid is withdrawn.

The amniotic fluid is processed to separate the cells from the fluid and then these cells are cultured. **Chromosomal analysis** is then carried out. It may take up to three weeks for the results to come back. A special technique called **fluoroscopic in-situ hybridisation (FISH)** can be used to confirm specific chromosomal abnormalities like Down syndrome. The results of this test can be obtained in 48 hours.

Risks of amniocentesis

Amniocentesis carries a small risk of causing a miscarriage in early pregnancy. This risk is less than 1 in 100. Rarely, the membranes surrounding the baby may give way and amniotic fluid may start leaking a few days to few weeks after the procedure. There is also a very small risk of an infection.

Chorionic villus sampling (CVS)

Chorionic villi are fingerlike outgrowths on the developing placenta. These are genetically identical to the foetus. Getting a sample of the chorionic villi helps in identifying specific abnormalities in the baby.

When is CVS advised?

A CVS sample can be used to rule out or confirm a chromosomal abnormality like Down syndrome. Blood diseases such as sickle-cell disease or thalassemia can also be diagnosed with CVS. Inborn errors of metabolism are caused by an enzyme deficiency, and direct enzyme analysis of the chorionic tissue can give a diagnosis. Single gene disorders, such as cystic fibrosis, haemophilia, thalassemia, Huntington's chorea and muscular dystrophy can be detected with the use of CVS.

How is a CVS done?

CVS is usually performed between 10 and 12 weeks under ultrasound guidance. Two routes are used, the transcervical route and the transabdominal route. In the transcervical route, the sample is obtained by passing a small catheter through the cervix (mouth of the uterus). The sample is obtained from the edge of the placenta. The chorionic villi tissue is then sent for analysis.

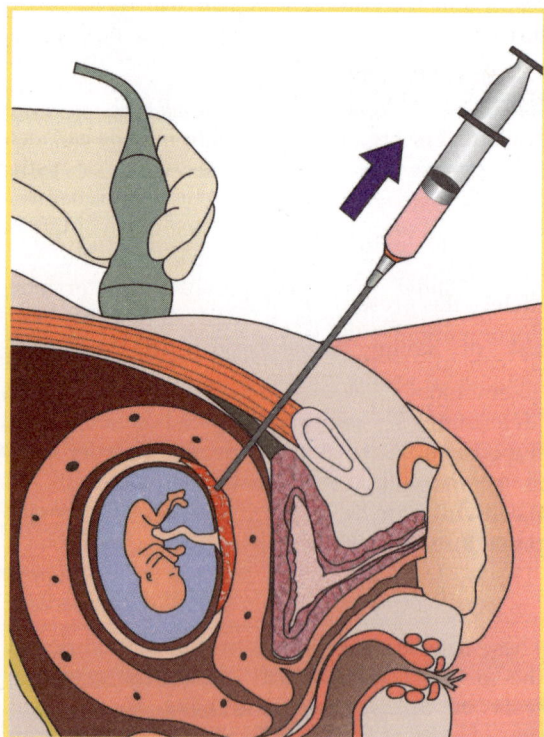

Transabdominal chorionic villus sampling

In the transabdominal route, the tissue is obtained using a needle inserted through the abdominal wall into the placenta.

The sample obtained is sent to a lab, where it is grown in a culture. This usually takes about seven days. The sample is then studied under a microscope to check for chromosomal defects. DNA analysis can also be done for inborn errors of metabolism or for other genetic abnormalities.

Risks of CVS

The risk of miscarriage following CVS is just one per cent higher than the spontaneous miscarriage rate. The advantage of a CVS is that it is done early in pregnancy and you do not have to wait too long to find out if the baby has an abnormality.

Foetal blood sampling (FBS)

Foetal blood sampling is a procedure where a sample of foetal blood is obtained from the umbilical cord of the foetus. This allows us to perform blood tests for the foetus. The blood can also be used for chromosomal analysis.

When is FBS advised?

Foetal blood sampling can be used for chromosomal analysis but is usually reserved for situations where the blood sample needs to be tested for specific blood related problems.

When a foetal infection is suspected with rubella, toxoplasmosis or cytomegalovirus, FBS can help detect the presence of infection. In cases of Rh incompatibility **(see Chapter 35: Rh factor: how it can affect pregnancy)**, assessing the baby's haemoglobin level is one of the methods to determine the severity of foetal anaemia and whether a blood transfusion is required for the baby while it is still inside the uterus.

How is an FBS done?

This test may be done at 18 weeks of pregnancy or later. Under ultrasound guidance, a needle is

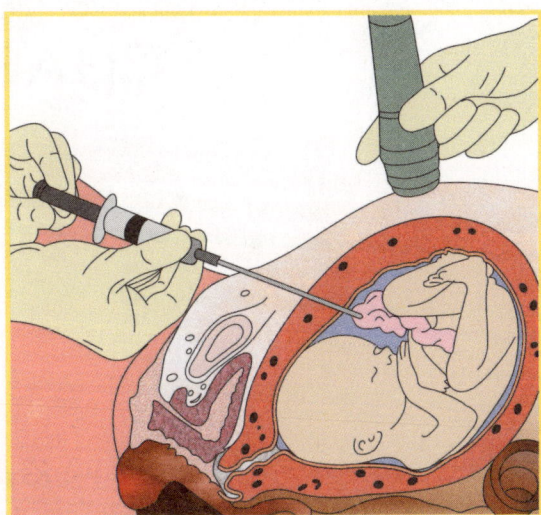

Foetal blood sampling

passed through the mother's abdomen and uterus into a blood vessel in the foetal umbilical cord. A small quantity of blood can then be drawn for testing.

Risks of foetal blood sampling

The risk of miscarriage is about 1-2 per 100.

Follow up of diagnostic tests

When a problem is detected following a diagnostic test, your obstetrician or a genetic counsellor will discuss the problem with you. Depending on the severity of the problem, a decision will need to be made about carrying on with the pregnancy. If the problem detected is so severe that the baby will not survive, you might be counselled about terminating the pregnancy. If the defect is compatible with life, you might be asked to meet a specialist who can give you more information about the implications of the defect. Sometimes, surgery or treatment is possible. You can then make an informed decision about the pregnancy. Testing can help prepare you so you can plan for any special care that the newborn may require.

CHAPTER 14

Birth defects

Supriya works in a school. She was coming home during the recent solar eclipse when she was stopped by an acquaintance. "Don't you know being out during the eclipse will cause the baby to be abnormal?" she was told. Supriya is genuinely concerned. Has she jeopardised her unborn child? She has no cause to worry. We know that birth defects are not caused by eclipses.

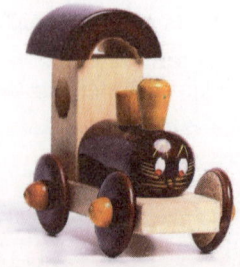

14 Birth defects

When you think about how just two cells, the egg and the sperm, combine to form a complex human being, comprising billions of cells, it is amazing to realise how many things can go wrong but do not. Just about every mother-to-be wants to know, "Is my baby normal?" **(See Chapter 11: Tests in pregnancy: How do I know my baby is normal?)** Luckily, most babies are born healthy. Out of every 100 babies born, only two or three have a serious defect. Some defects can be detected before birth, and a few can be prevented.

What is a birth defect?

A **birth defect** or **congenital disorder** is something abnormal that is present at birth. It can vary from mild to severe. A birth defect can be detected before birth, at birth or any time after birth. Some defects are easy to detect right away. Special tests may be needed to find others, such as heart defects or hearing loss. Some problems may not be detected until later in a person's life.

Types of birth defects

More than 3,000 different birth defects are known. They can be divided into several types, such as structural, genetic and those caused by exposure to an infectious disease or a harmful chemical agent. Some of these types overlap.

Structural defects

With a structural birth defect, some part of the baby's body is not formed properly. Such a defect can be internal such as a heart defect, or external such as a clubfoot or an extra finger. There is no single cause for structural defects.

Heart defects are the most common type of birth defect. Some of the problems are mild. Others are complex and may require surgery. **Neural tube defects** are another common structural birth defect. These result when the coverings over the spinal cord or brain do not close properly. Neural tube defects include spina bifida and anencephaly.

Genetic defects

Genetic defects can be caused by errors in one or more genes passed on by the parents (inherited defects), by a missing, damaged or extra chromosome (chromosomal disorders) or by a combination of factors (multifactorial defects).

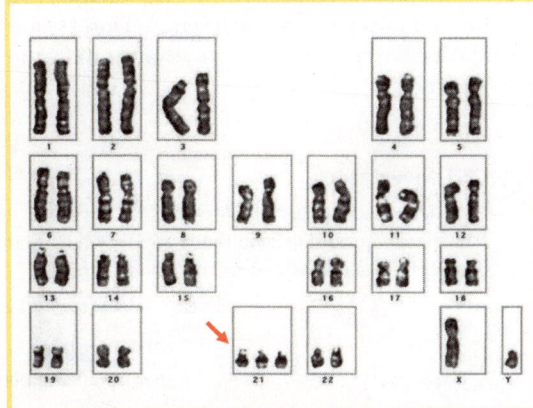

Chromosomal analysis showing trisomy 21 (Down syndrome). The red arrow indicates the three chromosomes 21.

Chromosomal disorders are most often the result of an error that occurs at the time of fertilisation. The risk of having a child with a chromosomal disorder increases with age. The most common chromosomal disorder is Down syndrome. In this condition, there are three chromosomes 21.

Exposure to infections

Some birth defects can occur when the mother develops an infection such as Rubella (German measles) during pregnancy, especially in the first three months.

Preventing birth defects

Most birth defects cannot be prevented. You do not have control over the way the baby is formed. However, the risk of a birth defect can be reduced by being careful about medications you take during the first three months of the pregnancy, the most susceptible time of the baby's development. If you are thinking about getting pregnant, visit your doctor first.

A pre-pregnancy visit is especially important for women who have medical problems, such as **diabetes** or **epilepsy**. Find out what changes in medication need to be made to bring your condition under control before you try to get pregnant. If diabetes is not well controlled at the time of conception, the baby has an increased risk of having birth defects.

Tell anyone who prescribes drugs for you that you are pregnant. That includes any doctors you see for non-pregnancy problems. Don't stop taking a prescribed medicine without talking to your doctor.

Folic acid

Taking folic acid supplements can help prevent neural tube defects like spina bifida and anencephaly. To do this, folic acid must be taken before you get pregnant and in early pregnancy. The time when the developing neural tube needs the folic acid often occurs before a woman knows she is pregnant. Therefore, all women trying for a pregnancy should take a daily supplement containing at least 0.4 mg of folic acid. Women, who already have a child with a neural tube defect, must take at least 4 mg of folic acid daily to prevent a recurrence in the next pregnancy.

Old wives' tales

A couple who has a child with a birth defect already faces a lot of anxiety and unnecessary guilt. Family and friends should refrain from apportioning blame on the mother by trying to come up with baseless, unscientific explanations for the birth defect.

Birth defects are **NOT** caused by:

- eclipses
- sewing during pregnancy
- being frightened by any incident
- having bad thoughts
- riding in autorickshaws
- using a cellphone
- eating certain foods
- using a microwave
- working on the computer for long periods of time
- flying in a plane

Genetic counselling

Shreyasee has a baby with thalassaemia major. Seeing her child having to undergo repeated transfusions, she wants to know if she can have a normal baby in her next pregnancy.

Susheela had a baby with cystic fibrosis. The child died at the age of five. She and her husband are worried. Will they have another baby with cystic fibrosis?

Shreyasee and Susheela both have had babies with a genetic disorder. They need to be seen by a **genetic counsellor.** In the 21st century, there is more and more knowledge being uncovered about the genetics of common diseases and how these diseases run in families. If there is a genetic disorder in the family, a genetic counsellor helps you understand your risk of having a baby with that disorder. If a couple has already had a child with an inherited birth defect, genetic counsellors can help them understand what their chances are of having another baby with the same genetic disorder. They can also help them learn what testing, surveillance or prevention strategies are available.

Do you need to see a genetic counsellor?

If you have a genetic condition, have a family history of an inherited disease, or have other risk factors for a genetic condition or birth defect, you may benefit from consulting a genetic counsellor. If your family history indicates the possibility of an inherited disease, your obstetrician may refer you to a genetic counsellor.

How does genetic counselling help?

The genetic counsellor takes a detailed family history. This allows her to draw up a family tree or **pedigree chart** which helps clarify the way the genetic disorder is being passed from generation to generation. This diagram also helps to determine your risk for inheriting that particular disease. If you do have an increased risk, the counsellor will make sure that you understand the basic genetic concepts that affect how the disease runs in families, educate you about the disease itself, and explain the level of risk for you and your family.

Let us take the case of Shreyasee and her husband. To assess their risk for having another baby with thalassaemia, the genetic counsellor discussed their family history. Shreyasee came from a community where there was a lot of intermarrying among close relatives. This increased the chance of both being **carriers** of the disease. (A carrier is a person who has both a normal and a defective gene. The carrier is therefore normal in all ways but can pass on the disease to the baby). The genetic counsellor tested Shreyasee and her husband to find out if they were carriers of thalassaemia. After DNA testing, both were found to be carriers of thalassaemia. The counsellor told them that they had a 25% (1 in 4) chance of having an unaffected (normal) baby, a 25 % chance of having an affected baby and a 50% chance of a baby who will be a carrier. With their next pregnancy, Shreyasee underwent a chorionic villus sampling **(See Chapter 13: Special tests in pregnancy).** This showed that the baby was a carrier but did not suffer from the disease. This meant that the baby had inherited a defective gene from one parent but also a normal gene from the other parent. The baby was born and has continued to stay healthy.

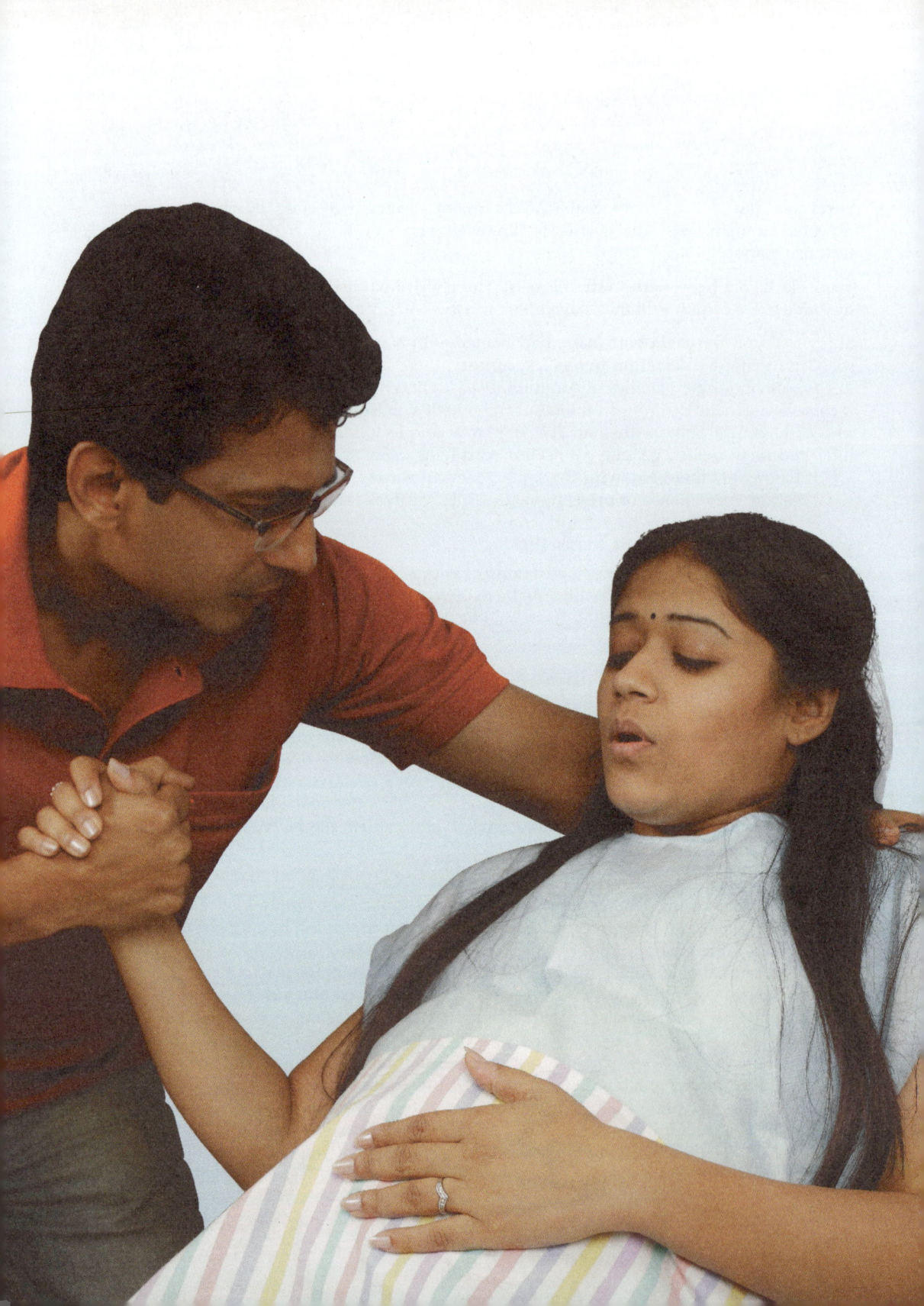

Labour and delivery

CHAPTER 15

Preparing for labour

Smriti worries constantly about being prepared for labour. There are certain steps that she can take to make sure that she is ready for going to the hospital. Being prepared will decrease the stress and anxiety which are present in the last weeks of pregnancy.

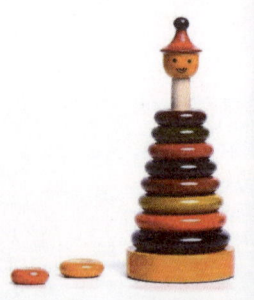

15 Preparing for labour

As you plan for the birth of your baby, you can take steps to go through your labour smoothly. It is best to discuss these questions about labour with your obstetrician before the time comes. Some of these questions probably have already occurred to you.

When should I call the doctor?

If your water bag breaks (rupture of membranes) or if your pains are coming regularly, call your doctor and inform her.

How can I contact the doctor or hospital after clinic hours?

Make sure you have all the phone numbers of your obstetrician and the hospital.

Should I go directly to the hospital or call first?

If you think you are in labour and the pains are coming at regular intervals, you can go directly to the hospital. Check with your obstetrician and the hospital that you are delivering at: knowing their protocols ahead of time will save you worry when you go into labour.

Are there any special steps I should follow when I think I am in labour?

Do not eat or drink anything if you suspect you are in labour. Once you have been examined and it has been determined that you are in labour, your obstetrician may allow you to drink liquids.

Why should you not eat or drink anything if you suspect you are in labour?

Once labour starts, digestion in the stomach comes to a halt. The food that you have eaten will stay in your stomach. In labour, you may have vomiting and if you have eaten a full meal, this can be uncomfortable for you. More important, if you have to have a caesarean, then having a full stomach can be a problem in case anaesthesia has to be given.

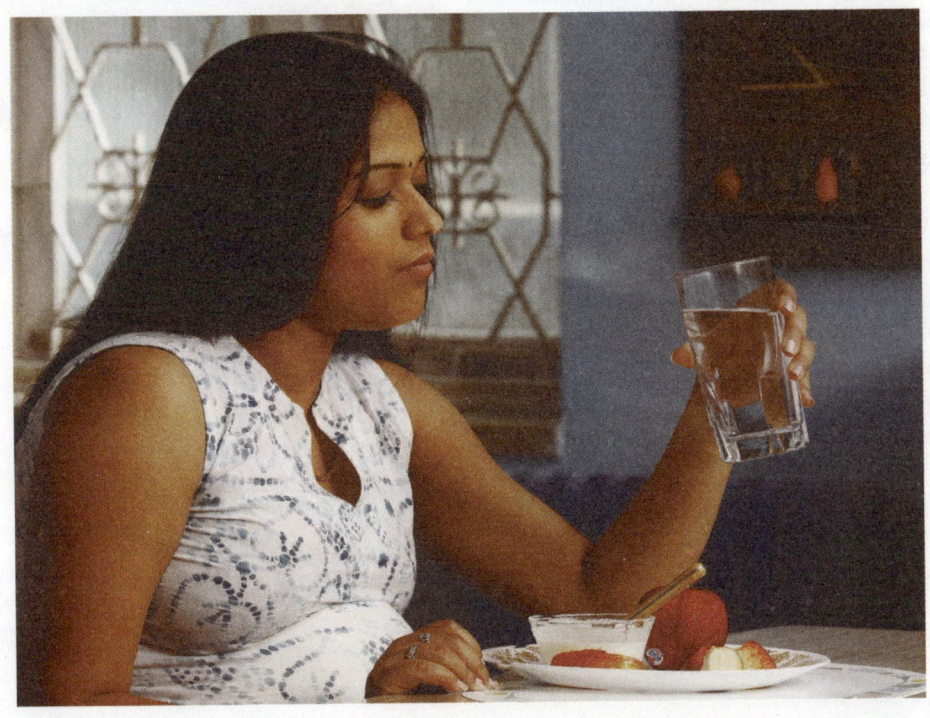

What to take to the hospital for childbirth

For mom-to-be

What will I need?

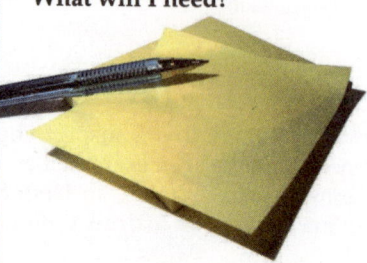

Consider packing the following things for yourself:

- three nightgowns with openings in front (front openings are helpful for breastfeeding and for examinations by the doctor)
- comfortable slippers
- three nursing bras (now available in any store selling women's clothing or newborn needs) as they are convenient for breast-feeding
- several pairs of panties, in case of blood stains (disposable paper panties are available in the market now)
- sanitary pads (you will not be able to use tampons for 6 weeks after your delivery)
- soap, shampoo and conditioner
- cosmetics (don't forget toothbrush and toothpaste!)
- comb / hair brush / nail clipper
- glasses (contact lenses will be removed during labour and in case of a caesarean section)
- books or magazines
- pad and pencil (good for writing down questions to ask doctors when they make rounds)
- change for phone in case you need to use a public phone
- your mobile phone charger
- phone numbers of friends and family to call after the delivery
- loose-fitting clothes and comfortable slippers to wear back home (you won't have your pre-pregnancy figure back yet)
- any prenatal reports, insurance information, and papers related to your stay at the hospital
- mosquito repellant (essential in India!)

Do not take large sums of money or valuables with you to the hospital.

For baby

What will I need for the baby?

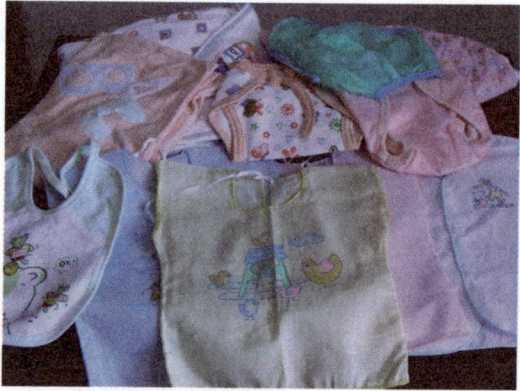

- jablas, simple cotton dresses
- blanket
- safety pins and rubber or nylon pants, if you are using cloth diapers
- disposable diapers and wipes
- cotton
- small cotton sheets to wrap the baby in
- plastic or rubber sheets to place under the baby
- mosquito net for the cradle
- baby soap, baby shampoo, baby lotion

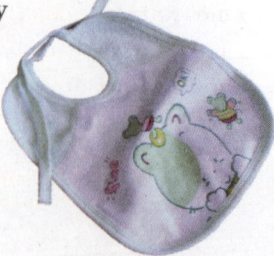

Where will the baby sleep?

While you are in the hospital, the baby may be kept in a crib in your room. When you get home, where are you planning to have the baby sleep?

Choice 1: Baby sleeping in your bed

Advantages of having the baby sleeping in your bed

- You don't need to buy a crib.
- You can feed the baby without getting up from the bed.

Disadvantages of having the baby sleeping in your bed

- It is difficult for you to sleep with the baby lying next to you.
- The bed can get soiled frequently. Make sure that you have rubber sheets or plastic bedding to place under the baby.
- You will always be worried that in your sleep you might roll over the baby or that the baby will roll off the bed. If you have no choice or if you really want the baby next to you, keep a pillow on either side of the baby after she falls asleep. This will prevent you from moving too close to the baby in your sleep and also will prevent the baby from rolling off the bed.
- You and your husband will find it difficult to resume intimate relations if you have the baby in the bed with you.

Choice 2: Baby bed, crib or cradle

Your family may already have a cradle which has been used for many babies in the family. There are also a variety of cribs and baby beds available in the market. Choose the one that suits your space and your budget. Before you spend too much money, remember that the baby will outgrow the crib in a few short months. Get something that will accommodate your baby as she grows for a few years.

What you should look for in a crib

Your baby will spend much time in the crib unattended, so you must make certain it is a safe crib. If you are using a crib or cradle with bars, make sure that the gap between the bars is not more than 6-7 cms apart. This is to make sure that the baby does not get an arm or leg caught between the bars.

There are cribs available which are covered all around. These covered cribs protect the baby against mosquitoes and flies.

The mattress should be firm and should fit the bottom of the crib well. It is better to place a waterproof (rubber or plastic) sheet between the baby sheet and the mattress.

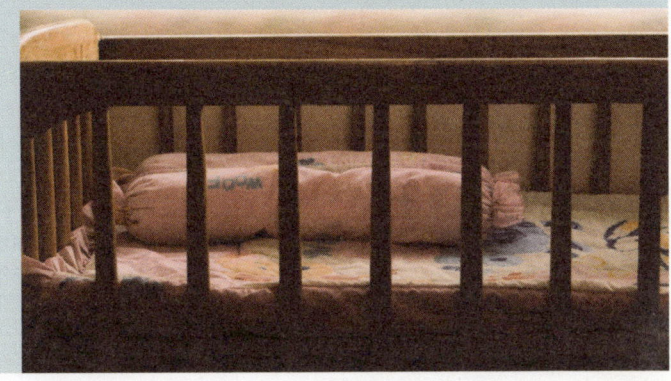

CHAPTER 16

Planning for labour

Sahana is ready and packed for the hospital. She knows that she may not have time to think about all the details once she is in labour. She has informed her office. She has also made arrangements in her home for the new baby. She is smart to be ready ahead of time.

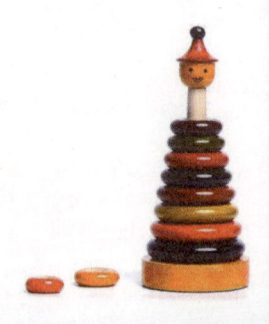

16 Planning for labour

Before it is time to go to the hospital, there are many things to think about. You may not have time to think about them once you are in labour, so it is best to consider them ahead of time.

Distance: how far do you live from the hospital?

If you stay close to the hospital where you are going to deliver, it will not make a difference. If you stay far from the hospital, it is important that you make arrangements to get to the hospital and know these arrangements ahead of time. Make sure you know how long it will take you to reach the hospital during the peak traffic hours so that you can give yourself extra time. When you are in pain, your husband and your family will get flustered if they feel it is taking too long to get to the hospital. Remember that it usually takes a few hours to deliver, so there is no need to panic.

How long will it take to get to the hospital?

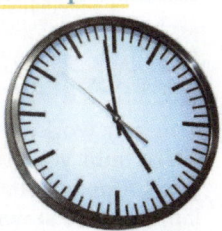

Check with your obstetrician if you need to be admitted before your due date. If you have a complication of pregnancy, you may be asked to get admitted before labour starts.

Occasionally, your obstetrician may suspect that you may have a fast labour and if you live far away, she may ask you to get admitted a few days before your due date.

Transportation: Is there someone who can take you to hospital at any time, or do you have to call and find someone? When you go into labour, any mode of transportation is safe to take to reach the hospital. If you have somebody who has offered to drive you to the hospital in their car at the time of labour, warn them before hand as you near your due date.

Time of day: Depending on where you live, it may take longer during rush hours than at other times of the day or night.

Calculate how long it takes to reach the hospital at different times of day. Plan the shortest route to the hospital. These measures will ensure that you and your family do not panic when labour pains start.

Home arrangements

Do you have other children to take care of at home, and do you have to make special arrangements for them?

In these days of the nuclear family, where both the husband and wife are working and live by themselves, you need to get yourself organised before you go into labour. You may need to inform the person who will be coming and helping with your home arrangements, well in advance.

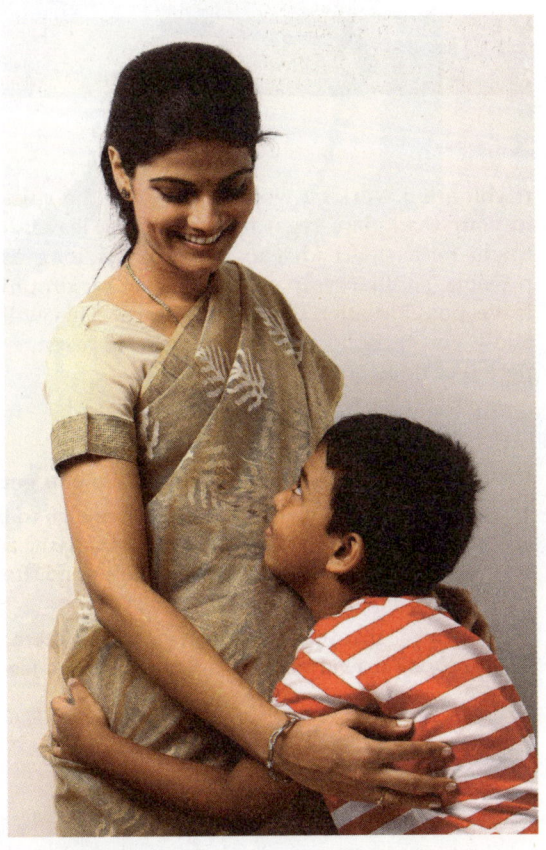

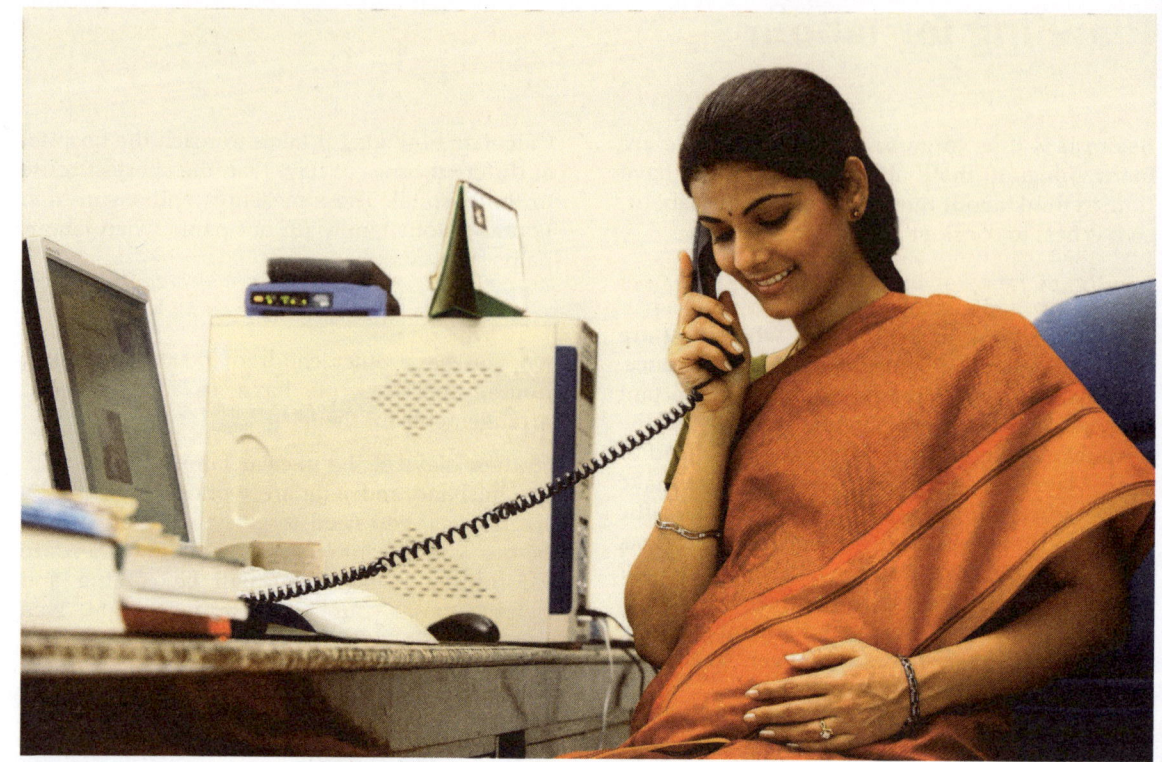

Work arrangements

If you are a working woman, find out the rules in your workplace regarding maternity leave. It might be a smart idea to work for as long as possible so that you can avail the maximum leave possible after the baby is born. This will allow you to bond with your baby for a longer period of time.

How long can you continue to work in the last few weeks of pregnancy?

You can work as long as you are comfortable. Make sure you have a colleague who will take you to the hospital in the event that you go into labour while at work.

Who will be there to help you when you get home?

In India, a new mother is usually lucky enough to have her mother or mother-in-law around to help with the baby. New fathers are also very enthusiastic and eager to help with the baby. Make sure that your husband is in the hospital with you during and after the delivery so that he can get used to the baby's feeding, sleeping and diaper changing routines.

Remember that your sleep patterns will be altered because of your baby's demands. It will help to have somebody around who will let you sleep for a few hours between the baby's feeds.

Readying your home for a new baby

The pregnancy has passed faster than you expected. It is almost time to bring the baby home. Are you sure that your home is organised and ready for the baby?

Once the baby arrives, you may have not much time to organise the house. Take a few days to plan what you need to do to keep everything ready. Will you be moving to your mother's home for a few weeks after the baby is born? Do you have everything there to take care of the baby? Are you planning to be in your own home after the delivery? Have you thought about where everything for the baby is going to be kept?

A place to sleep

A little time spent in planning everything will relieve you of a lot of stress and anxiety. You will need to prepare your room for the baby. You may purchase a crib to ensure that the baby sleeps in your room during the initial stages. The baby needs a crib that is comfortable and a soft firm mattress to sleep in.

Once the baby is a bit older you may consider moving him to another room or share a room with your first child, if you have one.

A place to change

You may need to decide where you will be changing the baby's diapers. If it is going to be on your bed, make sure that you have enough rubber or plastic sheets so that your bed does not get soiled. If you are going to use a table, then it has to be at a convenient height. The table has to be solid and wide enough for you to change the diaper comfortably. A soft blanket (covered with a plastic sheet) may be placed on top to make it comfortable for the baby too.

Where will the baby's supplies go?

Get one part of your cupboard cleaned out so that you can keep the baby's supplies there. There must be enough place to hold the baby's clothes, diapers, blankets, powder, soap, shampoo and creams.

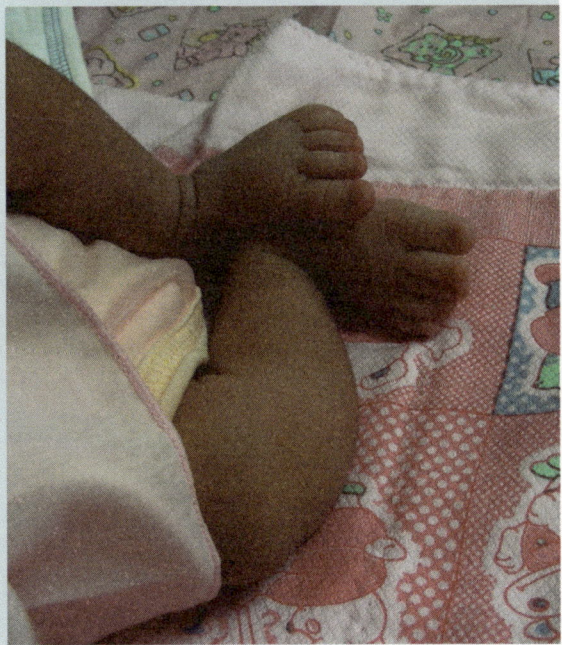

Getting your house ready

Once the baby is home, you will be so busy getting adjusted to the baby's schedule, that you may not have any time for regular household chores. Make sure that you have everything organised in your home so that you do not have to waste any time on routine chores. It will be better to find the right place for all items and to get into the habit of placing things in the place meant for them. This way the house may need little attention apart from regular cleaning.

CHAPTER 17

Labour and delivery

Sanjana and Ranjith look forward to the birth of their child. It is the culmination of months of hopes and dreams. Finally the time has arrived to go through the process of labour and be rewarded with a baby. But Sanjana is beset with mixed feelings. She is excited, but at the same time, filled with trepidation. After all, it is a mysterious process and the terms 'labour' and 'pains' evoke a sense of anxiety. It is important for her to understand the process so that she can undergo labour with the least amount of apprehension.

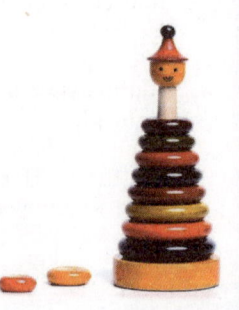

17 Labour and delivery

It is normal for a couple to be concerned about the hospital stay, the pain of labour and about how long the whole process will take. This chapter will give you the information needed to make you feel you are in control of your own body. It will give you the confidence to go through the entire birthing process, with the least anxiety.

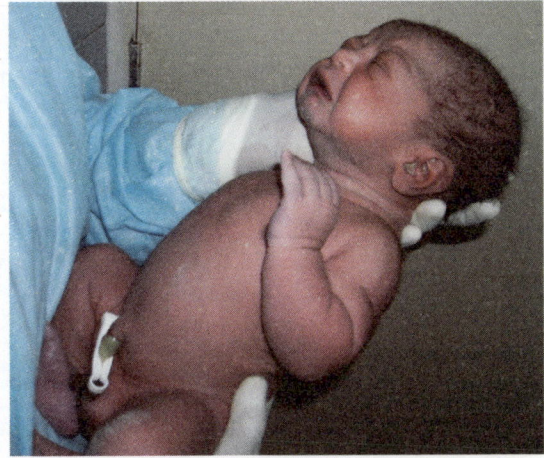

A human pregnancy usually lasts 280 days or 40 weeks. Once you complete the 37th week of pregnancy, you are considered to be at term. Most women will deliver a week before or a week after the due date. There is no need to panic if you have not delivered by your due date. Remember that only 4 per cent of pregnancies will deliver exactly on the given due date!

If any signs of labour occur before 37 weeks of pregnancy, the labour is considered **premature** or **preterm**. You should see your obstetrician immediately if you have any signs or symptoms of labour before 37 weeks. **(See Chapter 29: Preterm or premature labour).**

A normal pregnancy can also go beyond the due date which your obstetrician would have given you. This is not abnormal. When the pregnancy goes one week beyond the due date, it is called **postdated pregnancy.** If your pregnancy is progressing well and your baby is healthy, your obstetrician will wait 7-10 days after your due date and then plan on delivering you. **(See Chapter 30: Postdated pregnancy).**

Labour

It is the process by which contractions of a pregnant uterus cause birth. During labour, the cervix (mouth of the uterus) thins out. This is termed **effacement.** The gradual opening of the cervix is called **dilatation.**

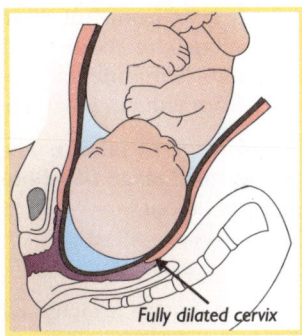
Fully dilated cervix

Delivery

It is the process which happens at the end of labour. The baby is born in the second stage of labour. A baby can be delivered either through the vagina or by a caesarean section.

Every labour is different. How long it lasts and how it progresses differs from woman to woman and from birth to birth. There are, however, general guidelines for labour that your obstetrician uses to decide whether it is progressing normally. If it is not progressing normally, you may need medical assistance or a caesarean delivery.

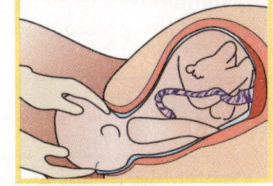
Head being delivered

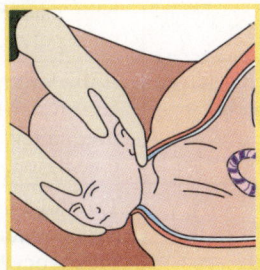
Head delivered

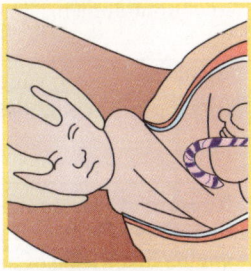
Shoulder being delivered

The three stages of labour

First stage of labour: At the beginning of labour, the cervix may be closed or partially open. In the first stage of labour, the dilatation progresses from a closed cervix (0 cm) or a partially open cervix, to full dilatation (10 cm). The first stage is the longest stage of labour.

Second stage of labour: The second stage of labour lasts from full dilatation of the cervix to the delivery of the baby. The second stage can last from 20 minutes to two hours. This time may vary from woman to woman.

Third stage of labour: The placenta is expelled in the third stage of labour. This is the shortest stage of labour.

What triggers labour?

No one knows exactly what starts the labour process. However, we do know that certain hormones such as **oxytocin** and **prostaglandins** cause uterine contractions and the thinning of the cervix. One theory is that the mother's pituitary gland begins to secrete oxytocin when the baby is fully developed and ready to be born. Oxytocin is the hormone that stimulates contractions.

Hormones from the baby also trigger labour by stimulating the mother's hormone production. The baby's lungs secrete an enzyme or chemical when they are fully developed. This causes prostaglandins to be released into the mother's system. The prostaglandins then trigger changes

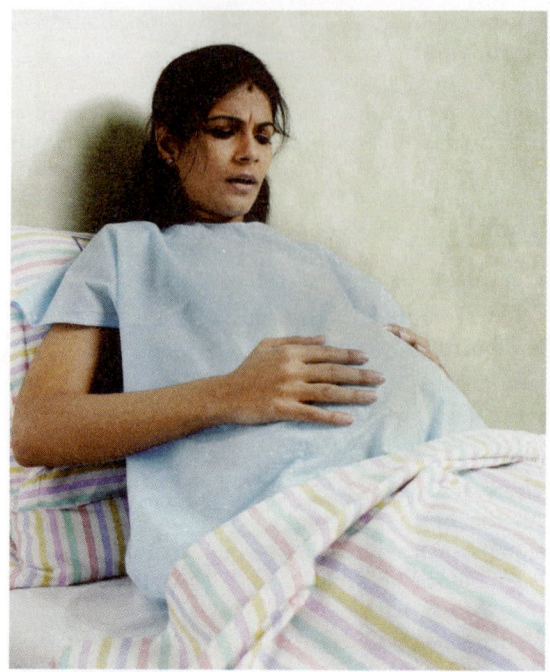

in the cervix and cause contractions. Another theory implicates the baby's adrenal glands. When the baby is ready to be born, the adrenal glands produce hormones. These hormones cause changes in the mother, which in turn set off the process that starts labour.

Is it time to go to the hospital?

You and your husband are nearing a special, exciting time. You have been preparing for weeks for the arrival of the baby. Although it is

Signs that you are approaching labour		
Sign	What is it?	When does it happen?
Lightening: feeling as if the baby has dropped lower down in your abdomen	This is known as 'engagement' or 'fixing' of the baby's head. The baby's head has settled deep into your pelvis.	From a few weeks to a few hours before labour begins.
Show: increase in vaginal discharge (clear, pink, or slightly bloody)	A thick mucus plug which has accumulated at the cervix during pregnancy is pushed out into the vagina.	From a few days before labour begins to the onset of labour.
Rupture of membranes: discharge of watery fluid from the vagina in a trickle or a gush.	The fluid-filled sac (membranes) that surrounds the baby during pregnancy breaks.	From several hours before labour begins to any time during labour.

not possible to know exactly when labour will begin, you can be prepared by knowing what to expect. Being prepared can make it easier for you to relax and focus on the arrival of your baby when the time comes.

Most first-time mothers are worried that they may not recognise labour when it starts. Even women who have had a baby earlier, may forget what it felt like when they went into labour the first time around!

Do not worry. It is almost impossible to go into labour and not know it. Most women can tell when they are in labour. Sometimes, however, it is hard to tell when labour begins.

There are some signs that labour will start soon. As the body prepares for labour it sends out signals. You may or may not notice some of them before labour begins.

Contractions or pains

When contractions start, you may have a regular pattern of cramps that may feel like a bad backache or menstrual cramps. These pains may occur every 15-30 minutes to begin with. Your uterus will tighten and relax. The frequency of contractions increases as labour progresses and the contractions may become more painful as the cervix opens and the baby moves down the birth canal.

Braxton-Hicks contractions

After the eighth month, you may start feeling occasional tightening of the uterus. This tightening is usually painless. These painless contractions are called Braxton-Hicks contractions. They are a normal occurrence but may be painful at times. When they are painful, you may panic and think that labour has started.

You may sometimes have false labour, or irregular contractions of your uterus, before true labour begins.

False labour

Sometimes it can be hard to differentiate false labour from true pains. Usually, false contractions are less regular and not as strong as true labour. In true labour, progressive changes will occur in the cervix which will ultimately lead to delivery. False labour pains will usually subside if you walk around or rest, and may be continuous as compared to true pains which will come and go. False pains are usually in the front and in the lower abdomen whereas true pains will travel from the top of the uterus to the lower abdomen or from the back to the front.

Sometimes, the only way to tell the difference is by seeing your obstetrician and having an internal examination done to find changes in your cervix that signal the onset of labour.

Differences between false labour and true labour		
Type of change	**False labour**	**True labour**
Timing of contractions	Often irregular and do not get closer together.	Come at regular intervals and, as time goes on, get closer together. Last about 30-60 seconds.
Change with movement	Contractions may stop when you walk or rest, or may even stop with a change of position.	Contractions continue, despite movement.
Strength of contractions	Usually weak and do not get much stronger (may be strong and then weak).	Increase in strength steadily.
Pain of contractions	Usually felt only in the front, especially lower abdomen.	Usually starts in the back and moves to the front. Moves from the top of the uterus downwards.

Occasionally, even after an examination, it might be difficult to tell whether you are in labour. You may then be admitted to the hospital and observed. If the pains go away and if your labour does not progress, you may be sent home.

True labour

Time your contractions

One good way to tell the difference between false labour and true labour is to time the contractions. Note how long it takes from the start of one contraction to the start of the next one. If you are having regular contractions, which seem to be increasing in intensity, labour may have started. Keep a record for an hour. It may be hard to time labour pains accurately if the contractions are mild. If you think you are in labour, go to the hospital as you have been instructed.

When should I go to the hospital?

If you have any one or more of these signs you should go to the hospital for a check-up and for confirmation of labour:

- Your contractions are coming at regular intervals and are increasing in intensity.

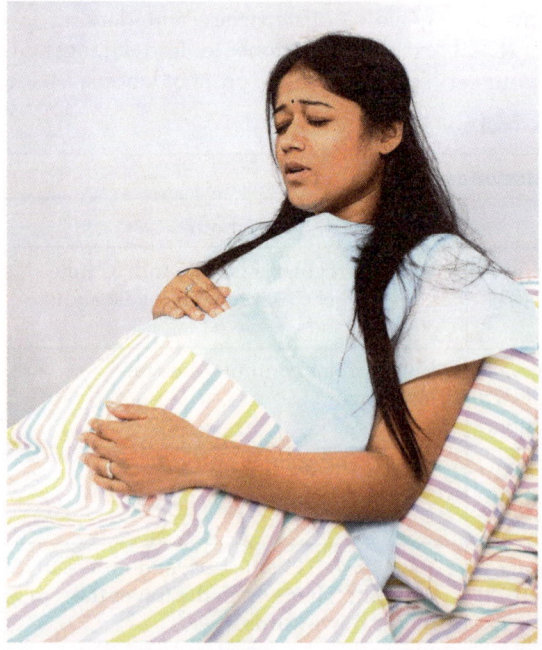

- Your membranes rupture (water runs down your thighs), even though you are not having any contractions.
- You are bleeding from the vagina (other than bloody mucus).
- You have constant, severe pain with no relief between contractions.
- You notice the baby is moving less often or not moving at all.

If any of these happens, contact your obstetrician right away.

> If you think labour has started, do not eat or drink anything until your obstetrician gives you further instructions.

On admission

When you reach the hospital, you will be examined by the obstetrician or the obstetric nurse. The most important decision that will be made at that time is whether you are in true labour. If it is difficult to determine whether you are in labour, you may be admitted for a few hours to see if the pains become regular and if labour progresses.

How will they know if it is true labour?

Contractions

You are observed to see if your contractions

- are occurring at regular intervals
- last for at least 30 seconds or more

Changes in the cervix

An internal examination is done to check the changes in the cervix. You are considered to be in labour if you have some or all of these changes:

- a discharge of mucus mixed with blood ('show')
- thinning of the cervix (effacement)
- opening of the cervix (dilatation)

Activity in labour

Depending on how strong your contractions are, you will be allowed to walk around your room or in the corridor. If the contractions get stronger, you may want to sit down or lie down in bed. You can be as active as you wish.

> **What should you eat?**
>
> When you are in active labour, it is best to avoid any solid food. As the cervix dilates, there is a tendency to vomit. Drink small amounts of water, buttermilk, milk or juices. You may be asked to have only sips of water or nothing at all, if the obstetrician suspects that you might require a caesarean section. This will prevent you from having a full stomach if an emergency caesarean section is decided upon. This makes it less risky to give you anaesthesia.

Enema

If you have not had a good bowel movement, then an enema might be given. A small amount of medication will be inserted gently into the rectum and this will make you pass motion. An empty rectum makes it easier for you when you have to push in the third stage of labour.

First stage of labour

At the beginning of labour, the cervix may be closed or partially open. In the first stage of labour, the dilatation progresses from a closed cervix (0 cm) or a partially open cervix, to full dilatation (10 cm). The first stage is the longest stage of labour.

The first stage of labour is divided into

- Latent phase
- Active phase
- Transitional phase

It is not uncommon for first-time mothers to make more than one trip to the hospital. If you are in early labour and have been sent home, try walking around, reading a book or watching a movie. This might make it easier to bear the pains.

Latent phase

Some first-time mothers experience a prolonged period of early labour with minimal or no change in their cervical dilatation. This is called the **latent phase of labour.** Support from your husband and the family will help you get through this frustrating part of early labour.

During the latent phase of labour, contractions will begin. They may begin gently but will gradually become stronger and more intense. The contractions will help the cervix change, becoming shorter and opening up more, so that the baby can begin its descent into the birth canal. This process is called effacement and dilatation.

This phase may be short or long and will differ from woman to woman and from one pregnancy to the other in the same woman. It can take some women as much as a few hours to dilate even a few centimetres.

Active phase

Once it is confirmed that you are in labour, you will be admitted to the hospital. In the beginning, while the pains are not yet strong, you may be encouraged to walk around. As the pains get stronger, you might want to sit down or lie down.

The active phase of labour is when things really progress. Once the cervix has dilated to 3 or 4 cm, the active phase is considered to have started. During this phase of labour, the cervix will change consistency. It will go from being firm to soft and stretchy. The contractions will start lasting longer. They may last up to 60 seconds and may occur every 3 to 4 minutes.

During the active phase of labour, the cervix (mouth of the uterus) thins out. This is termed **effacement.**

The gradual opening of the cervix is called **dilatation.** As labour progresses, the contractions become more frequent, longer and

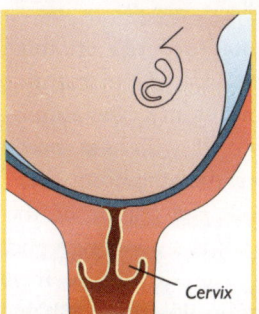
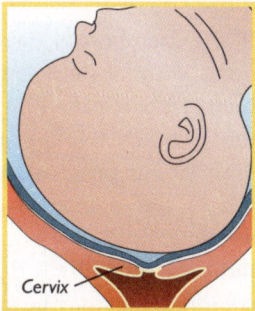

Uneffaced cervix   Effaced cervix

stronger, and the cervix begins dilating more quickly. Your obstetrician will examine you at regular intervals to assess how your cervix is dilating. The average woman in her first labour may dilate about 1 cm per hour during the active phase of labour. When the cervix has reached 10 cm it is considered to be **'fully dilated'**. Toward the end of active labour, the baby's head may begin to descend through the birth canal.

Cervical effacement and dilatation during labour

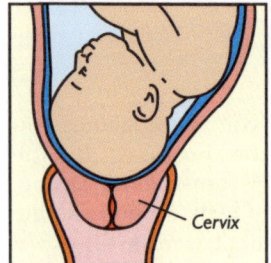

1. Cervix is not effaced or dilated.

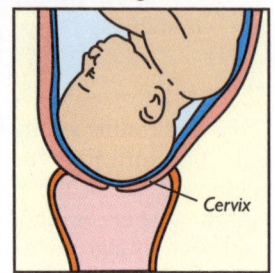

2. Cervix is fully effaced and dilated to 1 cm.

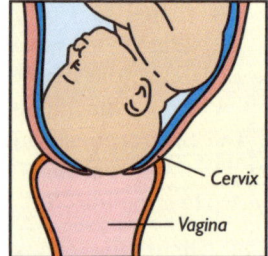

3. Cervix is dilated to 5 cm.

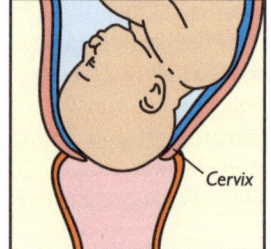

4. Cervix is fully dilated to 10 cm.

Rupture of membranes

The membranes may also rupture spontaneously during active labour and you may be aware of a gush of fluid from the vagina.

If the membranes have not ruptured on their own, your obstetrician may decide to rupture them. This is called an **amniotomy.** The amniotomy serves two purposes. It will help make your labour progress faster. An amniotomy also allows the doctor to check the colour of the amniotic fluid. If it is clear, it is a good sign and indicates the baby is doing well. If it is greenish coloured, this may be an indication that the baby has passed meconium inside the uterus. This may sometimes be a sign that the baby is facing difficulty inside the uterus.

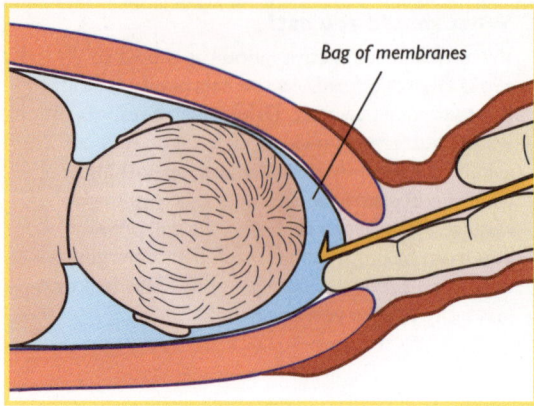

Amniotomy

How long does the active phase last?

The length of the active phase varies from woman to woman. In a first pregnancy, the active phase may last between 6-8 hours.

If you have had a previous vaginal birth, the active phase will be shorter.

In most cases, the frequency of contractions eventually increases to every two and a half to three minutes, although some women never have them more often than every five minutes.

Transitional phase

After the cervix is dilated to 8-9 cm, labour pains may ease off for a short period of time. This is called the transitional phase of the first stage of labour. But soon, the contractions become stronger and come at frequent intervals of 2-3 minutes. You might have an urge to push down. Your obstetrician might ask you not to push till the cervix is fully dilated. You will have to breathe rhythmically and try to relax so that you do not push at this point.

The husband's role is very important at this juncture. A woman who has reached this phase in her labour requires a great deal of emotional support.

Coping with the first stage of labour

- In the early part of labour, walking around might be useful

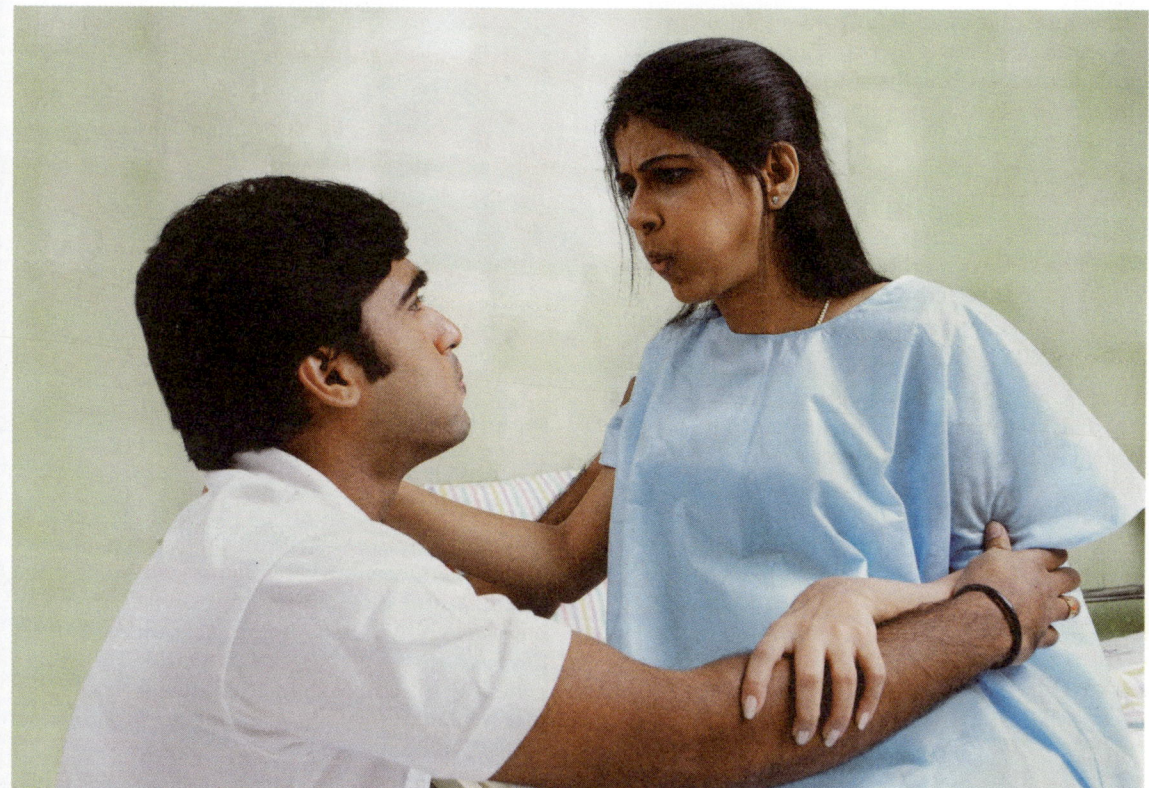

Breathing with the pains

- Later on, you might want to lie down. Choose whichever position is comfortable for you. Many women prefer to lie on their sides.
- Massaging your lower back may help. A hot water bottle may also be of use.
- Breathing exercises (see page 129) and relaxation techniques are taught to women in labour preparation classes. These might be useful in labour.
- You may choose to take an injectable pain killer.
- If epidural analgesia is available, it might make it much easier to go through labour **(See Chapter 20: Pain relief in labour and delivery)**.

Second stage of labour

The second stage of labour lasts from full dilatation of the cervix to the birth of the baby. After the cervix is fully dilated, the baby moves down the birth canal and is born. The second stage of labour is significantly shorter than the first stage. The second stage usually lasts from 1 to 2 hours, averaging about 90 minutes. This time may vary from woman to woman and may be as short as 20 minutes.

During the second stage of labour, the cervix is completely dilated. The baby's head now needs to come out of the birth canal. In addition to the uterine contractions, you will be asked to push so that the baby is born.

Pushing

This is the toughest part of labour. Your husband will be able to help you by supporting your head and neck as you push down. If you are lying on your back, the most effective way of pushing is to take a deep breath, put your chin on your chest and push down into your rectum. It is almost like being severely constipated and having to give terrific pressure.

Remember that there is always a gap of two to three minutes between each contraction. Just go limp, take deep breaths and relax during that time so you can gather up enough strength for the next push.

Crowning and delivery of the baby

When the mother has pushed for a while, the baby's head is seen at the opening of the vagina. This is called the 'crowning' of the baby's head. Soon, with a few more pushes, the baby will be delivered.

At this point, your obstetrician will decide whether you require an **episiotomy**. The baby's head will then be gently helped out of the birth canal. The shoulders and the rest of the baby will then follow very quickly. The obstetrician will guide the baby out, trying to avoid injury to your tissues.

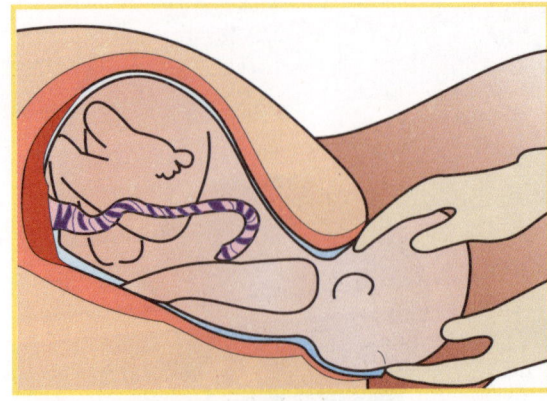

Delivery of the baby's head

Third stage of labour

You are almost done with the process of delivery! The final stage of labour occurs after the delivery of your baby. During this stage, the placenta and membranes are expelled from the body. There will be no more pain and you don't have to do any more hard work! This stage generally only takes 5 to 15 minutes. Rarely, the placenta may not detach from the uterine wall and the third stage may last a little longer.

Chances are that you may not pay much attention to this stage of labour because you will be busy holding your little bundle of joy!

Your obstetrician will make sure that the uterus has contracted well and that you are not having any excessive bleeding. She will also check to see if there have been any tears in the vaginal tissue.

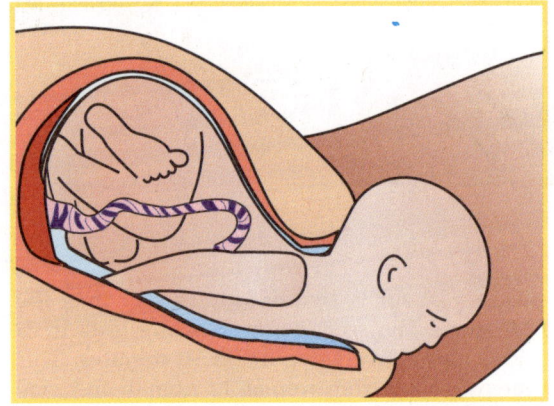

Crowning of the baby's head

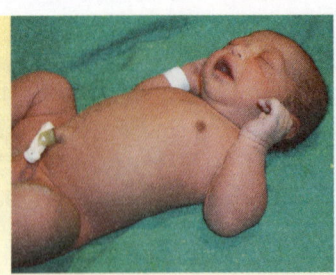

APGAR score

When the baby is born, your obstetrician will assign it an APGAR score. This is a good way of measuring the baby's response to its first few minutes of life after birth. The scores are given at 1 minute, 5 minutes and 10 minutes. A high score is indicative of a healthy baby which is responding well to birth. A low score at 5 and 10 minutes means that the baby has had trouble adapting to birth and may require admission to the newborn nursery.

    A = appearance (colour)
    P = pulse (heartbeat)
    G = grimace (reflex)
    A = activity (muscle tone)
    R = respiration (breathing)

Each of these is assigned a score of 2, 1 or 0, depending on the condition of the baby.

Episiotomy

An **episiotomy** is a surgical incision made through the **perineum,** which is the area below the vagina. This is usually done to enlarge the vagina and assist the delivery of the baby. It is one of the most common medical procedures performed on women.

In a first delivery, the tissue of the perineum may be not be very lax and may tear during the delivery. If your obstetrician feels that an episiotomy might cut short the second stage of labour or if she feels that you will have more damage to your pelvic tissues if the cut is not made, she might perform an episiotomy.

An episiotomy is usually done under local anaesthesia. It is sutured after the delivery of the baby. Most women will not feel the episiotomy being done, especially if it is done during a contraction.

If you have had a baby before, the vagina may be more lax and it might be possible to deliver without an episiotomy.

After care for the episiotomy

An episiotomy can be painful for a few days after the delivery. Usually, the pain will peak around the 4th or 5th day and then will gradually become less.

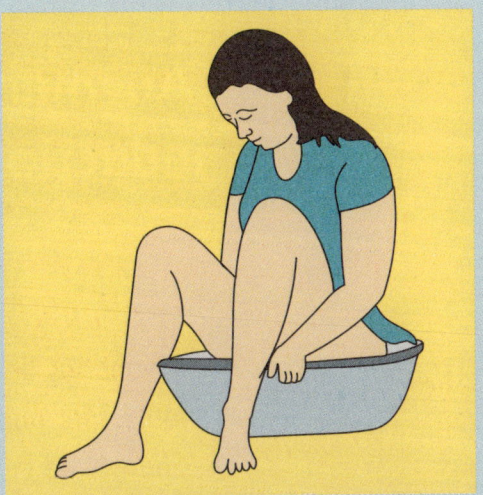

Sitz bath

There is no need for any oral antibiotics to be taken just because you have had an episiotomy. You need not apply any ointment on the episiotomy.

For pain relief, you can take a pain killer like ibuprofen. You may also be given a Sitz bath which is basically a basin filled with warm water in which you can sit. This is soothing for the pain. An infrared lamp can also be used on the episiotomy to relieve the pain.

CHAPTER 18

Augmentation and induction of labour

Shivani has been in labour for five hours. Her pains are not effective. She will be getting medication to augment labour so that she can deliver without further delay.

Sangeetha is 41 weeks pregnant. Her obstetrician has advised her to get admitted to the hospital. She will be undergoing induction of labour.

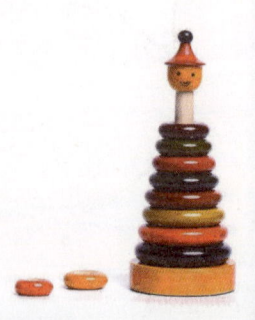

18 Augmentation and induction of labour

What is labour augmentation?

Occasionally, labour may not progress as rapidly as it should. Sometimes the contractions continue to be irregular and are not effective in dilating the cervix and moving the baby down the birth canal. At this point, your obstetrician may decide to **augment** labour.

Your obstetrician will carefully assess the pattern of the **contractions,** how much your cervix is dilated, and how far your baby has descended. The baby's heart rate is also closely monitored. If the baby's heartbeat is normal (both during and immediately after the contractions), she will proceed with augmentation of labour. This will ensure stronger, more effective contractions so that you deliver your baby faster and safely.

What is induction of labour?

Sometimes, labour may be **induced** if the health of the woman or baby is at risk.

This means that the obstetrician may use medication or other methods to make the woman go into labour. Whether the labour will be induced depends on the condition of the mother and the baby, the week of pregnancy, the status of the cervix and other factors.

Augmentation of labour

An **amniotomy** is the most common form of augmenting labour. If the membranes have not ruptured on their own, your obstetrician may decide to rupture them. The amniotomy will help make your labour progress faster.

An amniotomy also allows the doctor to check the colour of the amniotic fluid. If it is clear, it is a good sign and indicates that the baby is doing well. If it is greenish coloured, this may be an indication that the baby has passed meconium inside the uterus. Sometimes this may be a sign that the baby is facing difficulty inside the uterus.

Augmentation with oxytocin

The most common drug that is used for augmentation is a synthetic form of the hormone oxytocin. You will receive it through an intravenous (IV) drip.

Augmentation is usually started with a small dose, and the dose is gradually increased until your uterus responds appropriately. The aim is to have about three contractions in ten minutes.

Your pains will be monitored till you are having effective contractions. It is also important to make sure that your pains are not too frequent or too strong. Effective contractions will cause your cervix to dilate and will help the baby's head descend into the birth canal.

While your labour is being augmented, the baby's heartbeat will be monitored regularly to make sure the baby is tolerating the labour well.

Induction of labour

Induction of labour is the use of artificial means, such as a medication, to start the process of childbirth. This is done if the health of the woman or baby is at risk.

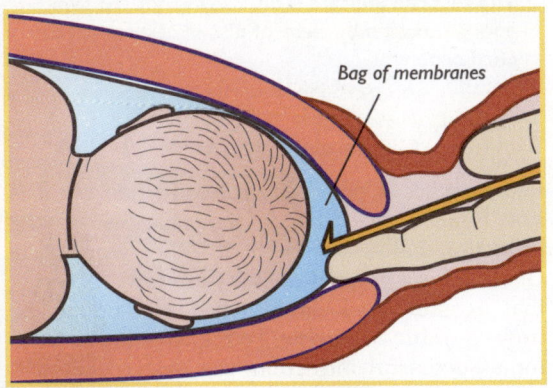
Amniotomy
Bag of membranes

Reasons for inducing labour:

- Postdated pregnancy i.e. pregnancy that has continued at least 7 to 10 days past the due date
- Rupture of the membranes before labour has started
- Pregnancy induced hypertension (PIH) i.e. the mother has high blood pressure caused by the pregnancy
- Diabetes in pregnancy (especially if the mother is taking insulin to control the sugar levels)
- If the baby is small due to growth restriction
- Infection of the amniotic sac (chorioamnionitis)
- Separation of the placenta (abruption) from the inner lining of the uterus
- Logistical reasons (for example, the pregnant woman lives too far from a hospital or there is a history of fast labour)
- Death of the baby before birth (intrauterine foetal demise)

Optimising induction of labour

Once a decision is made to induce labour, the obstetrician ascertains if the conditions are right for induction.

Checklist for mother

The induction has more chances of succeeding if

- the cervix has thinned out
- the cervix has started to dilate
- the baby's head has descended into the birth canal

Checklist for baby

The baby will tolerate induction better if

- the water around the baby (**amniotic fluid**) is adequate. This is assessed by an ultrasound examination.
- the baby has adequate reserves – this is assessed by doing a test known as a **non-stress test** where the baby's heart rate is monitored electronically.

Foetal non-stress test (NST)

This is a simple, non-invasive test performed in pregnancies over 28 weeks. It is done to check the well-being of the foetus. Since there is no stress placed on the foetus during this test, it is termed a "non-stress" test.

How is a NST performed?

Using an electronic foetal monitor placed on the mother's abdomen, the baby's heart beat is recorded for 20-30 minutes. The way the baby's heart beat reacts to the baby's movements gives an indication of the baby's well being. Healthy babies will respond with an increased heart rate during times of movement, and the heart rate will decrease at rest. When the baby is receiving less oxygen for any reason, the baby's heart beat will not respond normally. Sometimes the baby may be sleeping and may not move much. The nurse or doctor may then shake the baby or use a loud noise to make it move.

A **reactive non-stress** test indicates that blood flow (and oxygen) to the foetus is adequate. A **non-reactive non-stress** test may need further testing or immediate delivery of the baby.

Indications for a NST

A NST may be performed if:

- you have felt that the movements are less than usual
- you are past your due date
- the foetal growth is inadequate
- there is reason to suspect that the placenta is not functioning well
- there is a complication in the pregnancy

The test can indicate if the baby is not receiving enough oxygen because of placental or umbilical cord problems.

Ripening of the cervix

If the cervix is not ready for induction i.e. it is not effaced or dilated, the chances of the induction failing are high. In other words, the chances for a vaginal delivery are low. A cervix that is still thick and closed is said to be **unfavourable** or **unripe**. To improve the chances for a successful induction, the obstetrician will proceed with **ripening of the cervix**.

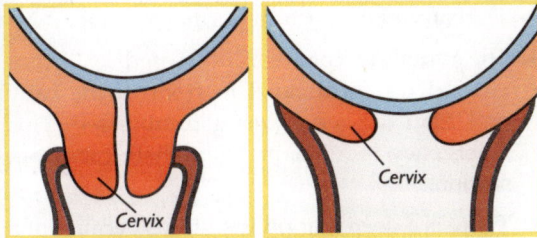

Unfavourable or unripe cervix   *Favourable or ripened cervix*

Stripping of the membranes is a procedure where the obstetrician inserts the examining finger through the opening of the cervix and gently detaches the membrane of the amniotic sac from the wall of the uterus. This may help start the process of ripening.

Ripening of the cervix is better achieved by using **prostaglandin gel** placed in the cervix, or **prostaglandin tablets** placed in the vagina or given orally.

Methods of inducing labour

Amniotomy

If the cervix is favourable (thinned out and dilated), an amniotomy is often resorted to. Though it may not be an effective method for labour induction by itself, it works well in combination with medications like oxytocin and prostaglandins.

During an internal examination, the obstetrician identifies the thin membrane lying over the baby's head and ruptures it with a special instrument. When the membrane is opened and the amniotic fluids start coming out, uterine contractions may start within a short period of time.

Amniotomy is usually avoided if the baby's head is too high and has not descended into the birth canal.

Oxytocin

The commonest drug used for induction, the world over, is oxytocin. Oxytocin is the hormone that the body produces in spontaneous labour. It makes the uterus contract. For induction, a synthetic form of the drug is given intravenously (IV).

The dosage of oxytocin is always low to begin with and then gradually increased till adequate and effective contractions set in. The contractions are monitored carefully to make sure that they are not stronger than what is safe for the mother and baby.

As with any procedure, induction of labour with oxytocin must be done according to standard protocols. This will help avoid any risk to the mother and baby.

Prostaglandin tablets

As an alternative to oxytocin, prostaglandin tablets may be given orally. The dose is increased gradually till contractions start. Once labour has started, the contractions may be made stronger and more effective with the use of oxytocin given intravenously (IV).

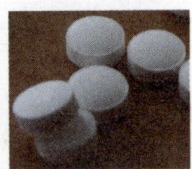

> Prostaglandin tablets or gel are best avoided if the woman has had a previous caesarean section. Their usage may sometimes result in the previous scar giving way.

Risks of labour induction

When monitored properly, induction of labour is safe. But as with any procedure, induction of labour may carry some risk for the mother and baby. To minimise these risks, the contractions are monitored carefully. The amount of drug given is also increased gradually. The medication is reduced or stopped completely if there is any problem.

In some cases, there is a small risk of complications such as:

- **Foetal distress** which results in an abnormal foetal heart rate. This can result from contractions that are too strong or frequent. This can also be due to compression of the umbilical cord. If this happens, the oxytocin infusion will be turned off and the baby's heart rate will be monitored carefully. If the baby's heart rate is back to normal, the oxytocin may be restarted at a lower dose.
- A tear or **rupture** of the uterus.

- A **caesarean section** which may need to be done if the induction is not successful or if there is foetal distress.

When should labour not be induced?

Induction of labour is not attempted when

- There is a placenta praevia i.e. the placenta lies very low in the uterus, and is lying in front of the baby's head. The opening of the uterus is partially or completely covered by the placenta.
- The baby is lying in an abnormal position.
- The umbilical cord has prolapsed i.e. it has entered the birth canal in front of the baby and is in danger of being compressed. This emergency requires an immediate caesarean section.
- There is a deep scar on the uterus because of a previous surgery like a caesarean or removal of a fibroid.

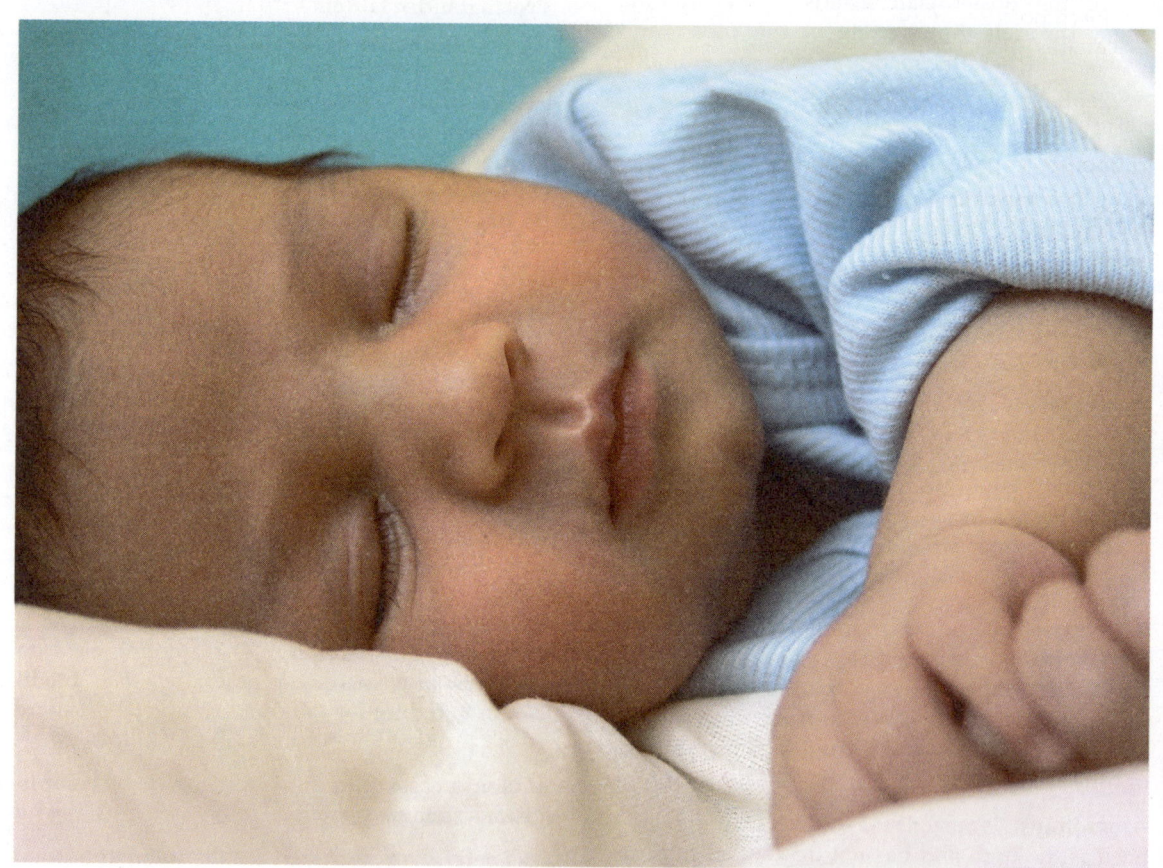

Terms you will hear in the labour room

Amniotic fluid
Amniotic fluid consists mostly of foetal urine and water and fills the sac surrounding the foetus.

Breech presentation
When the foetus has not turned to the head-down position and is coming through the birth canal with its buttocks or feet first.

Cephalopelvic disproportion(CPD)
The baby is too large to safely pass through the mother's pelvis.

Caesarean section
An incision through the abdominal and uterine walls for extraction of the foetus.

Contractions
There is tightening and relaxation of the uterine muscle at regular intervals. These contractions push the baby through the birth canal.

Dilatation
The cervix (mouth of the uterus) opens to let the baby through. This opening of the cervix is called dilatation. It is measured in centimetres, with full dilation being 10 centimetres.

Effacement
This refers to the thinning of the cervix in preparation for birth and is expressed in percentages. The cervix will be 100% effaced and fully dilated when you begin pushing.

Epidural
An excellent method of pain relief used during labour. It is inserted through a catheter which is threaded through a needle, into the dural space near the spinal cord.

Episiotomy
An incision made on the perineum to widen the vaginal opening for delivery.

Foetal distress
This is a condition when the baby is not receiving enough oxygen or is experiencing some other complication. It is recognised by abnormalities in the baby's heart beat.

Forceps
Stainless steel instruments which may be placed gently on either side of the baby's head and used to help guide the baby's head out of the birth canal during delivery.

Meconium
This is the greenish-black substance that is present in the bowels of a growing foetus and is normally discharged shortly after birth as the baby's first few bowel movements. Occasionally, this is discharged during labour and may suggest that the baby is having foetal distress.

Neonatologist
A paediatric specialist who cares for newborns.

NICU
Neonatal Intensive Care Unit.

Oxytocin
Hormone secreted by the pituitary gland that stimulates contractions and the milk reflex. In the synthetic form, this hormone is used to induce or augment labour.

Placenta
The tissue that connects the mother and foetus to transport nourishment and take away waste.

Vacuum cup
A vacuum cup is an instrument used to assist the delivery of the baby.

CHAPTER 19

Forceps delivery and vacuum-assisted birth

Sudarshana has been in labour for five hours. For the past one and a half hours, she has been trying to push the baby out of the birth canal. She is exhausted.
She needs help. Her obstetrician will assist her birth by applying a vacuum cup to the baby's head and easing it out of the birth canal.

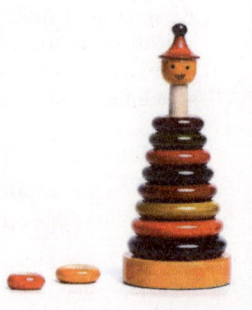

19 Forceps delivery and vacuum-assisted birth

What is an instrumental delivery?

Occasionally, the obstetrician may use a forceps or vacuum cup to help the mother deliver the baby. These instruments are placed on the baby's head so that it can be gently eased out with the least trauma to the mother and baby.

Instrumental delivery might be required when

- the woman is having a difficult time pushing the baby out through her birth canal
- the woman may have become too tired and exhausted to continue pushing
- the woman has had an epidural and may not have the urge to push
- the woman should not push too long because of a medical condition (e.g. heart disease)
- the baby may need to be delivered quickly because it is showing signs of being in distress
- the second twin might require assistance in delivery

What are forceps?

Forceps are stainless steel instruments which are placed gently on either side of the baby's head and are used to cradle the head. Holding the baby with the instrument, the obstetrician will apply traction and lift the baby out of the birth canal.

What is a vacuum-assisted birth?

The vacuum cup is attached by a flexible rubber tube to a small vacuum pump. The cup, which fits on top of the baby's head, may be made of metal or silicone plastic. The soft silicone cups are less likely to cause damage to your baby's head, and are more commonly used now. The obstetrician applies gentle traction on the tube attached to the cup, and lifts the baby out of the birth canal.

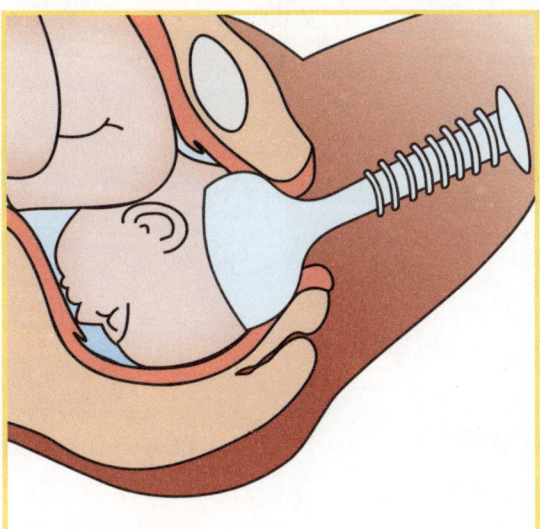

Vacuum-assisted birth

After your baby is born

Even after a normal vaginal delivery, the baby's head may be a little elongated and conical. This happens because the baby has to mould itself to the shape of the birth canal.

In babies born with the help of a forceps or a vacuum extractor, the head may be a little more conical or there may be a prominent bulge where the vacuum cup was applied. This will usually

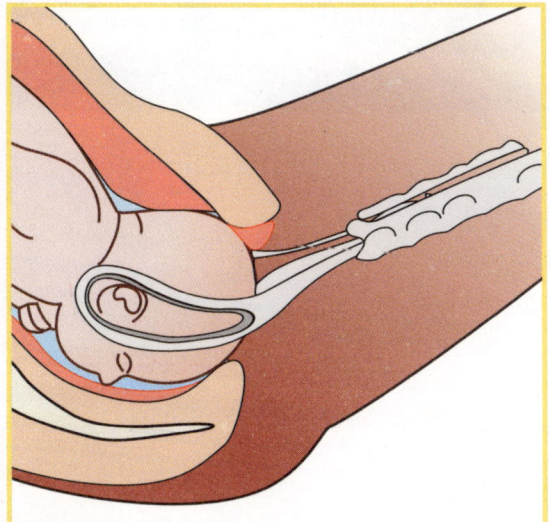

Forceps delivery

subside in a few days. There is no need to massage the head - it will get back to a normal shape on its own.

Babies born using a vacuum cup are not more likely to need phototherapy (a treatment for **newborn jaundice**) than babies born using forceps.

Some women are worried that a forceps delivery or a vacuum-assisted birth can harm the baby. This is not true. When a child is born with cerebral palsy or mental retardation, parents are sometimes quick to blame the use of instruments. In reality, instrumental deliveries cannot result in a baby being born with mental retardation.

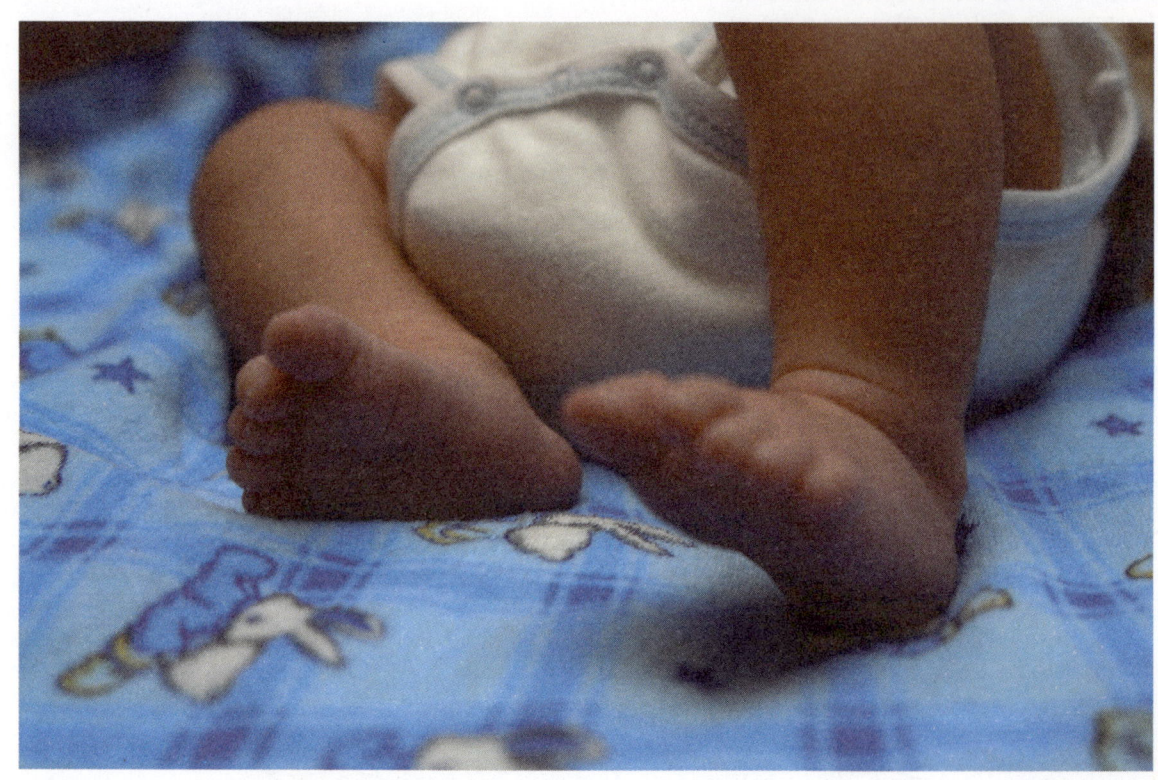

Umbilical cord blood banking

What is umbilical cord blood banking?

Once considered a waste product that was discarded with the placenta, umbilical cord blood is now known to be rich in potentially life-saving **stem cells**. When used for stem cell transplantation, umbilical cord blood offers several distinct advantages over bone marrow or peripheral stem cells.

In many parts of the world, including India, private companies have aggressively marketed the need for the storage of umbilical cord blood. The marketing definitely plays on the guilt of parents and grandparents who feel that if they do not store their baby's cord blood, they have not done something essential to safeguard the baby's future.

Public cord blood banks allow this valuable product to be stored and used by anybody, much like blood banks store units of blood which can be used to save anyone's life, not just the donor's.

How is cord blood collected?

After the delivery, the placenta is removed from the uterus, the cord is cleaned and a needle is inserted into a cord blood vessel. Lab technicians run the blood through a battery of tests, extract the stem cells from the sample, and prepare the sample for the freezer, where the cells remain until they are needed.

Should every parent store their baby's cord blood?

In India, collection, processing and storage of cord blood in a private company can cost between Rs 80,000 and Rs 1,00,000 to the parents.

The American College of Obstetricians and Gynecologists and the American Academy of Pediatrics categorically state that in most cases, private storage of cord blood is unwise. No accurate estimates exist of the likelihood that children will need their own stored cells, but estimates range from 1 in 2,700 to 1 in 200,000. It is interesting to note that in seven years of operation, one of the leading private cord blood storage banks in America has not used a single unit of stored blood!

To date, approximately 7000 stem cell transplants have been done around the world. The vast majority of cord blood stem cell transplants have been done using cells from unrelated donors from public banks. About 300 transplants have involved sibling donors while approximately 14 have been done using a child's own cells.

Will your child need its own cord blood in the future?

Most parents are terrified that their child might develop a condition in the future that might be only curable with its own stem cells. They are particularly concerned about genetic diseases or leukemia. But if a child has a genetic disease or childhood leukemia, his or her own cord blood would be useless in treating it because the cells will be chromosomally or genetically abnormal. A sibling's cord blood or an unrelated donor's cord blood might help.

For marketing purposes, many companies are stating that cord blood stem cells will be useful in the future for treating diabetes, heart disease, nerve diseases and arthritis. There is no scientific basis for this at present. What is more concerning is that the amount of stem cells present in the unit of cord blood stored will not be sufficient for treating an adult. Using two or three units from a public cord blood bank might be more efficient.

Stem cell transplants from a donor are as effective as from the same individual. Donating the cord blood to a public blood bank will be more useful and cost-effective than storing it for one individual.

CHAPTER 20

Pain relief in labour and delivery

Shraddha is due to deliver in another week. She is very apprehensive. She has heard tales of horror from many of her friends and dreads the pain of labour. Though her mother has reassured her that labour pains are tolerable, she is still concerned. Shraddha should talk to her obstetrician about the options available for pain relief in labour.

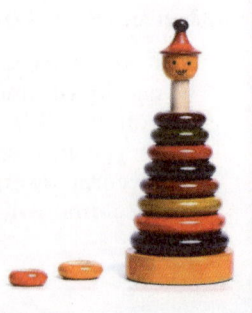

20 Pain relief in labour and delivery

In every language in the world, the words childbirth and labour are synonymous with pain. The joy of giving birth is always coloured with the fear of pain during labour. Pain is a natural part of labour and every woman is unique in the ability to handle the level of pain. Pain tolerance varies from woman to woman. Some women dread childbirth to the extent of demanding a caesarean section instead of going through natural childbirth.

You may be filled with apprehension. Your friends and relatives may have used some ill-chosen words to describe the travails of labour. You may be really frightened about going through labour. You need not worry. Modern obstetrics offers you many choices for pain relief in labour and delivery.

Why is labour painful?

There are several reasons for pain during labour and delivery.

Uterine contractions

The pregnant uterus is one of the largest muscles in the body. As the uterus contracts, the blood supply to the muscle is cut off. This causes intense pain. The other reason is that during the contraction, the muscle stretches and this results in pain.

Cervical dilatation

The stretching of the cervix as it dilates causes pain.

Pressure on the pelvic nerves

As labour progresses, there is pressure on the pelvic nerves causing intense pain.

Dilatation of the vaginal and perineal tissues

As the baby's head descends through the vagina and pushes against the skin at the opening of the vagina, the stretching results in pain.

Pain management in labour

Pain relief offered during labour is safe for both the mother and the baby. There are many ways

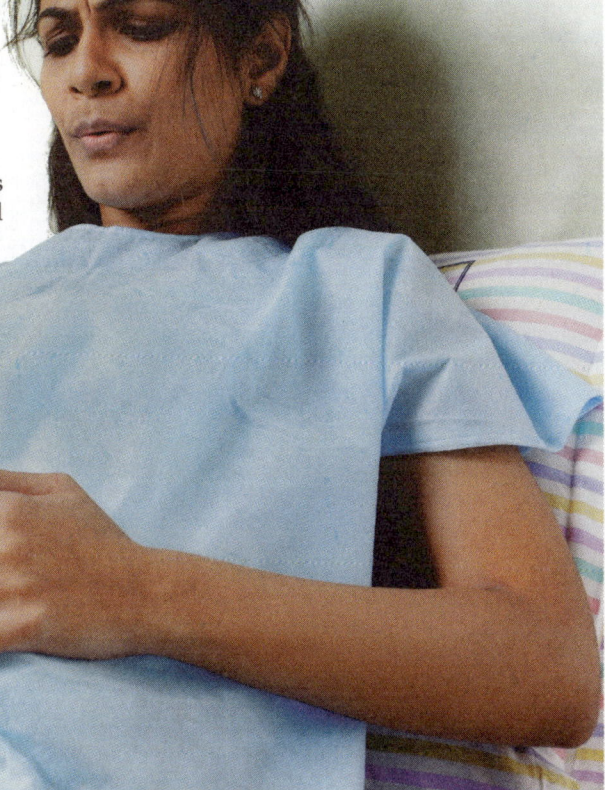

to lessen pain during labour and the birth of the baby. Being prepared with knowledge of the birth process is the first step towards being able to handle labour pains. Labour preparation classes for the couple are, therefore, important.

The common methods of pain relief are

- Breathing and relaxation techniques
- Pain-relieving drugs that can be given as an injection
- Newer methods include epidural analgesia and pain relieving gas mixture.

The type of pain relief that is right for you depends on your pain threshold. Some women can tolerate pain to a greater extent than others. Some women have a low threshold for pain and this, combined with the fear of labour pains, can make them very intolerant of the slightest pain. A woman's physical fitness, attending labour preparation classes, the length of labour, the intensity of labour pains and the size of the baby play a role in the ability to handle the pain of labour.

Drugs used for pain relief

Narcotics (such as Pethidine or Tramadol) may be used during the first stage of labour to help you relax. Narcotics are usually injected into a muscle (IM) or into a vein (IV). These drugs generally take about 20 minutes to start working.

Narcotics lessen the pain and can help you feel less tense or anxious. You may actually feel drowsy with Pethidine. The effects usually last for about two to four hours. If needed, the injection can be repeated.

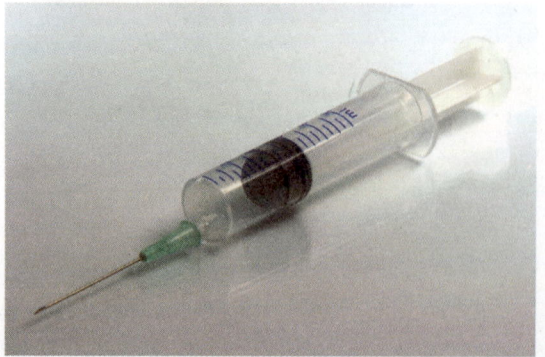

The effects of the drugs, such as drowsiness, can be passed on to the baby. It is, therefore, not given if it appears that the baby will be delivered very soon.

Remember, an injection of Pethidine will not eliminate the pain completely. It will only take the edge off the pain so that you can deal with it more easily.

Regional analgesia (epidural)

A regional block lessens or completely blocks the pain in a specific part of the body. The goal of regional analgesia is to reach a balance between easing the pain and still feeling the urge to bear down to actively participate in delivering your baby.

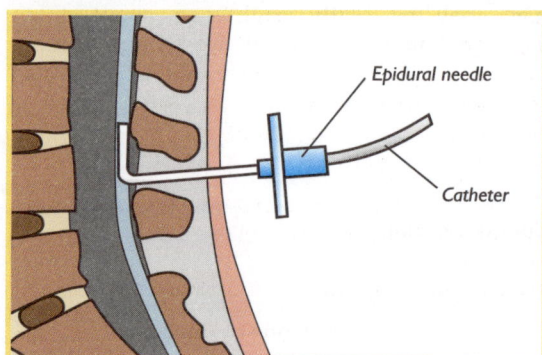

Epidural catheter in place

The **epidural block** is a commonly used type of regional analgesia during labour. A woman in labour may reach a point where narcotics are no longer giving her adequate pain relief. At this point, she may opt to go ahead with epidural analgesia. With epidural analgesia, there is no loss of consciousness, so the mother can actively participate in the process of delivery.

(**Spinal anaesthesia** is also a regional block but is used only for a caesarean and not for pain relief during labour).

What is an epidural block?

An epidural block is given in the lower back into a small area (the epidural space) below the spinal cord. You will be asked to sit or lie on your side with your back curved outward and to stay this way until the procedure is completed.

The position may be a little uncomfortable but it is only for a short while.

After the epidural block is given, you can lie down and still move from side to side. You may not be allowed to walk around.

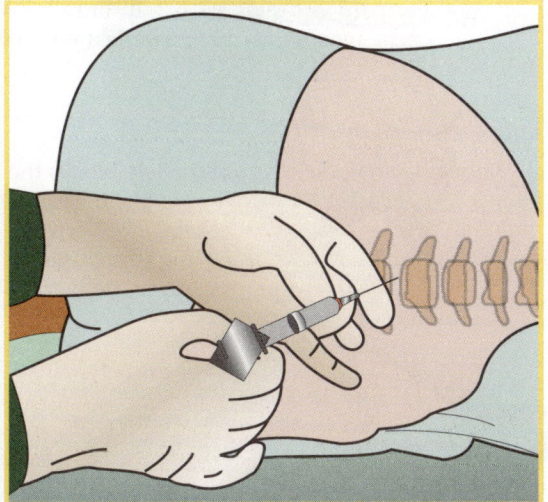

Epidural catheter being inserted

Before the block is performed, your skin will be cleaned with an antiseptic solution. Local anaesthesia will be used to numb the area of your lower back where the needle will be inserted. After the epidural needle is inserted, a small tube (catheter) is introduced through it, and the needle is withdrawn. In some cases, the catheter may touch a nerve. At this point there may be a brief tingling sensation down one leg.

You might notice a bit of temporary numbness, heaviness or weakness in your legs.

Small doses of the medication are then given through the catheter to reduce the discomfort of labour. The medication can also be given continuously.

The effect of the epidural may take a few minutes to be felt because the medication needs to be absorbed. Pain relief will begin within 10–20 minutes after the medication has been injected.

Low doses are used because they are less likely to cause side effects for you and the baby. In low doses, an epidural block eases the pain of contractions and numbs the birth canal during labour and delivery. The pressure of the contractions is still felt with an epidural block but the pain component will be minimised. In higher doses, an epidural may be used for caesarean sections.

Pushing with an epidural block

Although an epidural block will make you more comfortable, you still may be aware of your contractions. You will also continue to have some degree of discomfort when you are examined to see if the cervix is dilating. The anaesthetist will adjust the degree of numbness for your comfort. When it is time to push, the epidural will be allowed to wear off a little bit so that your urge to push is not suppressed.

Are there any risks of these methods of pain relief?

Because a narcotic like Pethidine affects the entire body, both the mother and the baby may have mild side-effects from this drug. Drowsiness and feeling dizzy are the most common side-effects. Pethidine is usually not used when the baby is just about to be born because the baby may be drowsy immediately after birth.

The medicines used in epidural analgesia are less likely to pass to the baby or affect the baby because they do not enter the bloodstream.

An epidural block may cause the mother's blood pressure to drop. This may in turn cause the baby's heartbeat to slow down. To help prevent this from happening, fluids are given to the mother through an IV drip before the epidural block is given.

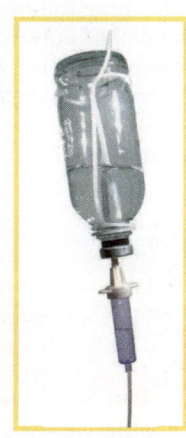

Pain relieving gas mixture

Pain relieving gas is often used to relieve labour pain. Gas mixtures will help to relieve pain but will not remove it completely. It is a mixture of oxygen and nitrous oxide. It provides good pain relief without causing undue sleepiness. The gas

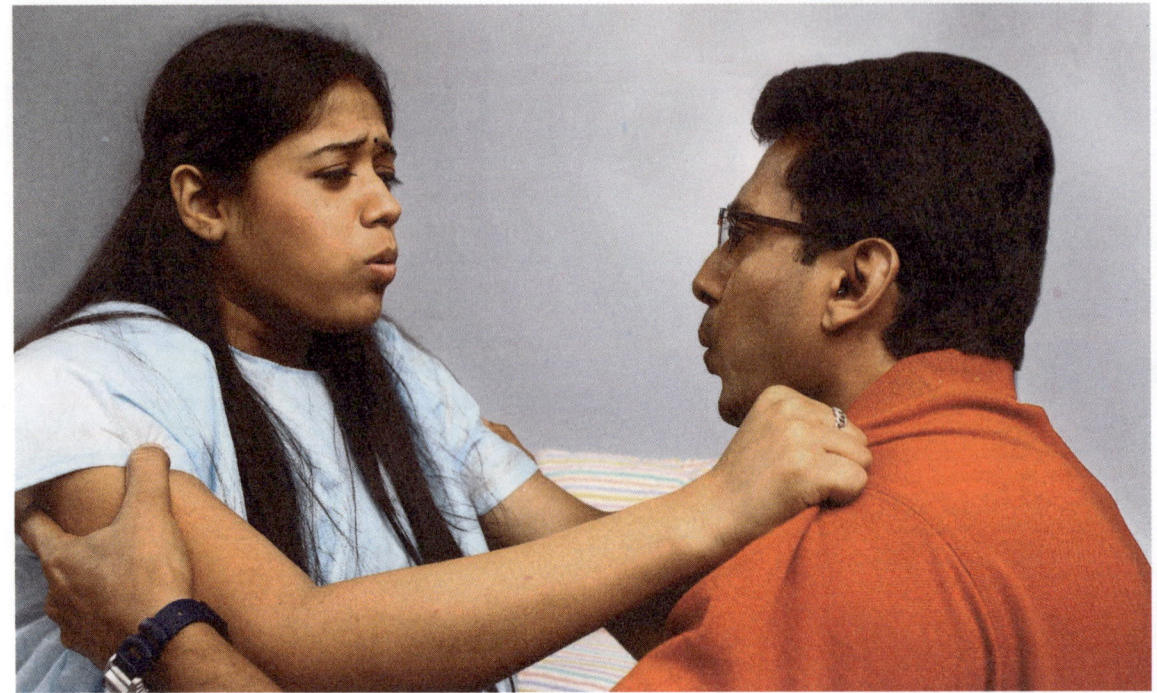

works quickly, but takes about 30 to 45 seconds to have the pain relieving effect.

As you feel a contraction start, you can start breathing the gas through a mask. You have total control of how much you want to inhale and how much pain relief you are comfortable with. The gas mixture crosses the placenta but is not known to have any effect on your baby. Since nitrous oxide is an anaesthetic gas, you may feel a little dizzy.

How can pain during labour be relieved without drugs?

- Each woman has a different threshold for pain. How a person deals with the pain depends on her attitude to labour. Attending labour preparation classes helps relieve the anxiety about labour. Breathing exercises are an important part of pain relief during labour.
- Your husband's presence in the labour room is also important. Your husband can encourage and support you as you go through labour. It is a strong bonding experience.
- You and your husband can take classes to learn about childbirth, body conditioning exercises and methods of relaxation. All of these techniques can be used with other treatments for labour pain.

Can an epidural cause back pain?

Many women are apprehensive that an epidural can cause back pain which will persist for years. This is not true. Recent studies have shown that you are no more likely to get a backache after having an epidural for labour than if you deliver without an epidural.

Very rarely, a slow leak of spinal fluid can occur after an epidural and this may lead to a headache. You might be advised to lie flat for a day or so until the leak seals itself. If needed, a second injection may be given to seal the leak.

Most women find that an epidural makes their labour much more enjoyable.

Breathing techniques in labour

When that first strong pain hits, most women are taken by surprise at its intensity. It is important to learn and practise breathing techniques well ahead of time so that you can use them when the pains start becoming uncomfortable. If you can attend a **labour preparation class** with your husband, both of you will be ready to handle labour.

Breathing techniques give you something to focus on. When the pains get stronger, many women lose control. Breathing rhythmically enables you to feel in control. Most importantly, proper breathing ensures that you and your baby get an adequate supply of oxygen in labour.

Different breathing exercises can be useful during the different stages of labour.

Breathing techniques in early labour

During the initial stage of labour you should focus on slowly inhaling and exhaling throughout your contraction. Inhale through your nose and then exhale slowly through your mouth. When you are exhaling, it helps to purse your lips and blow out your breath. Face your husband, focus on his eyes or mouth and hold his hands as you go through the breathing together.

Breathing in the active stage

With the beginning of each contraction, continue to inhale through your nose and exhale through your mouth as you were doing during the earlier part of labour. As the intensity of the contraction increases, you can start to take shallower, quicker breaths. As the contraction reaches its peak, it may help to breathe in and out through your mouth as if you were panting. When the intensity of the contraction begins to lessen, resume rhythmic inhalation: in through your nose and out through your mouth.

Closer to delivery you may get a strong urge to push. If you are not fully dilated, your doctor may ask you not to push. Concentrate on your breathing and try not to push at this time.

Breathing and pushing

Once your cervix is fully dilated, you will be asked to push the baby through the birth canal. For effective pushing, use the following breathing technique:

Take a deep breath and hold it. Push down into your rectum, as if you were severely constipated. After a good push, take a deep breath again and push again if the pain is still there. Once the pain subsides, take a few deep breaths and then relax.

Practise the breathing techniques

Start practising the breathing techniques with your husband, in the last month of pregnancy. Once you are in labour, it will be difficult to follow rhythmic breathing unless you have practised them before.

CHAPTER 21

Monitoring the baby's well-being during labour

Sanjana has been in labour for the past four hours. She has high blood pressure which started in pregnancy. She is concerned. Will her baby tolerate labour well?

There are many ways of making sure that the baby is doing well during labour. It is important to monitor the baby's well-being during the process of labour.

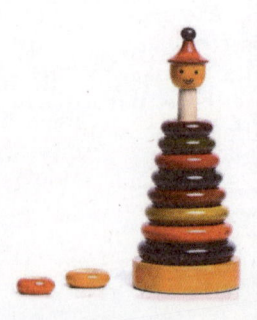

21 Monitoring the baby's well-being during labour

When you are in labour, your obstetrician has to take care of two individuals, you and your baby. While checking how your labour is progressing, she will also constantly check to see if the baby is tolerating the labour well.

Foetal heart rate

The best way of telling whether the baby is handling labour well is to monitor the heart rate. Most babies will have some changes in their heart rate during labour. Your doctor knows which changes are considered to be normal. Abnormal heart rate patterns alert the doctor that a problem may be present. At this point, steps will be taken to help the baby.

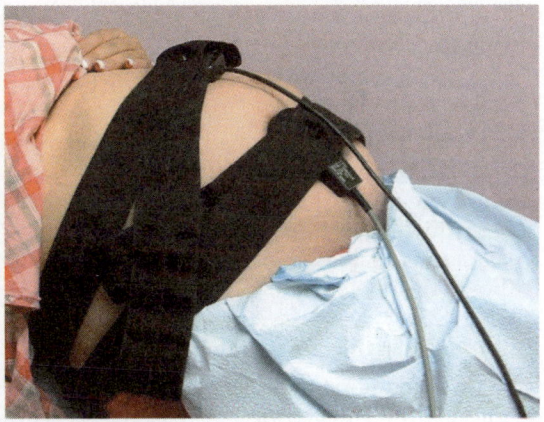

Listening to and monitoring the foetal heart rate is an important component of good obstetric care. In labour, the baby faces a lot of stress due to contractions of the uterine muscle.

The foetal heart rate is monitored at least every half to one hour in the first stage of labour. In the second stage, the nurse or doctor will listen to the foetal heart more frequently. The heart rate will be particularly monitored during and immediately after the contraction so that any stress to the baby is picked up.

Colour of amniotic fluid

Another indicator of foetal well-being is the colour of the amniotic fluid which surrounds the baby. When the membranes rupture spontaneously or if they are ruptured by the obstetrician, the colour of the fluid is checked. When it is clear i.e. it looks like water, then the baby is usually not having any problems. When the fluid is greenish, it means that the baby has passed motion inside the uterus. This can be indicative of decreased oxygenation to the baby. The decision to continue with a vaginal delivery or proceed with a caesarean section at this point, depends on a number of factors. Your obstetrician will decide which is best for both you and your baby.

Methods of monitoring the foetal heart rate

Auscultation is a method of listening to the foetal heartbeat using a **foetoscope** or a **hand-held Doppler instrument**.

When there is a doubt that there may be a problem with the heart rate, **electronic foetal monitoring** may be used. For this, special electronic equipment is used to record the heartbeat of the foetus. This equipment also records the contractions of the mother's uterus during labour.

Auscultation

Auscultation simply means listening to the baby's heartbeat during labour. As mentioned earlier, the number of times that the baby's heartbeat is listened to depends on which stage of labour you are in, the frequency and strength of your contractions and any risk factors for the baby. If abnormal patterns are found with auscultation, electronic monitoring may be done.

Foetoscope

A special device called a foetoscope is most commonly used to listen to the foetal heartbeat. The broad end is pressed on your abdomen and the nurse or doctor can hear the baby's heartbeat and will be able to count the heart rate. The foetoscope allows your baby's heartbeat to be heard clearly.

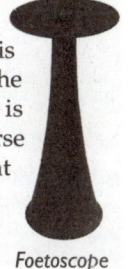

Foetoscope

Hand-held Doppler device

This is a small device that is pressed against the abdomen to hear the baby's heartbeat. This device uses a form of ultrasound to convert sound waves into signals of the baby's heart. The heartbeat can be heard clearly because it is amplified - you can hear it too!

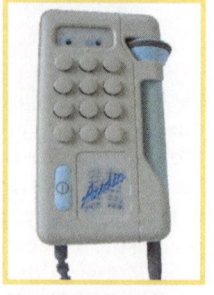
Hand-held Doppler

Electronic foetal monitoring

Just like adults have an ECG taken to diagnose abnormalities in the heart, electronic foetal monitoring uses special equipment to provide a record of the foetal heart rate. A graph records the baby's heartbeat and this record is read by the doctor or the nurse. The pattern of the foetal heart rate can reassure the doctor that the baby is tolerating the labour well. On the other hand, abnormalities in the heart rate pattern can alert the obstetrician that the baby is in distress.

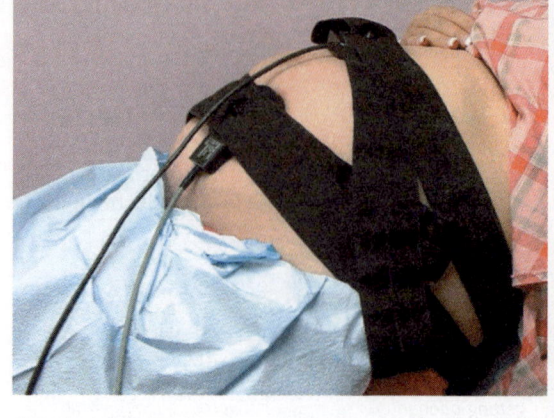

A pair of belts is wrapped around the mother's abdomen. To one is attached a device which uses Doppler to detect the foetal heart rate. This information is transmitted to the machine and the heart rate pattern is recorded. The other device measures the frequency and duration of the uterine contractions.

Foetal heart rate patterns

The foetal heart rate normally varies between 110 and 150 beats per minute. (This is much faster than an adult's heart rate). A healthy foetus which is tolerating labour well will have accelerations of the heart rate i.e. the heart rate will periodically increase.

Abnormal foetal heart rate patterns

Certain changes in the heart rate pattern may denote a problem for the baby. A foetal heart rate which **becomes flat (lacks variability)** or is **too slow** (less than 110 beats per minute) or **too fast** (more than 160 beats per minute) may signal a problem.

The changes in the foetal heart rate are correlated with the timing of the contraction. The seriousness of the abnormal heart rate changes depending on its relation to the contraction. If there is a serious change in the foetal heart rate pattern, the baby is said to be having **foetal distress**.

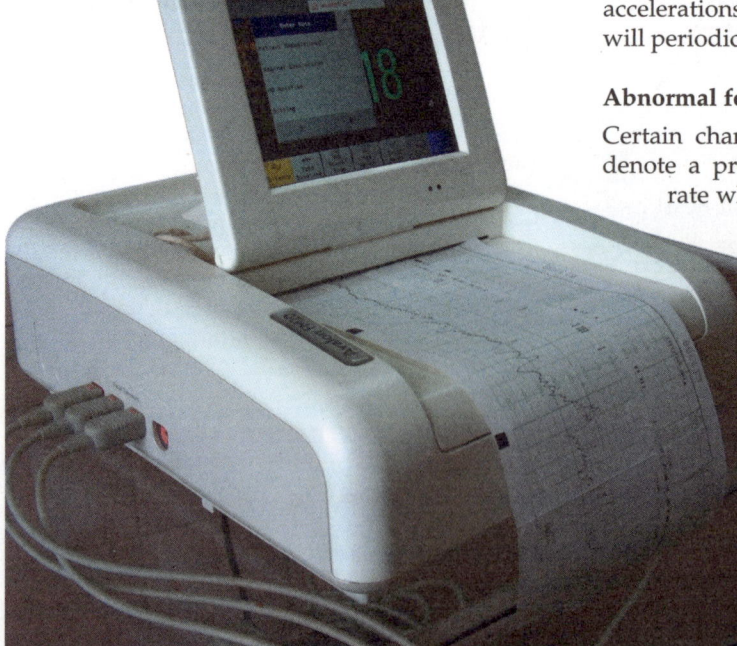
Electronic foetal monitor

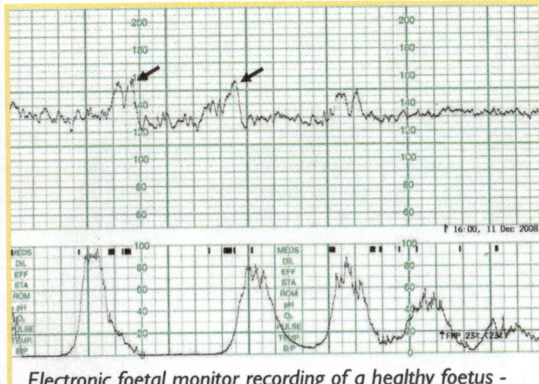

Electronic foetal monitor recording of a healthy foetus - arrows indicate accelerations which means the foetus is getting adequate oxygen and is tolerating labour well.

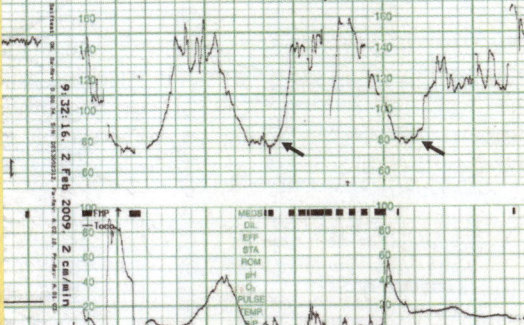

Recording of a foetus which is showing signs of distress. Arrows indicate decelerations which mean that the foetus is not getting adequate oxygen and is not tolerating labour well.

Managing abnormal foetal heart rate patterns

If there is an abnormal foetal heart rate pattern, certain steps may be taken to help the baby.

You may be

- asked to change positions - this may take the pressure off the cord if it is getting compressed
- given oxygen through a mask or a small tube in the nose - this is useful for the baby
- given intravenous (IV) fluids
- given medication to lessen the contractions and relax the uterus

What happens if abnormal foetal heart rate patterns persist?

Your obstetrician will make a decision about the abnormal foetal heart rate pattern depending on:

- The severity of the abnormality
- How close you are to delivery
- The size of the baby
- The colour of the amniotic fluid

If conditions are favourable and delivery is expected soon, then the obstetrician may proceed with a **forceps** delivery or a **vacuum-assisted birth.** If the baby has a problem, and it does not look like the delivery will happen soon, then the doctor may have to proceed with an immediate **caesarean section.**

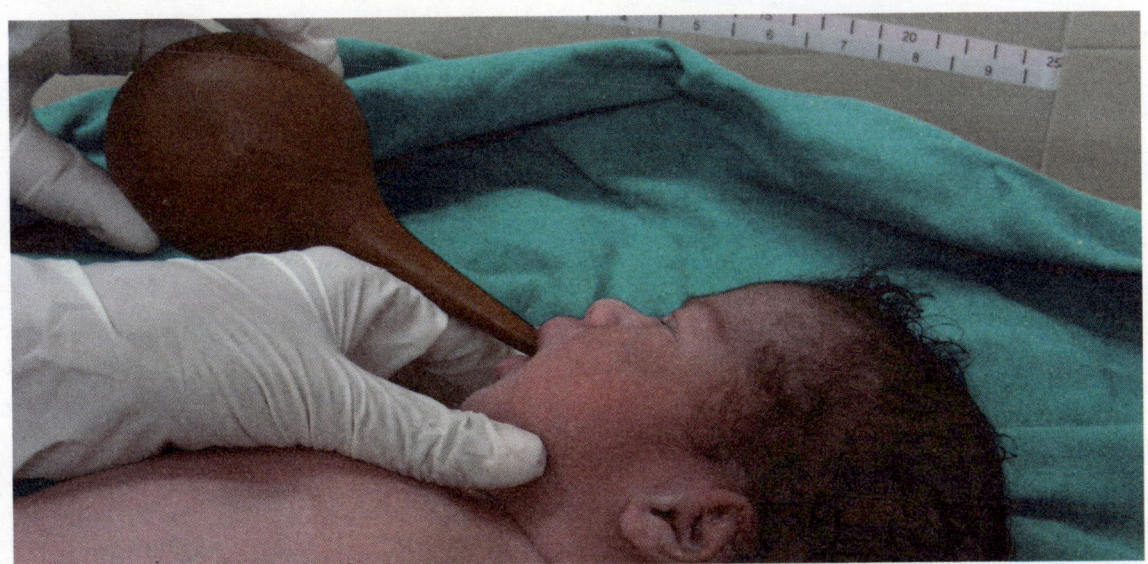

Suctioning the baby's mouth after delivery

CHAPTER 22

Complications in labour

Sunanda and her husband have been looking forward to a normal vaginal delivery. They both attended the labour preparation class and have practised relaxation techniques. Unfortunately, she has developed a complication in labour. The baby's heartbeat has started slowing down.

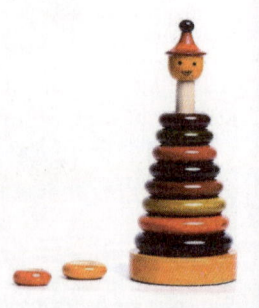

22 Complications in labour

Unfortunately, not every woman has a smooth labour. Some problems may be anticipated before labour starts. For example, your obstetrician may suspect that the baby may be too large for your pelvis and you may have trouble delivering. Sometimes, the baby is too small and may face problems during labour.

On the other hand, your obstetrician may be expecting you to have a vaginal delivery but a complication might crop up during labour which may result in your having a caesarean section.

When can problems be anticipated?

- If your baby is large, but there is still a chance for a normal vaginal delivery, your obstetrician may allow you to labour, and if the labour does not progress normally, may then opt for a caesarean. This is known as a 'trial of labour'.
- On the other hand, babies which are much smaller than expected for that stage of pregnancy (growth restricted) may also develop problems during labour which may result in a caesarean section.
- If you have gone more than one week beyond your due date, then problems may be anticipated.
- If you have hypertension or diabetes complicating your pregnancy, there may be an increased chance of having a caesarean section.
- Women older than 35 and younger than 18 also have a higher chance of caesarean section.
- If the labour has been induced for any reason, then the chance of undergoing a caesarean section increases.

What are unanticipated problems?

Failure of labour to progress

Sometimes, a problem can arise due to one or a combination of events. If the labour contractions are not strong enough, your obstetrician may give you medication to make the contractions stronger. In spite of this, the labour may fail to

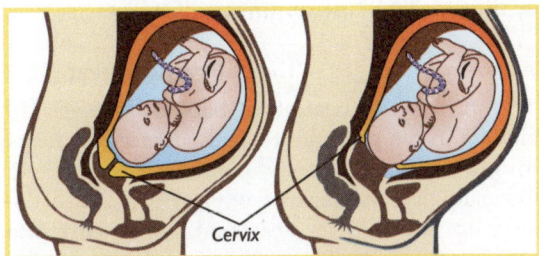

During normal delivery, the cervix will dilate completely and allow the foetus to come through. In cervical dystocia, the cervix fails to dilate after a certain point.

progress. This could be due to the cervix (mouth of the uterus) not dilating. This condition is called **cervical dystocia.**

Cephalo-pelvic disproportion

When the foetus is too big to fit through your pelvis or if your pelvis is too small for your baby to pass through, it is called **cephalo-pelvic disproportion (CPD).** Cephalopelvic disproportion can cause **a failure of descent** (when the head of the baby is unable to come down the birth canal) or **failure of dilatation** (when the cervix does not dilate).

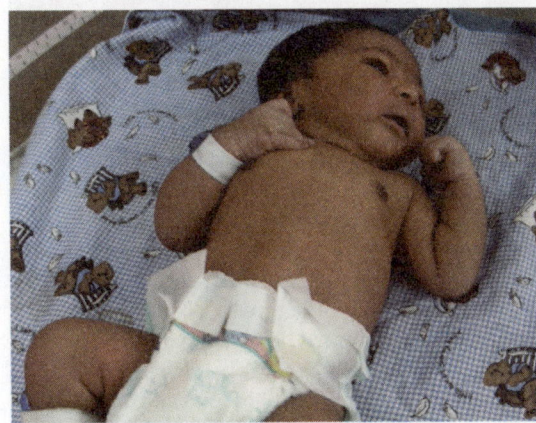

Large baby born by caesarean section

Foetal distress

This can be an unexpected problem leading to a caesarean section. When the foetus shows signs which indicate it is not getting enough oxygen, the foetus is said to be in distress. The two common signs of foetal distress are:

- changes in the baby's heartbeat
- the passage of meconium inside the uterus

Abnormal changes in the baby's heartbeat

The normal heartbeat of the baby is between 110 and 150 beats per minute. If the heartbeat drops to 110 or below, foetal distress is suspected. Occasionally, the lack of oxygen can cause the baby to push up its heartbeat, so a heart rate above 160 can also be a sign of foetal distress.

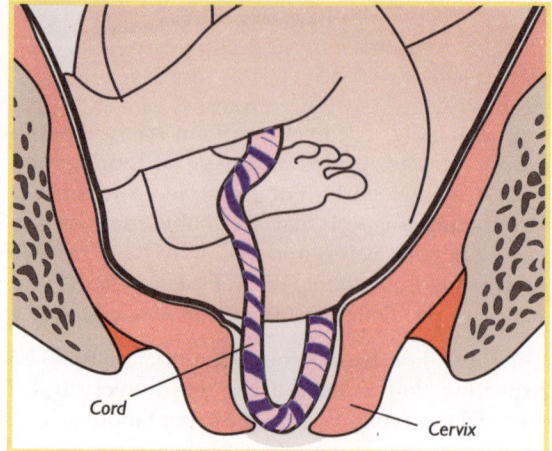

Cord prolapse

A cord prolapse is an emergency situation and can cause problems to the baby if not recognised and treated immediately. Compression of the cord can occur leading to foetal asphyxia i.e. the baby does not get enough oxygen to its brain. It occurs most commonly in the following situations:

- When the fluid around the foetus is abnormally increased (polyhydramnios).
- During delivery of the second baby in a twin pregnancy.
- The foetus is lying crosswise in the uterus (transverse lie).
- The foetus is in the breech position.
- When the membranes rupture spontaneously or when the doctor ruptures the membranes during a vaginal exam before the foetal head has descended into the pelvis.

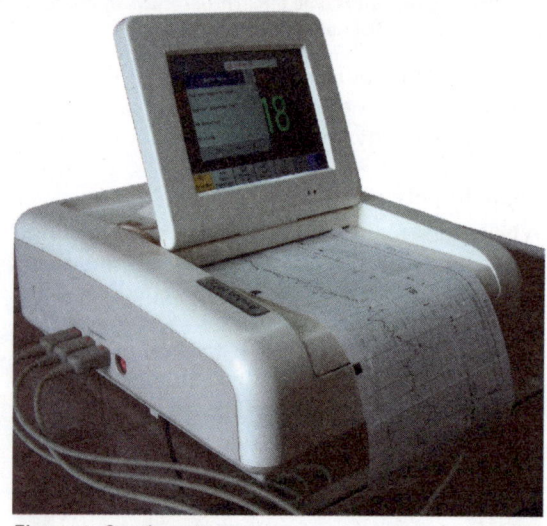

Electronic foetal monitor

Passage of meconium

The baby usually does not pass motion inside the uterus. When the baby's oxygen supply through the placenta and the umbilical cord are compromised, then the baby may pass motion as a reflex. The motion is greenish coloured and can turn the amniotic fluid green. When meconium is seen during labour, the heartbeat of the baby is carefully monitored. Your obstetrician may take a decision to deliver the baby by caesarean.

Cord prolapse

Foetal distress may also occur if the umbilical cord slips out of the cervix ahead of the baby's head. This is a rare occurrence and is called cord prolapse.

Shoulder dystocia

When the baby has broad shoulders, the baby's head will deliver but the shoulders will get caught in the birth canal. This is called **shoulder dystocia.**

As the obstetrician tries to deliver the rest of the baby, the baby may have trouble breathing because the chest is compressed by the birth canal. As a result, oxygen levels in the baby's blood decrease. This complication is more common with large foetuses, particularly those of diabetic mothers.

When this complication occurs, the obstetrician quickly tries various techniques to free the shoulder so that the baby can be delivered vaginally. In extreme circumstances, if the techniques are unsuccessful, the baby may be pushed back into the vagina and delivered by caesarean section.

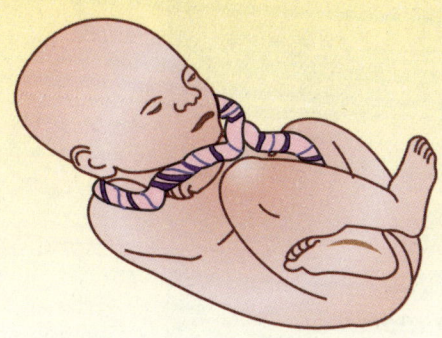

Cord around the neck

Many people are under the impression that the baby will have problems if the cord is wrapped around the baby's neck. **Remember that the umbilical cord is wrapped around the foetus's neck in one out of three deliveries.** Normally this does not harm the baby in any way.

Sometimes, an ultrasound done before the delivery may reveal that the cord is around the neck. **This does not automatically mean that you need a caesarean section.**

There is an old wives' tale that you should not reach above your head with your arms or you should not turn from side to side while lying down because this may cause the cord to wrap around the baby and jeopardise the baby. **This is not true!**

Postpartum haemorrhage

Postpartum haemorrhage is excessive bleeding following the birth of a baby. The average amount of blood loss after the birth of a single baby in vaginal delivery is about 500 ml. The average amount of blood loss during a caesarean section is approximately 1,000 ml. When the blood loss exceeds these amounts, you are considered to be having postpartum haemorrhage. Most postpartum haemorrhage occurs immediately after delivery, but it may occur after a few hours or even days.

Causes of postpartum haemorrhage

Once a baby is delivered, the uterus contracts to compress and control the bleeding from blood vessels. Medications are given to help the uterus contract. Occasionally, in spite of these medications, the uterus will not contract. This is called **uterine atony.** This is the most common cause of postpartum haemorrhage. Sometimes the bleeding occurs if there are pieces of placenta left behind in the uterus or if there are tears in the vaginal area due to the baby passing through.

CHAPTER 23

Caesarean section

Shameem is in her eighth month of pregnancy. Her best friend just had a baby and underwent a caesarean section. Shameem is keen on having a normal vaginal delivery. She wants to know if there is anyway she can ensure that.

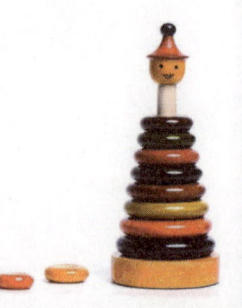

23 Caesarean section

There are various reasons why a caesarean section is done. Sometimes, the foetus will not fare well if put through the stress of a vaginal delivery. Sometimes, the caesarean is done to protect the mother from unnecessary harm.

It is important to know that caesarean section rates may vary from hospital to hospital. One of the ways you can ensure that you have the best chances for a normal, vaginal delivery is to ask for the caesarean section rates for the hospital or obstetrician you are consulting. On an average, 20-25 women out of 100 may undergo a caesarean section. If it is a first pregnancy, you have crossed 37 weeks of pregnancy and the baby is lying in a head down position, you should have a 82-85 per cent chances of a normal, vaginal delivery.

In India, the rate of caesarean section has climbed drastically. Recent articles in medical journals have placed the rate as high as 45 per cent. This is unacceptable. Health care professionals in India have been alarmed by the rising rate of caesarean sections and strategies are being designed to decrease these rates.

What is a caesarean section?

A caesarean section is an abdominal operation performed to deliver a baby when vaginal delivery is not possible or safe. A cut is made through the mother's abdomen and uterus to remove the baby. This procedure is also called a C-section. Caesarean sections can save the lives of newborns and their mothers or prevent the potential complications of a delayed vaginal birth.

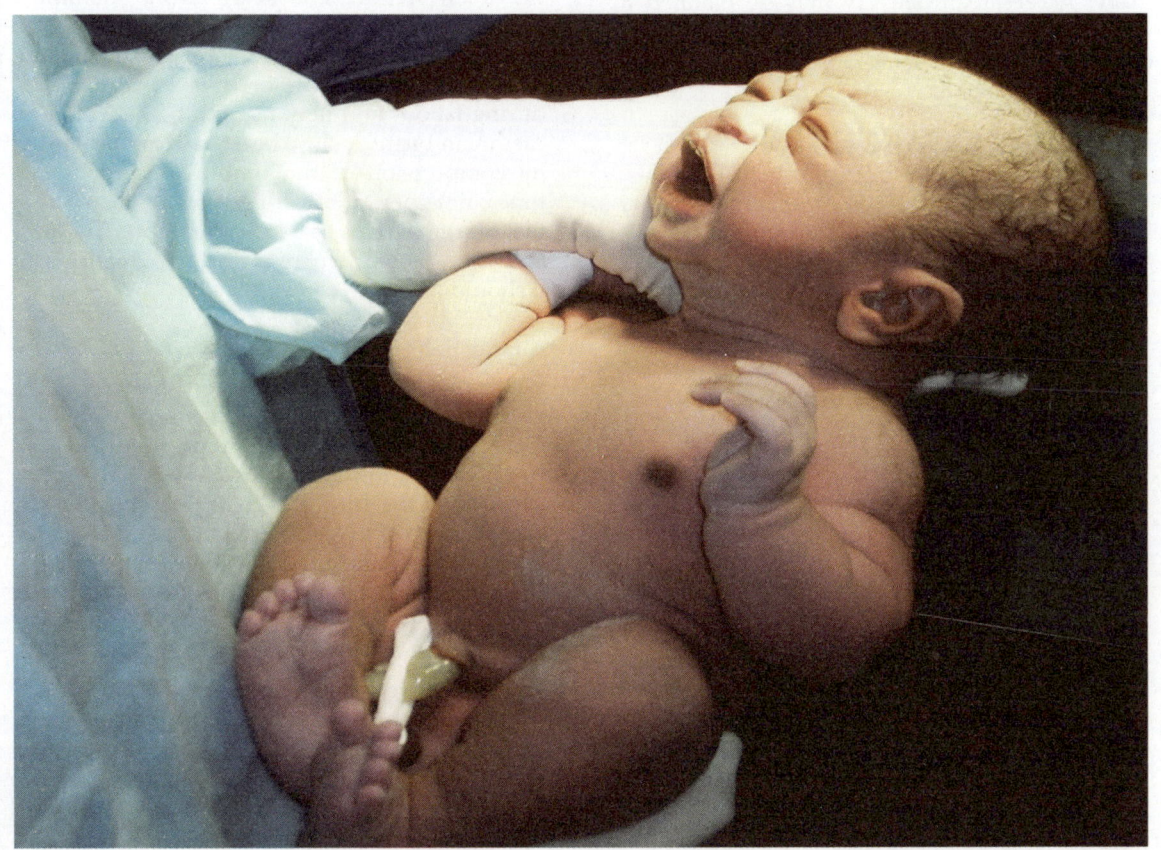

Elective caesarean section

A caesarean section may be performed before labour begins if there are medical reasons for not allowing labour or a vaginal delivery. For example, the health of the mother or the baby may be in jeopardy if the pregnancy continues, or vaginal delivery might be impossible or unsafe. This is called a **planned or elective caesarean section.**

Emergency caesarean section

A caesarean section may be done when labour begins or during labour if certain problems occur, either for the mother or the baby. This is called an emergency caesarean section.

When is a caesarean needed?

There are many reasons why a caesarean section may be opted for to deliver your baby. It may be a good medical decision for both you and your baby. A caesarean delivery may be planned in advance when certain conditions are known. In some cases, if problems arise, the decision is made during labour.

> **Reasons for doing a caesarean**
> - Failure of labour to progress
> - Foetal distress
> - A large baby
> - Breech presentation
> - Problems with the placenta
> - Previous caesarean section
> - Multiple pregnancy
> - Maternal infections

Failure of labour to progress

About one third of caesarean sections are done because labour does not progress normally. In a normal labour, as the pains get more frequent and stronger, the cervix will gradually open till the baby can pass through. In some women, there may be a failure of labour to progress. This means that the cervix does not open normally. If this is because of poor contractions and labour is progressing slowly, the obstetrician can speed up labour with medication. It may take a number of hours to determine whether labour is

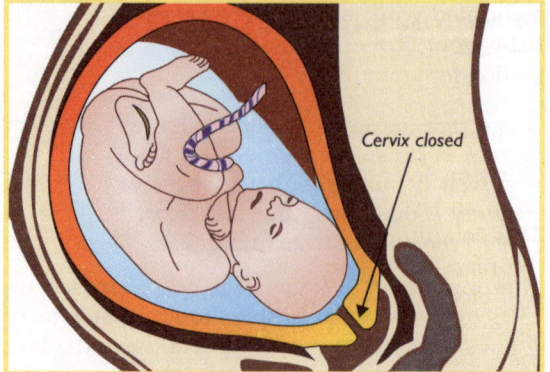

Failure of the cervix to open

progressing well or not. Your obstetrician may watch for several hours before deciding on a caesarean section.

Foetal distress

This is one of the common reasons for a caesarean section. The heart rate is monitored periodically during labour. When there is an abnormal change in the baby's heart rate, it could indicate that the baby is having trouble during labour and may need to be delivered by caesarean birth. A slow heart rate can be caused by compression of the **umbilical cord.** Sometimes, not enough blood flows to the baby from the **placenta.** This is particularly possible in a post-date baby or where the baby is smaller than it should be.

A large baby

When there is a misfit between the size of the baby and the size of the mother's pelvis, it can result in **cephalo-pelvic disproportion (CPD).** In simple terms, this means the baby is too large to fit through the birth passage. Occasionally, the baby may be of average size but the mother may be small built and may not have enough space for the baby to fit through.

Breech presentation

Normally, by 37 weeks, the baby is in a head down position. About 4 per cent of babies will not get into this position. They will come down into the pelvis with their feet or their buttocks presenting first. This position is called **breech.** Because of some complications which are associated with the vaginal delivery of a breech baby, your obstetrician might advise a caesarean section for you.

Problems with the placenta

Occasionally, the placenta is placed below the baby and covers the cervix partly or entirely. This condition is called **placenta praevia.** When the placenta lies in front of the baby's head, it will block the baby's exit from the uterus. It can cause severe bleeding. Another condition that may present as an emergency is **placental abruption.** This happens when the placenta separates before the baby is born and cuts off the oxygen supply to the baby. Placenta praevia and placental abruption can both cause heavy bleeding and may require a caesarean delivery. **(See Chapter 28: Bleeding in pregnancy).**

Previous caesarean section

Having had a caesarean section with a previous pregnancy plays a part in whether you will need to have one again. Many women who have had a caesarean birth before may be able to give birth vaginally. This depends on the reason for which the caesarean was done the first time. If the reason does not exist in this pregnancy, your obstetrician might suggest trying for a vaginal delivery, also known as **vaginal birth after caesarean** or **VBAC.** However, a vaginal delivery after a previous caesarean delivery may not be a good option for a woman when the baby is very large, not in the proper position or there is an interval of less than two years between the previous caesarean and this pregnancy.

> Having a caesarean once does not always mean that you have to have a caesarean again – discuss this with your obstetrician.

Multiple pregnancy

Most women carrying twins can usually have a vaginal delivery. A caesarean delivery may be required if the babies are preterm (being born too early) or if the first twin is not in a head down position. The likelihood of having a caesarean birth increases with the number of babies a woman is carrying.

Maternal infections

Maternal infections such as **human immunodeficiency virus (HIV)** or **herpes** may require a caesarean delivery. The baby can be infected if it comes through the birth canal. To reduce the risk of transmission to the baby, a caesarean delivery is recommended in women who are HIV positive or have an active herpes infection at the time of delivery.

> **Can you request a caesarean delivery?**
> This is a complex decision that should be carefully considered and discussed with your doctor. Remember that a vaginal delivery is probably the best way to have a baby. Having a caesarean does not guarantee that the baby will not have any problems. So, if you are under the impression that a caesarean section will prevent all risks for you or the baby, and are requesting an elective caesarean section based on this, remember that this is not true. Though it is an excellent option when done to save the baby or the mother, like any surgery, a caesarean also carries some risk, albeit small.

Being prepared for a caesarean

When do you need to go to the hospital?

If you have been scheduled for an elective caesarean section, you will normally be asked to get admitted the previous day to the hospital. Sometimes you may be advised to get admitted at least a day or two prior to the caesarean in case you need to be observed and treated for complications of pregnancy. This is particularly true with diabetes or hypertension complicating pregnancy.

What happens after admission?

After admission, the admitting nurse will take you to your room and check your temperature, pulse and blood pressure. She will also record your baby's heartbeat. You will be advised **not to eat or drink for 6-8 hours before the scheduled time of surgery.** This will ensure that you have a smooth surgery and recovery.

Your obstetrician or one of her team will come and see you on admission. The size and position of your baby as well as your baby's heartbeat will be recorded. Your medical record file will be checked. Some blood tests may be done if necessary. A sample of blood will also be drawn so that blood can be reserved for you in case you require blood transfusion during or after the caesarean section. The doctor will also discuss the caesarean section with you. You will be asked to sign a consent form allowing the doctor to proceed with the caesarean section.

The anaesthetist will be informed about your admission and will be told about the time of the caesarean. In most hospitals, a paediatrician will be present at the time of the caesarean section. The same paediatrician will take care of your newborn during your stay in the hospital. You may opt to follow up with him after discharge.

What happens on the day of the caesarean section?

If the doctor has prescribed any medication for the morning of the operation, the nurse will give it to you with a sip of water.

You may be given an enema to empty your bowels. You will also be asked to take a bath with a medicated liquid soap. Avoid using any creams, talcum powder or cosmetics. You will be given a gown to wear and asked to remove all jewellery and leave it with your attendant.

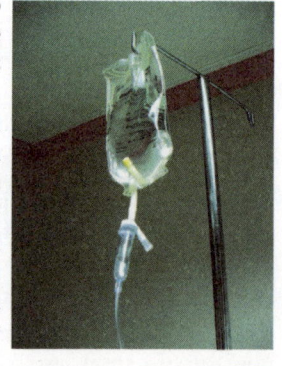

You will be taken to the operating theatre at least 45 minutes before your operation. IV fluids will be started and you will be given some medications. These pre-anaesthetic medications will make you feel a little drowsy and they will ensure smooth anaesthesia and recovery for you.

What happens in the operating room?

You will be asked to lie down on your back on the operating table. You will not have much space to move and turn on this bed, but you will be comfortable. A blood pressure cuff and other devices will be attached to you so that your heartbeat and blood pressure can be monitored throughout the procedure.

A small tube (catheter) will be passed through the passage where you pass urine, to empty your bladder. This tube may be kept in place for 12-24 hours.

What sort of anaesthesia will be given?

You are given a regional (spinal or epidural) or general anaesthetic. A **regional anaesthetic** numbs part of your body, preventing you from feeling pain while you remain awake. A **general anaesthetic** relaxes your muscles, puts you to sleep and also prevents you from feeling pain.

> You may have a choice of spinal, epidural or general anaesthesia for the caesarean section. Discuss this with your obstetrician / anaesthetist.

What happens during the procedure?

The obstetrician makes a cut below your navel and into the lower part of the uterus to deliver the baby. The obstetrician then removes the placenta and membranes and then sews the uterus and abdomen closed.

> Usually, a transverse (side-to-side) incision is made on the skin. This is commonly called a 'bikini cut'. Occasionally a vertical incision is used.

Once the doctors have started your caesarean, your baby is usually born within 2 to 3 minutes. The whole operation will take between 30 to 45 minutes. Your baby will be examined by a paediatrician and will be kept in the nursery for an hour or two, till you are ready to start breastfeeding.

What happens after the procedure?

You may stay in the hospital about 3 to 5 days, depending on your condition.

After you return home, you can gradually resume normal work so that by the end of one month after the operation, you should be able to perform most of your normal housework. You can climb stairs two weeks after the caesarean section.

You will be on a normal diet a day or two after the operation. There are no food restrictions. You

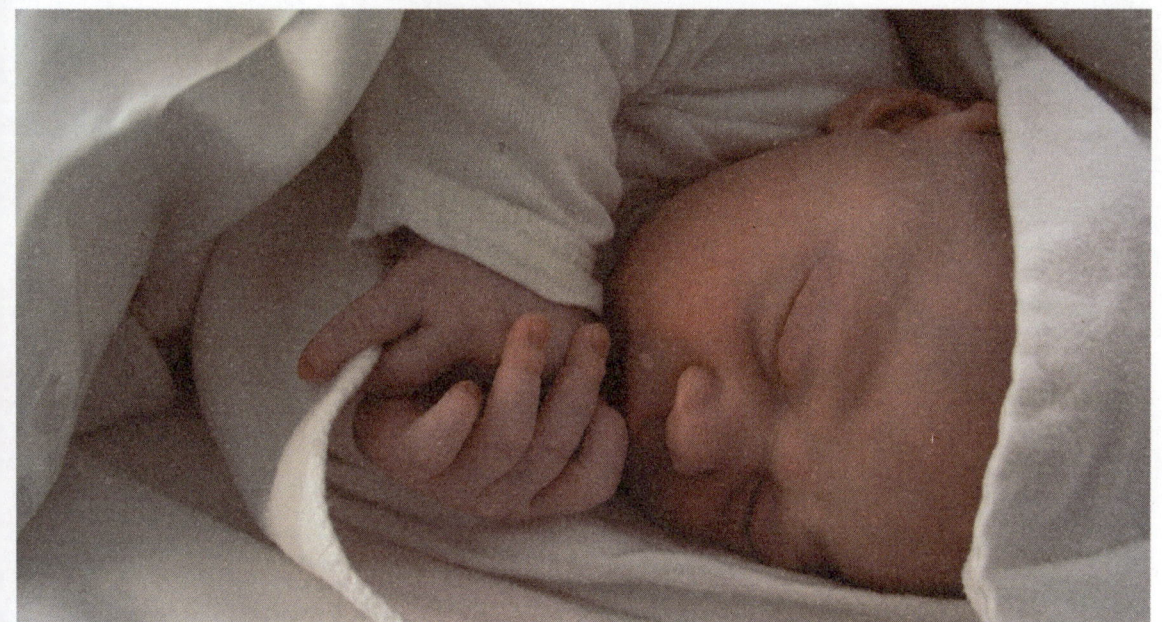

should concentrate on taking a balanced diet with a good amount of proteins. Avoid fat like ghee or butter because they have no dietary benefit and the weight that is gained during pregnancy and immediately afterwards is difficult to shed.

Avoid lifting heavy things for six weeks. Intercourse also should be avoided for at least six weeks.

After 4-6 weeks, you may begin an exercise programme to regain abdominal muscle tone. Join a fitness programme which will help regain your muscle tone, especially of your abdominal muscles. There is no need for an abdominal belt. **(See Chapter 26: Diet and exercise after delivery).**

What are the risks associated with this procedure?

Most caesarean sections are safe. Occasionally, there can be complications which are inherent in any surgery.

- You may have excessive bleeding during or after the caesarean section.
- You may develop an infection
- Rarely, the cut in the wall of the abdomen may leave a weak part in the wall. This may result in an incisional hernia.
- You may still be allowed to have a vaginal delivery with your next pregnancy. However, chances for a repeat caesarean section increase depending on the reason the caesarean was done in the first place.

Old wives' tales

- If you sweep and swab and do heavy physical labour during your pregnancy, you can avoid a caesarean. **Not true!** Just be active; it is important in any pregnancy.
- Eating fish, or 'cold' food like curds (yogurt) and fruit juice can cause pus in the wound. **Not true.** Infections are caused by bacteria, not food.
- You should not lift anything heavy for six months after the caesarean. **Not true.** You can be completely normal in 3-4 weeks and can lift anything heavy six weeks after a caesarean section.

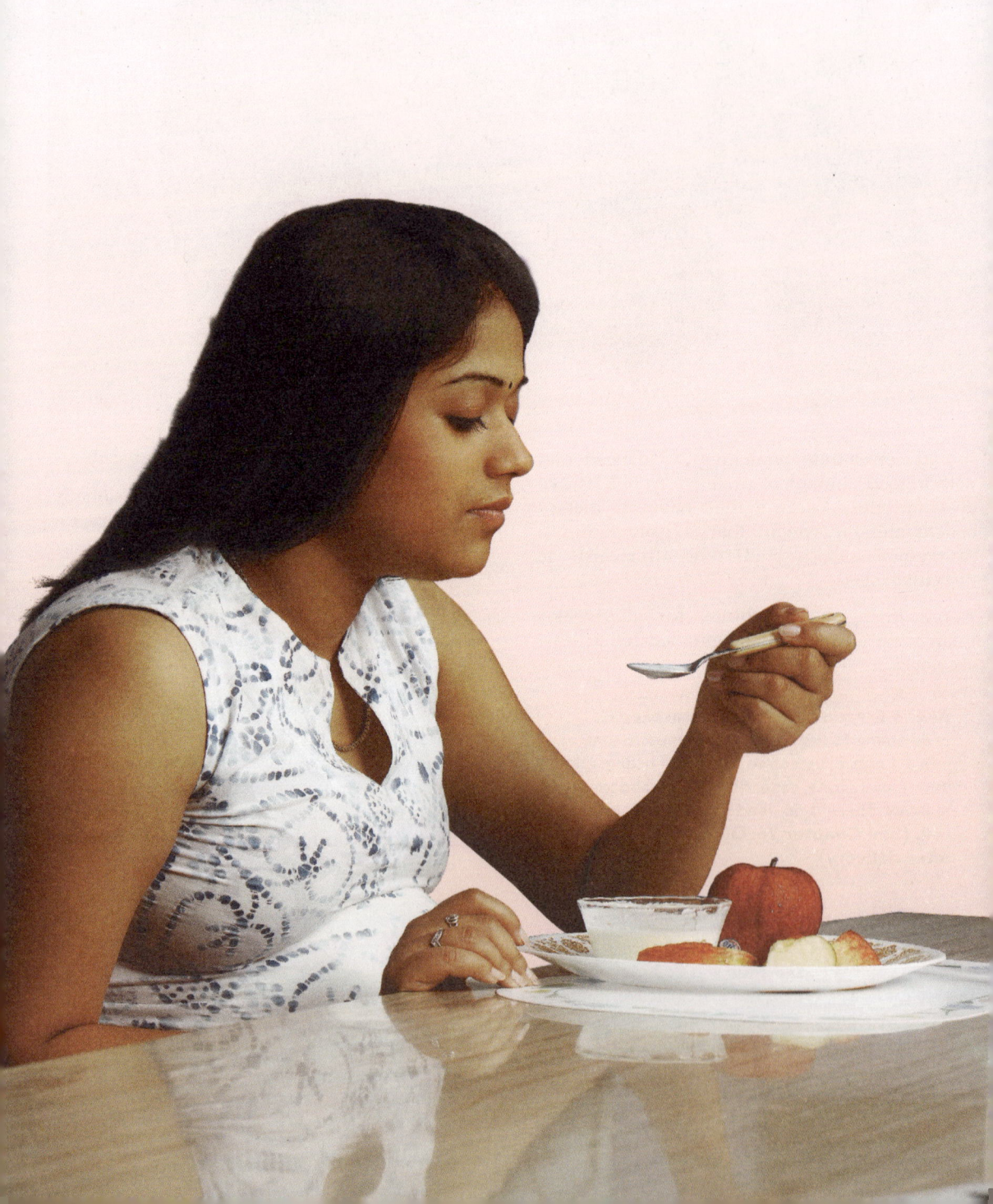

After the delivery

CHAPTER 24

After delivery care

Whether you have had a vaginal delivery or a caesarean section, it is important to regain your health. Taking care of yourself by eating the right food and starting exercises early will go a long way in bringing you back to your pre-pregnancy state.

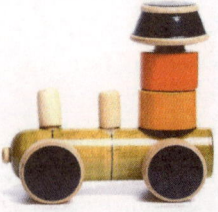

24 After delivery care

After a vaginal delivery

Changes in the uterus

Your uterus was stretched to accommodate your baby during the pregnancy. Now it has to contract and reach its normal size. In the first few days after delivery, you might find a hard round lump in the lower part of your abdomen - this is the uterus which has contracted to half the size it was just before your delivery. The uterus will shrink rapidly in the next few weeks.

You might have some cramping occasionally, especially when you breastfeed. That is why breastfeeding is good for you: it helps the uterus contract.

Bleeding

It is normal to have vaginal bleeding for 2-6 weeks after the delivery. The discharge from the vagina after a delivery is called 'lochia'. The amount of bleeding may vary from day to day. The colour will change from bright red to watery red/pink. After a few weeks, it will change to a yellow/white/clear colour. The type of sanitary napkin you use will depend on the amount of bleeding you have. **You cannot use tampons.**

Heavy bleeding: Occasionally, you might have heavy bleeding after the delivery. If it is immediately after the delivery (while you are in the hospital), it might be due to your uterus not contracting. You might be given medicines to help the uterus contract. If the bleeding becomes heavy after you go home, you can call your obstetrician. You might be prescribed an oral medication which will help the uterus contract.

Bladder and bowel function

Bladder function

For months, the uterus was pushing on the bladder. During delivery too, there would have been pressure on the bladder. This can cause the bladder to lose sensation or become 'numb'. You might not always have the sensation that your bladder is full even though it is. It is important for you to pass urine at least every two to three hours. Drink plenty of fluids.

> **Atonic bladder**
>
> Sometimes, the bladder becomes so 'numb' after the delivery that it might keep filling up without your realising it. After a few hours, your bladder might be overdistended. You might need to have a catheter inserted to empty your bladder. The best way to avoid an atonic bladder is to make sure that you pass urine within six hours after your delivery and then at least every 2-3 hours after that.

Bowel function

You might have your first bowel movement two to three days after your delivery. You might be scared that it will be painful because of the episiotomy. There is nothing to be worried about. Make sure you take food high in fibre and drink plenty of fluids so that your stools are not hard. If needed, your obstetrician may give you a stool softener.

> **Haemorrhoids or 'piles'**
>
> In pregnancy, it is common to develop haemorrhoids. Due to the pushing during delivery, they can become bigger and painful. Make sure that your stools are soft after the delivery. If the haemorrhoids are large and painful, Sitz baths (sitting in a basin of warm water) will help. You can also take stool softeners and use a local anaesthetic ointment. Remember that most haemorrhoids will shrink after a few weeks though you may always continue to have a small, painless swelling near your anus.

Eating healthy after a delivery

In India, there are a lot of misconceptions about the food that can be eaten after a delivery. It is important to remember that there are no dietary restrictions after a delivery. No particular food will prevent the healing of the uterus or the episiotomy.

It is also important to remember that if you put on too much weight after the delivery, you will find it difficult to shed the extra kilos. The excess weight gain after a delivery may lead to lifelong obesity.

Eat foods from the four food groups, especially those with iron (meat, beans, green leafy vegetables, dried fruit), calcium (milk, curds, cheese) and protein. **Avoid all fatty foods especially ghee, butter and deep fried food.**

Drink enough fluids to satisfy your thirst. Continue taking your prenatal vitamins and any iron supplements prescribed by your obstetrician. Discuss weight management with your obstetrician at your postnatal check-up.

> **'After pains'** is the term used to describe the pain that you experience as the uterus shrinks. 'After pains' occur with any delivery but may be mild with a first delivery and can be worse after subsequent deliveries. These cramps can be relieved with a painkiller like ibuprofen. A hot water bag can also be used.

Resuming normal activity

You can start moving around your room in the hospital as soon as you feel up to it. You can walk to the bathroom. You can have a bath the very next day after your delivery. You can wash your hair in a few days and as often as you want after that.

You might feel tired and exhausted after the delivery because you are still not used to the baby's schedule. Rest whenever the baby is sleeping.

Once you are home, you can resume normal activity gradually.

You can climb stairs. One month after the delivery, you should be able to completely resume all your normal activities, including driving your vehicle.

Fluid retention

It is normal to see an increase in the swelling in your legs during the first one or two weeks after delivery. Remember that the body can retain up to 6 litres of water during a pregnancy! After delivery, this might tend to collect in your legs. In a few weeks, this swelling will come down by itself, as your body gets rid of this excess fluid.

Kegel's exercises

Kegel's is a specific type of exercise for the muscles that support the rectum, vagina and the urethra. Strengthening these muscles can help bladder control after a vaginal delivery, and decrease the risk of getting a prolapse.

To learn how to contract the right muscles, try to stop the flow of urine when you are urinating. Do this several times. Once you know how to squeeze the muscles to stop the flow of urine, you know how to contract the right muscles.

You can then start doing these exercises anytime, anywhere, preferably while sitting down. Squeeze the pelvic muscles for 10 seconds and repeat 20-30 times. You can do this 3 times daily. Make sure you empty your bladder before doing the exercises. Check with your obstetrician, if you are not sure how to do them. (Also see pages 161-162).

Handling pain after delivery

Perineal pain

It is common to have pain near the vagina and over the episiotomy. In the first 24 hours after delivery, you may even be given an injectable painkiller if you find the pain unbearable. After that, you should be able to manage with painkillers like ibuprofen.

Sitz baths and infra red lamps can also help in relieving the pain of an episiotomy. **(See Chapter 17: Labour and delivery).**

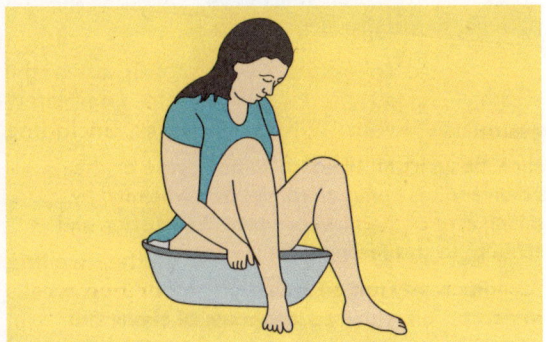

Sitz bath

Sexual intercourse

After a vaginal delivery, it is usually safe to resume intercourse six weeks after birth. By that time, you would have had your postnatal check-up and your obstetrician would have made sure that you have healed well. You may be a little apprehensive about pain the first few times but you will be comfortable soon.

Remember that even if you have not resumed your periods or are breastfeeding, you can still become pregnant. Birth control should be used shortly after birth. Talk to your obstetrician about the safest and most suitable birth control option for you. **(See Chapter 43: Methods of birth control).**

After a caesarean section

Activity after a caesarean section

While you are in the hospital

You will be encouraged to get up and try to go to the bathroom within the first 24 hours after surgery. When you get up for the first time, you may feel a little dizzy. Sit up for a few minutes and then get up from bed only after the dizziness has passed.

Urinating after the catheter is removed can sometimes be uncomfortable - the nurse attending on you will help you.

You may need help in changing your sanitary pads soon after the surgery because of the incision pain. After 1 or 2 days, you will be able to manage by yourself.

Soon you will be able to stroll in your room and in the hospital corridor. Walking helps in relieving the gas pain that you may experience.

After you get home

Your activity level should be gradually increased. In the first week after you get home, you can walk around the room and take care of your baby. Over the next week, you can start walking around the house. In the third week, you can start resuming small domestic chores, like cutting vegetables and making coffee or tea. A month after you are home, you can resume your normal work, including cooking and washing. You can start climbing up and down stairs two weeks after your surgery.

It is important not to lift very heavy objects till six weeks after the surgery.

Care of the incision

The incision should be kept clean and dry. You may wash the incision with soap and water after the dressing is removed. It is recommended that you wear cotton underwear and no tight fitting clothing. The incision itself will heal in a few days, but it takes 6-8 weeks for the complete healing of all the layers of the abdomen and uterus that were cut.

Bathing

You can bathe every day. Let the water run over the suture line. You can gently apply soap over the wound. There is no need to apply any lotion or cream over the wound. You can wash your hair once a week.

Sexual intercourse

After a caesarean section, it is usually safe to resume intercourse six weeks after birth. By that time, you would have had your postnatal check-up and your obstetrician would have made sure that you have healed well. You may be a little apprehensive about pain the first few times but you will be comfortable soon.

Remember that even if you have not resumed menstruating or are breastfeeding, you can still become pregnant. Birth control should be used shortly after birth. Talk to your obstetrician about the safest and most suitable birth control option for you.

Exercise

After 4 to 6 weeks, you may begin an exercise programme which will help you regain your pre-pregnancy figure. Join a fitness programme which will help you get back your muscle tone, especially of the abdominal muscles.

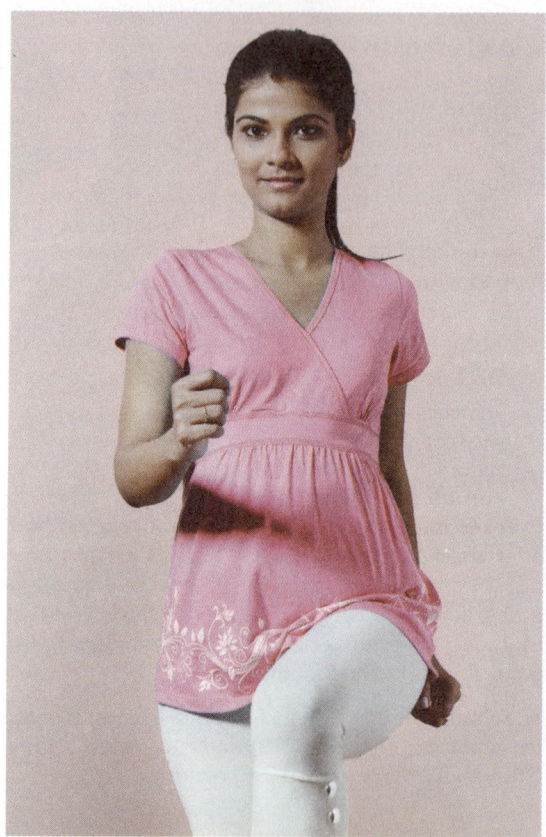

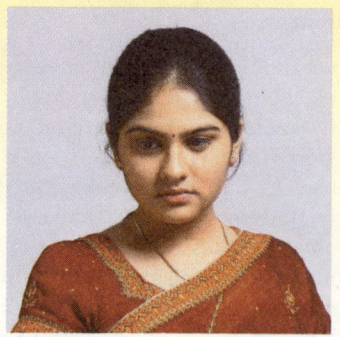

Post-partum depression

Most women experience 'postpartum blues' to some degree or the other. Soon after the delivery it is common to feel overwhelmed by the responsibility of taking care of the newborn baby. Exhaustion and sleeplessness can contribute to this feeling of helplessness.

In some women, this condition may not be temporary. It can progress to severe post-partum depression with frequent bouts of crying and irritability, no desire to see or touch the child and uncontrollable anger. This period could last from a few days to a few months. This is the time for strong family support and understanding. In severe cases, professional counselling may be required.

Reasons to call your doctor

- You should not have a fever after you get home. If you have a fever of more than 100°F (38°C), for more than 24 hours, you should call your doctor
- Sudden onset of pain in the abdominal area, accompanied by tenderness
- Foul smelling vaginal discharge
- Sudden onset of pain over the incision area along with redness and discharge of pus. This might be a sign of infection in the wound
- Burning urination or blood in the urine which may indicate a urinary infection
- Extremely heavy bleeding that soaks a maxi pad within an hour or the passage of large clots
- A sore, red, painful area on the breast that may be accompanied by fever. This might be the beginning of a breast abscess
- Feeling anxious, panicky, and/or depressed may be a sign of 'postpartum blues'. This is common and you might feel down for a while. If this feeling persists and worsens and you are unable to cope, you might require professional help
- A swollen, red, painful area in the leg might be indicative of a rare condition where there is a blood clot in the veins of the leg
- Severe headache that begins right after birth and does not let up in intensity. This is rare but might be an indication of a blood clot in the brain

Do I need to wear an abdominal belt after delivery?

Immediately after the delivery, the abdominal muscles are flabby and without any tone. Most women are very concerned that they will never regain their muscle tone. Somebody might advise you to bind your abdomen tightly with a piece of cloth or to buy an expensive abdominal belt. **These methods are completely worthless.** The only way you can regain the tone of your abdominal muscles is by exercising. **(See Chapter 26: Diet and exercise after delivery).** Regular abdominal exercises can be started 4 weeks after a vaginal delivery and 6 weeks after a caesarean section.

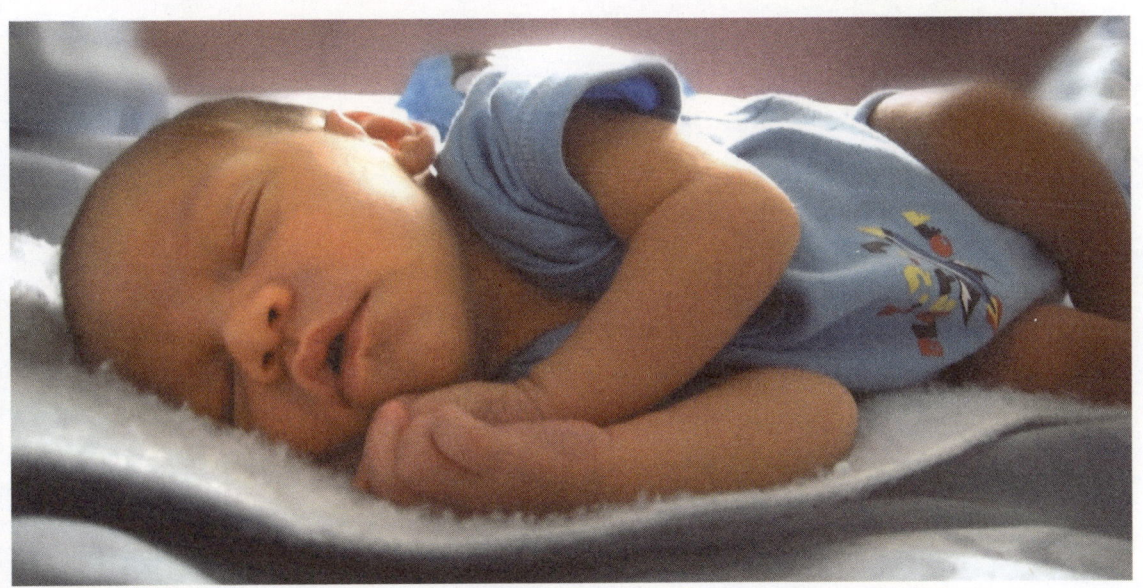

CHAPTER 25

Breastfeeding

Stella is in the final weeks of her pregnancy. She is very keen on breastfeeding her baby because she knows that mother's milk is the best for the baby. She wants to do whatever is necessary to make sure that her baby gets enough milk from her.

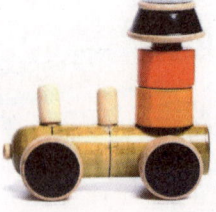

25 Breastfeeding

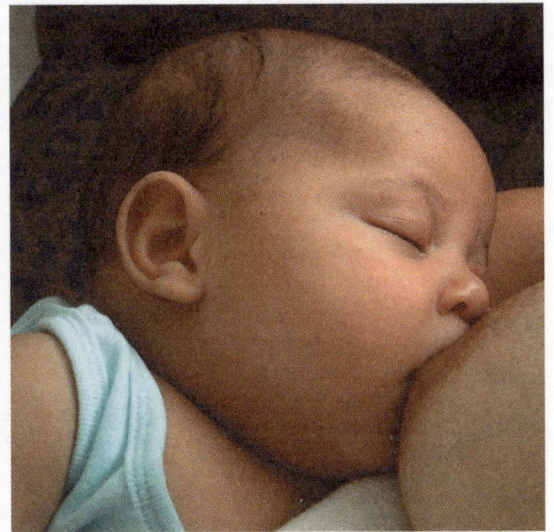

One of nature's miracles is the ability of a woman to sustain her baby with her breast milk. There is no question that babies who are breast-fed have fewer infections and allergies during the first year of life than babies given milk supplements. Breast milk is specially made for the new born and contains the correct proportion of nutrients. It also contains important antibodies which protect the baby before it develops immunity to infections.

Unfortunately, most mothers are so anxious when they start breastfeeding that it will seem as if everything is going wrong. The baby keeps crying, does not seem to latch on and does not seem to be getting enough milk. Sometimes, overzealous relatives try to convince the mother that she does not have enough milk and should give milk supplements. Remember that most mothers, even those who have had a caesarean section, will be able to feed their babies. All it requires is patience and perseverance.

Breastfeeding the baby up to a year after birth provides the baby with good nutrition. If you are a working woman, and have to get back to work, try to feed the baby for as many months as possible.

Why early breastfeeding?

Nursing as soon as possible after birth has advantages for a mother who has had a caesarean section just as it does for a mother who has delivered vaginally. Early breastfeeding

- promotes bonding
- provides stimulation to help the milk start flowing sooner
- releases the hormone oxytocin to help the uterus contract
- provides the baby with the immunological advantages of **colostrum** (the thin colourless fluid which is secreted in the first few days, before the actual milk starts flowing)

Should you be giving anything other than breast milk?

It is absolutely important to give only breast milk to the baby. Do not give sugar solutions or commercially available milk supplements unless there is an overwhelming reason and your paediatrician advises you to do that.

Will you have enough milk?

Do not let anybody persuade you to give milk supplements "because you may not have enough milk." People might make you feel guilty that you are "starving" the baby. Don't worry. All mothers will be able to produce enough milk for their babies. In a few weeks, you will know that you have enough milk because the baby will start gaining weight.

When does the milk start flowing?

For the first three days, you will produce only a thin, watery secretion which is called **colostrum**. The baby needs this because it is rich in antibodies and protects the baby against infection. Milk will start flowing on the third or fourth day after the baby is born.

Once lactation is established, you may find that the milk may leak from your breasts even if you hear the baby cry. This is Nature's way of making sure your baby has milk when it needs it.

How often should you feed?

When you first start breastfeeding, you can start feeding every one and half to two hours. As the milk starts flowing, you should continue to keep this interval. This way the baby will get hungry and suckle better. Some people recommend 'demand feeding' which means you feed the baby whenever she cries. This might be exhausting and feeding the baby at regular intervals might be easier. In a few weeks, the baby will settle into a pattern. At nights, you can wait without giving a feed for up to 3-4 hours, if the baby is sleeping.

How long should you feed?

In the beginning, you might find that the baby may feed for only 5 to 10 minutes at each breast. Within a few days, the baby will start suckling for 15 to 20 minutes at each breast. The more the baby suckles, the more the milk will flow. You can tell your baby has finished on a breast when the suckling slows down and the breast becomes soft. Then, offer the second breast to your baby. Change the breast you start with each time you nurse.

What if your milk flow does not get established?

Occasionally, a mother might find that she has difficulty in establishing milk flow. You might be prescribed drugs called galactagogues, which stimulate your brain to produce **prolactin,** which is the hormone which helps you produce milk. Two of the commonly used galactagogues are domperidone and metoclopramide. These medicines must be taken only with a prescription from your doctor.

> **Releasing the breast from the baby's mouth**
> Do not pull the baby's mouth off the nipple. The suction from the baby's mouth will cause the nipple to become sore. Insert your little finger gently between the baby's gums, release the suction and then move your baby away from the breast. Doing this will help prevent sore nipples and cracks.

Does the food you eat affect the baby?

New mothers are often worried that the food they eat may affect the baby by passing through the milk. You need not worry. Make sure you eat a balanced diet. What you eat will not affect the baby but a healthy diet can improve the quality of milk.

Do the medications you are given affect the baby?

Many mothers are worried that the medications prescribed for them after delivery will adversely affect their babies. The medications used for pain relief are usually not a problem, and are routinely given to the mothers of newborns. If an antibiotic has been given at the time of the caesarean section, it too will not affect the baby. Although these medications do pass into the milk in very small amounts, the volume of colostrum or milk produced during the first few days of nursing is small, so the amount ingested by the baby is minimal.

Breast feeding after a caesarean section

Having had a caesarean will not have an adverse effect on breastfeeding. Even the initiation of breastfeeding need not be delayed. Though there will be some discomfort because of the pain of the stitches, you will be encouraged to start breastfeeding as soon as possible.

As soon as you are fully conscious and alert and able to hold the baby, you can begin breastfeeding. Mothers who have epidural or spinal rather than general anaesthesia will generally be able to hold the baby sooner and nurse her. Ensure that the baby is brought to you as soon as you are awake enough to be able to hold the baby. You will, of course, need assistance for the first few times. The earlier that you start breastfeeding, the sooner you will master the art of holding and satisfying your baby.

Having the baby's father or another person staying with you in the hospital room can be a great help in lifting the baby, changing position, changing diapers, and so forth. You can be up and about soon after the caesarean, but for the first few days your ability to move around is restricted. Having a person in your room to assist you can help establish breastfeeding early.

Positions for breastfeeding

It might a little difficult to find a completely comfortable position for breastfeeding after a caesarean section. The nursing staff can be a great help in lifting and positioning the baby initially, so that there is no pressure on the incision.

The movements of one of the arms may be restricted due to the placement of the IV fluids. Usually, the IV fluids will be removed after the first 24-48 hours and you will then find it easier to hold and manipulate your baby.

The side lying position

This position is the most preferred in the first few days after surgery. You should turn slowly on your side, and put a rolled up towel next to the incision in case the baby kicks. The baby should be placed on her side, facing your body.

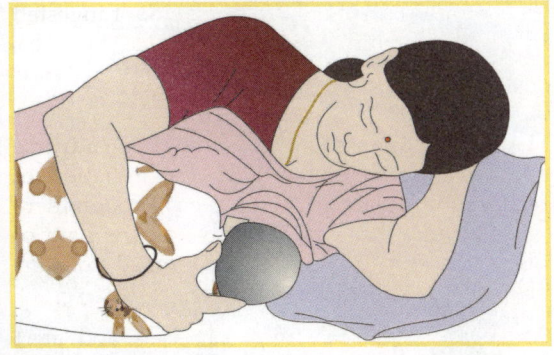

She should always be directly facing the breast so that she won't have to turn her head to nurse. A rolled up towel placed behind the baby can help keep her from pulling off the breast as she relaxes during the feeding.

Cradle hold

If the cradle hold is used, the baby can rest on a pillow. This is particularly useful after a caesarean section because the pillow will cover the tender incision. Many mothers find the cradle hold more comfortable after the first few days of recovery from surgery, but not in the very beginning.

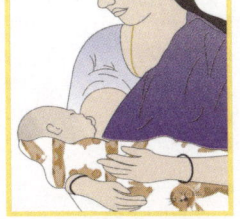

Breastfeeding: "latching on"

Latching on

It is important to make sure the baby is latched on correctly. Making sure that the baby opens its mouth wide and latches on well behind the nipple and not just on the tip can help avoid nipple soreness and facilitate effective milk transfer.

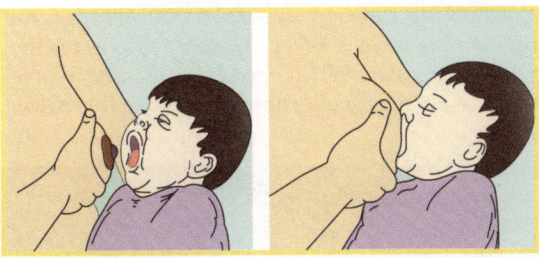

Support your breast with 4 fingers below and the thumb above. Place your fingers far enough behind the areola (the dark area surrounding the nipple) so that the baby will have enough place to hold on to.

Once your baby opens her mouth wide, pull her quickly towards your breast and make sure that she grasps not just the nipple but most of the areola too. Her tongue should be well applied to the under surface of the nipple.

Problems during breastfeeding

Breast engorgement

It is common to have your breasts become heavy, hard and painful, especially soon after delivery. This is called **engorgement** and happens because the baby has not suckled adequately and the milk is distending the breast. Hot fomentation or ice packs are both effective in relieving the pain. You might also get relief by feeding the baby often. A mild painkiller like ibuprofen will help.

Nipple pain and cracks

In the beginning, since the nipples are still soft, there may be a certain amount of discomfort when the baby starts suckling. If the baby's mouth is positioned properly, there should be no pain. If the baby does not latch on properly, the nipples can be very painful during feeds and can develop cracks. Nipple creams and a nipple shield can be used for temporary relief but learning the proper method of latching on is the best treatment.

Breast abscess

Occasionally, bacteria from the baby's mouth can enter the breast and cause an infection. The breast can become painful and there may be a hard, red patch. In the early stages, this is called **mastitis**. You might develop severe tenderness of the breast and have a fever. Mastitis might resolve with antibiotics. When the infection gets worse, there may be a collection of pus in the breast called a **breast abscess**. The only treatment would be to remove the pus either by aspiration through a needle or by a surgical incision.

Breast care

Clean your nipples with water only. Make sure the nipple is completely dry before putting the bra on again. Wear a supportive bra. Apply a nipple cream if soreness, cracking or redness develops. Change breastfeeding positions to lessen soreness. Avoid deodorants and perfumes for a while.

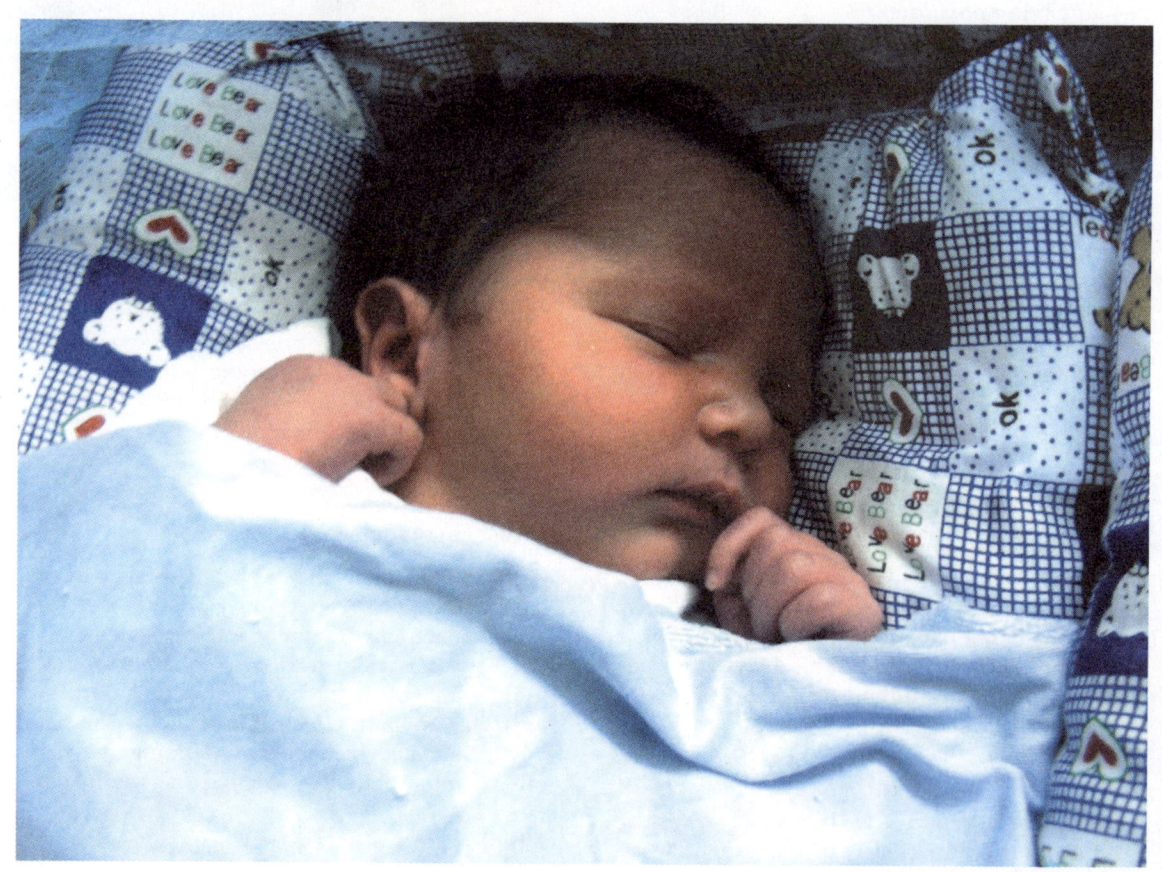

Why breast milk is the best milk

The ideal nutrients

Breast milk is rich in the nutrients that are essential for brain growth and nervous system development. Breastfed babies perform better on different kinds of intelligence tests as they grow older. They also develop better eye function. Certain fatty acid chains present only in human milk and which are not available in artificial formulas, are responsible for this.

Bio-availability of nutrients

It is not enough for the nutrients to be present in the milk: they should be present in the right quantity and the right form so that the baby can use them. This is called bio-availability. The bio-availability of nutrients in human milk is perfect for human babies.

Easy digestion

It makes sense that human milk is the most easily digested food for human babies. Because breast milk is easily broken down in the baby's delicate digestive system, the baby is able to get all the components in the milk which are important for its growth and development.

Help in boosting immunity against infections

Human milk is rich in antibodies and immunity-boosting factors. This helps the baby's ability to resist mild to severe infections. Babies, who are exclusively or almost exclusively breastfed, have significantly fewer gastrointestinal, respiratory, ear, and urinary infections. Antibodies in human milk directly protect against infection. Breast milk also appears to have properties that help boost a baby's own immune system. If the baby does develop an infection, then it will be milder if the baby has been breastfed.

Giving milk substitutes

Breastfeeding is no doubt the best option for babies. Unfortunately, in certain circumstances, the mother may not be able to feed the baby.

Cow's milk is not easily digested by babies so is not recommended. Commercially available milk formulas are manufactured under sterile conditions. They try to reproduce mother's milk using a complex combination of proteins, sugars, fats, and vitamins. The disadvantage of milk substitutes is that they do not contain the antibodies and immunity boosting properties of breast milk. They are also very expensive.

Sterilising bottles and rubber nipples

Bottles and nipples need to be sterilised before the first use and then washed and sterilised again before every use. Bottles and nipples can transmit bacteria if they are not cleaned and sterilised properly.

Any milk that a baby does not finish must be thrown out. Bottles left out of the refrigerator longer than 1 hour should not be used.

Present day milk powders do not require very hot water for mixing. After pouring warm water into the bottle, add the milk powder and then shake the bottle. Do not mix the formula in a separate tumbler and then pour it into the bottle. This can lead to infection.

CHAPTER 26

Diet and exercise after delivery

Shonal just had a baby. Her family is asking her to eat a lot because she is breastfeeding. Is this necessary? She is concerned about putting on weight. She also wants to regain her pre-pregnancy figure.

If Shonal eats a balanced, healthy diet and follows a strict exercise regimen, she can be fit and not put on unwanted weight.

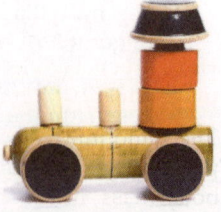

26 Diet and exercise after delivery

Diet

So you have had your baby! Suddenly, all the necessary and unnecessary advice you got throughout your pregnancy from friends and relatives seems to have doubled. When you reach out for that piece of mango, your mother-in-law is horrified. "You can't eat that", she says, pulling the fruit away. "You have just delivered!" Your mother wants you to have a tablespoon of ghee with each meal. An aunt who has come to see the baby checks with your mother if you are getting a special mix of dried fruits and nuts.

Who should you listen to? Having just delivered, do you really need to have a special diet? Can you eat normal food or does everything have to be specially prepared for you? If you have had a caesarean section, will certain kinds of food affect the wound?

Indian culture places a great deal of misplaced importance on food and its effects on a woman who has just delivered. Common sense should dictate what you eat after a delivery.

A balanced diet with plenty of fruits and vegetables is important for you.

After the delivery, you will find that you have lost more than half of what you had put on during pregnancy. You still have to lose a few kilos to regain your pre-pregnancy weight.

It is important to eat a balanced diet and at the same time, lose the excess fat that you have accumulated during the pregnancy.

> Obesity in women starts very often in pregnancy. If you don't lose all the excess weight after the delivery, you will put on even more in a subsequent pregnancy. This additional weight tends to accumulate each year.

How much weight should you have gained in pregnancy?

The amount of weight you should gain in pregnancy depends on your pre-pregnancy body-mass index (BMI). BMI is calculated as your weight in kilos divided by your height in metres^2.

If you have gained the ideal amount of weight in pregnancy, then you will find it easier to reach your pre-pregnancy weight. If you have gained more than you should have, then you will have to work harder to shed that weight.

BMI before pregnancy	Ideal weight gain in pregnancy
Less than 18 (underweight)	12-14 kilos
18-25 (normal weight)	10-12 kilos
25.1–29.9 (overweight)	8-10 kilos
30 or more (obese)	6-8 kilos

A balanced diet after delivery

You do not have to eat large quantities because you are breast feeding. It is important to eat a balanced diet. There are no foods that will affect the baby.

There are no foods that you should not eat after the delivery. There are many old wives' tales that restrict what a woman can eat after the birth of a baby but these have no scientific basis.

Dairy products

When you are breastfeeding, you should drink two glasses of milk and have two cups of curds (yogurt) a day. If you have gained too much weight in pregnancy, you can drink low fat or skim milk. Even the curds can be made from low fat or skim milk.

Dairy products are an excellent source of protein and calcium. Cheese and paneer are good

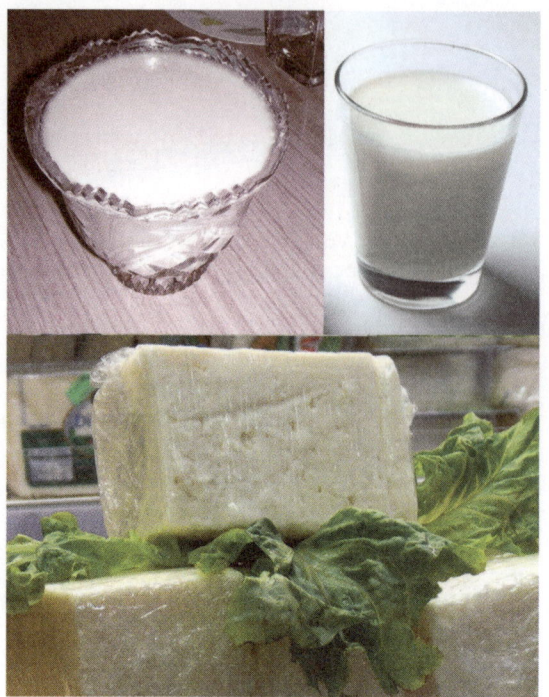

Carbohydrates

Carbohydrates provide you with energy. When taken in larger quantities, you will only get empty calories. You need not increase the quantity of rice that you normally take. Substitute chapathis for rice at one meal, if you are not shedding enough weight.

Vegetables and fruits

Vegetables provide vitamins, minerals and roughage. Try to include 3 to 4 servings per day. A salad with fresh vegetables is highly recommended. About 2 to 3 servings of fruit should be included daily. The old wives' tale of not eating papaya, pineapple and mangoes after a delivery has no basis in science.

Greens prevent constipation and therefore, reduce the chance of bleeding from haemorrhoids (piles) which may have developed during the pregnancy.

A rainbow of vegetables and fruits on your plate provides excellent nutrition!

sources of milk protein. Avoid ice-creams because remember, you may love fat-containing foods, but unfortunately, they love you back!

Protein

Proteins are the building blocks for the baby. Make sure your diet includes dairy products, grains, nuts, pulses, eggs, meat, fish or poultry.

Avoid deep fried food.

Vitamins and minerals

Many women of childbearing age have low iron stores. It is important to be on a combination supplement of iron, B-complex and folic acid for a few months after a delivery. Calcium requirements double during pregnancy and lactation. A mother's body adapts to absorb more calcium from the foods eaten and so keep up your intake of dairy products.

Old wives' tales:
- Eat plenty of ghee. It will help the uterus heal. **Not true!** You will only put on unnecessary weight. Ghee is very unhealthy since it is a saturated fat.
- Avoid spicy food and hot or cold drinks because it will harm the baby. **Not true!**
- Eat lots of garlic, it will increase milk flow. **Not true!** Garlic by itself does not increase the flow of milk. It makes the milk smell which may tend to make the baby suckle more.
- Ajwain water is good for you. **Not true!**
- Avoid certain kinds of lentils, root vegetables and certain fruits. **Not true!** There is no food that you should specifically avoid. If you find that the baby gets colicky after you eat a particular food, then you can avoid it.

Exercise

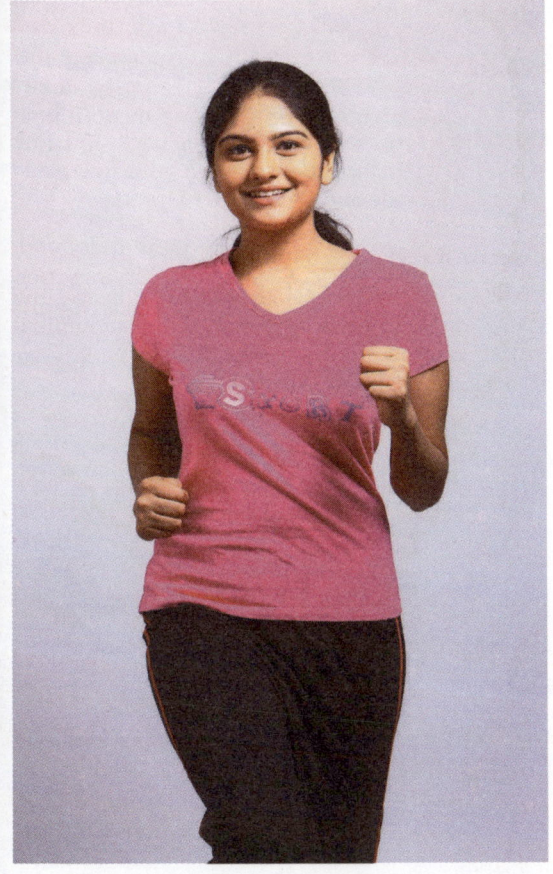

Postnatal exercises are as important as antenatal exercises. To begin with, you can start slowly but within a month after a vaginal delivery, you should be able to push up your activity level comfortably.

If you have had a caesarean section, it would be normally recommended that you start light exercises a month after the surgery. Six weeks after the surgery, you should be able to start postnatal exercises, after having obtained a clearance from your obstetrician.

In the beginning, you can restrict the duration of the exercise to 15 minutes but slowly can work your way up to 30 to 45 minutes a day.

Remember that walking is a great form of exercise and should be resumed when you are comfortable and pain free.

Tips for healthy exercising

- Exercise twice a day
- Repeat each set of movements about ten times in every session
- Remember to keep your breathing slow and smooth
- Work up your stamina gradually
- Try and take a few classes with a physical trainer or watch a video and learn the exercises

Why do postnatal exercises?

Postnatal exercises have many benefits. They help in:

- Strengthening the pelvic floor muscles which prevent leaking of urine
- Preventing lower back pain
- Restoring your body to a healthy shape - that flabby abdominal wall has to be worked on!
- Boosting energy levels

When should I start postnatal exercise after delivery?

Remember that after a vaginal delivery, there is no reason that you cannot start walking around the house in a day or two. After a month, you can start a good fitness regimen.

After a caesarean, you can gradually increase your activity. After six weeks, you can start an exercise regimen after getting a clearance from your obstetrician.

A sampler of exercises

Pelvic floor (Kegel's) exercises

Kegel's exercises are specifically focussed on the pelvic floor muscles which support the uterus, bladder and bowel. They are useful both for prevention and treatment. By keeping the pelvic floor muscles toned, the risk of urinary leakage with aging can be reduced. Kegel's exercises can also help control urinary leakage.

Kegel's exercises are recommended both during pregnancy and after delivery. Well-toned pelvic floor muscles make it less likely to develop prolapse of the uterus.

To learn how to identify and contract the pelvic floor muscles, the best method is to try and stop the flow of urine as you are urinating. You may not succeed initially, but with practice, the basic move can be mastered. Stopping and starting the urine stream should only be used initially to learn the technique, and should not be done all the time - it may lead to bladder dysfunction. Another technique is to insert two fingers inside the vagina and to attempt to squeeze the surrounding muscles. The vagina can be felt to tighten around the fingers and the pelvic floor will be felt to move upward. When the muscles are relaxed, the pelvic floor can be felt moving down to the starting position.

Once the pelvic floor muscles have been identified, the exercise can be done in a sitting or standing position. The exercises can be done while watching television, working on the computer or whenever there is some free time. The exercises should be done three times a day. The bladder should be emptied. The pelvic muscles should be contracted for 10 seconds and then relaxed for 10 seconds. This sequence should be repeated a total of 20-30 times at each session. Care should be taken not to contract the muscles in the abdomen, thighs or buttocks. Breathe freely while doing the pelvic floor exercises.

Back and abdominal exercises

Hold each position for 10-20 seconds. Repeat each set at least 10 times. Use an exercise mat for greater comfort.

Exercise 1

Lie on your back and bend your knees with your feet slightly apart. Breathe out and tighten your abdomen. Press your pelvis downwards to flatten your low back against the floor.

Exercise 2

Lie on your back. Bend your knees and keep them together. Tighten your abdomen and flatten your low back against the floor. Bring both knees to the right side so as to let your right knee touch the floor as far as possible. Return to the starting position and rest. Repeat on the left side.

Exercise 3

Lie on your back and bend your knees. Tighten the muscles of your hips, upper back and low back. Lift your hips to straighten your low back. Hold for a while and lower your hips slowly.

Exercise 4 - cat stretch

Kneel on all fours, keeping both hands and the knees on the floor. Tighten your abdominal muscle and round your back. Then flatten your back slowly.

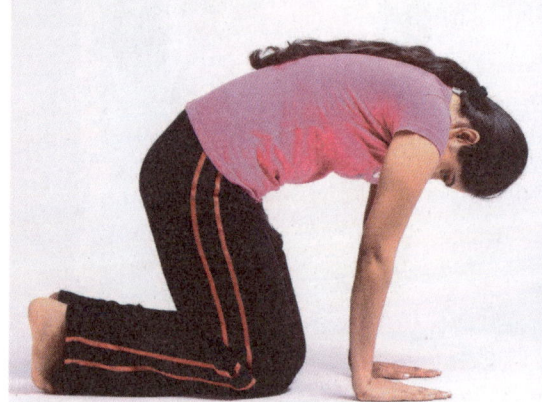

Cat stretch position 1

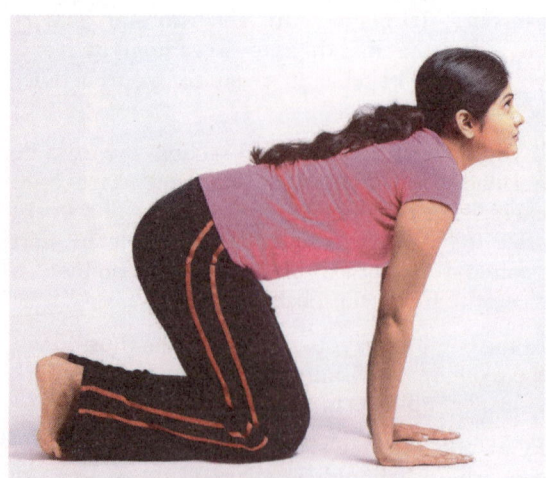

Cat stretch position 2

Exercise 5

Lie on your back and bend your knees, keeping your feet together. Tighten your abdomen, and press your pelvis downwards to flatten your low back against the floor. Lift your head and shoulders just off the floor with both hands touching the knees, hold for a while, and lie down slowly.

Exercise 6 - abdominal crunch

Lie down with hands crossed over the chest or behind the head and feet on the floor, knees bent. Contract the abs and lift the head and shoulders off the floor, bringing the rib cage towards the lower belly. Lower slowly back to start and repeat.

Exercise 7 - oblique crossover crunches

Lie on your back and cross the left foot over the right knee. Place your right hand under your head. Lift the shoulder blades off the floor and twist to the left, bringing the right shoulder and elbow towards the left knee. Lower back down and repeat for all reps before switching sides.

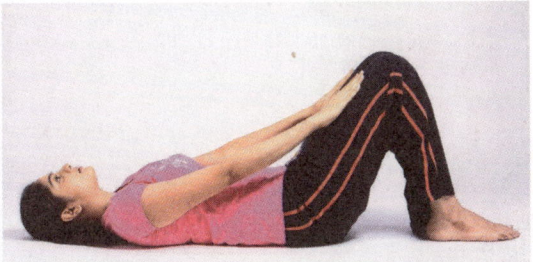

Exercise 5 Position 1

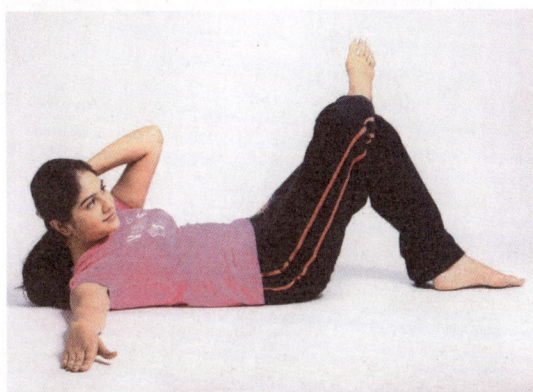

Oblique crossover crunch

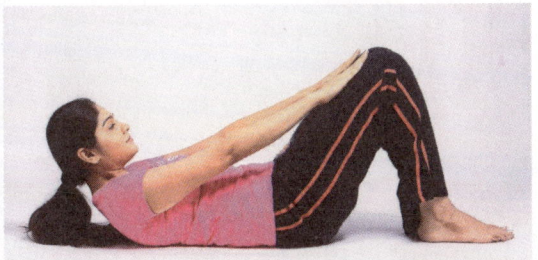

Exercise 5 Position 2

These are just a few suggestions for exercising your abdominal muscles. You need to have determination and discipline to regain your pre-pregnancy shape. Exercise will help you keep fit and boost your energy levels.

Towards a flat abdomen

The disadvantage of Indian clothes is that they hide many body flaws! Do not hide behind loose clothes after the delivery. Always be aware of your abdominal muscles. Make it a point to keep pulling in your tummy muscles. Walk with a good posture, with your shoulders pulled back and your tummy tucked in. Encourage the return of a flatter abdomen by pulling in your deep abdominal muscles whenever you think about them, when walking, when cooking, when driving, when working and even when you feed your baby.

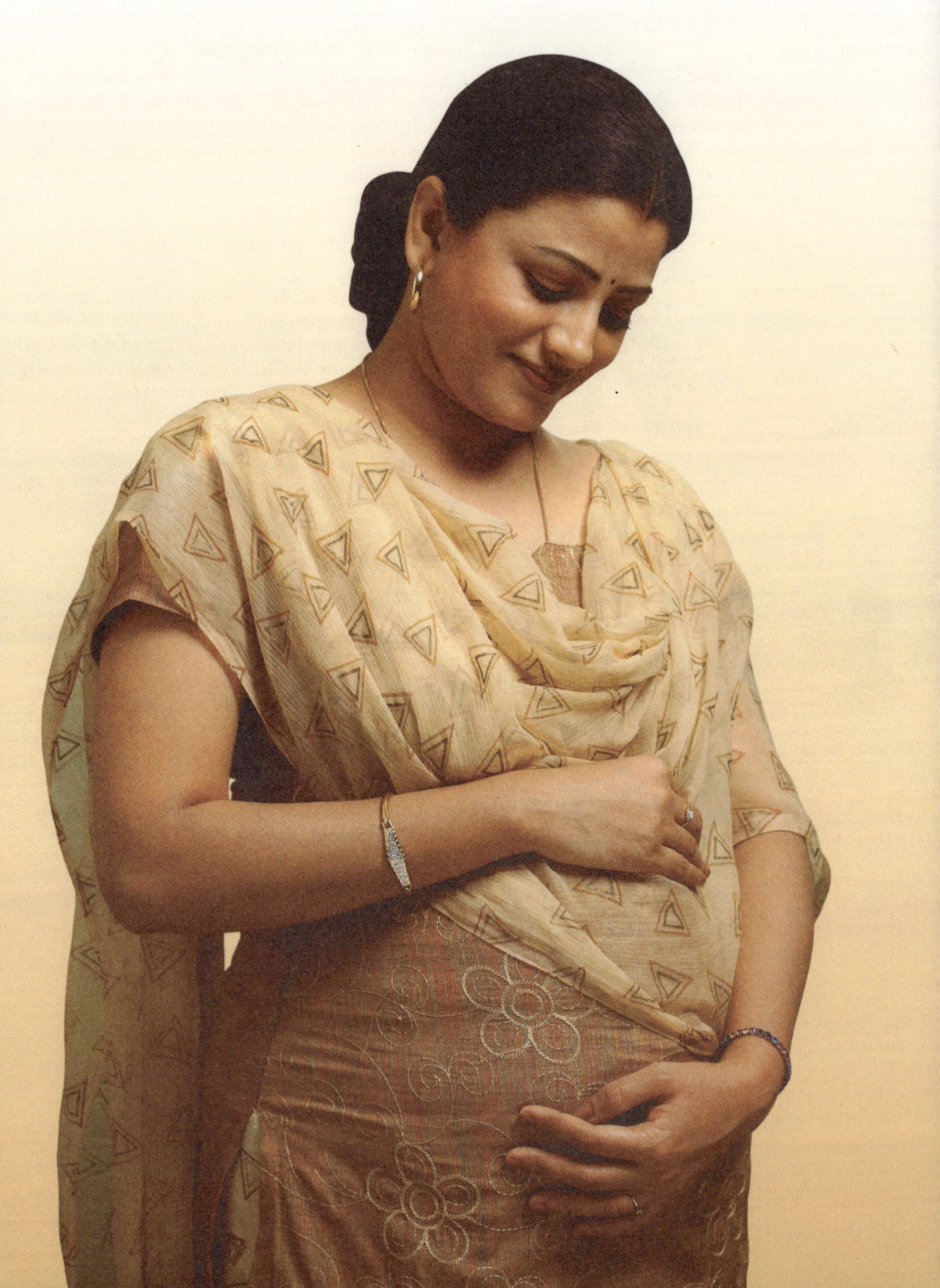

When things go wrong

CHAPTER 27

Miscarriage (abortion)

Shantha is fighting back tears. She is holding on tightly to her husband's hand. He too, is looking stunned. At their routine third month check-up, their obstetrician has told them that the baby inside the uterus has not grown beyond two months. Shantha has had a missed abortion.

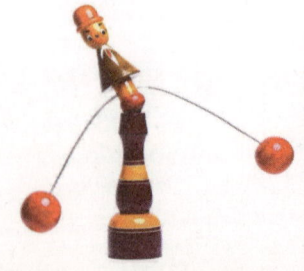

27 Miscarriage (abortion)

Being told that you are undergoing a miscarriage (abortion) is distressing. Even more disturbing is the lingering feeling that you may have in some way caused it. To compound this needless guilt, misinformed relatives and friends give you a list of things you may have done that places the blame of the miscarriage squarely on your shoulders.

It is important to realise that miscarriage is a natural process and cannot be caused by something you did or didn't do. **About 15 to 20 per cent of women who conceive will lose their pregnancy in a miscarriage.** There is no reason why you will not be able to have a baby the next time you try.

What is a miscarriage?

A miscarriage is the spontaneous ending of a pregnancy before the 5th month (20th week) of pregnancy. The medical term for miscarriage is **spontaneous abortion.**

Most miscarriages occur during the first 16 weeks of pregnancy. Many occur within the first 10 weeks. Some women miscarry even before they know they are pregnant.

How does it occur?

It is often difficult to pinpoint the exact cause of a miscarriage. However, most miscarriages are caused by problems that occur during fertilisation, when the sperm and the egg fuse to form an embryo. The commonest cause of a miscarriage is an abnormal number of chromosomes - either too many or too few. Often, the foetus does not develop at all, or it may develop abnormally. In such cases, miscarriage is the body's way of ending a pregnancy that is not developing normally.

A fall by the mother seldom causes miscarriage. The baby is well protected within the uterus. In addition, there is no evidence that emotional stress, physical overactivity or sexual activity causes miscarriage in a normal pregnancy.

What are the symptoms?

Possible symptoms include:

- Bleeding, which can range from a few drops of blood to a heavy flow. The bleeding may start with no warning or there may be a brownish discharge first.
- Cramping pain in the lower abdomen.
- A gush of fluid from the vagina without bleeding or pain. This may mean that the membranes have ruptured.
- A clot-like tissue may pass out of the vagina. Try to keep this material so the doctor can examine it.

Sometimes, it happens that there is minimal or no bleeding and pain, but the foetus has died and symptoms of early pregnancy have disappeared. The diagnosis is made only when an ultrasound examination is done. This condition is called a **missed abortion.**

How is a miscarriage diagnosed?

Your doctor may do a pelvic exam to check the size of your uterus and find that the size of the uterus does not correspond to the duration of pregnancy. You might have bleeding and cramping. An ultrasound scan will confirm an abortion.

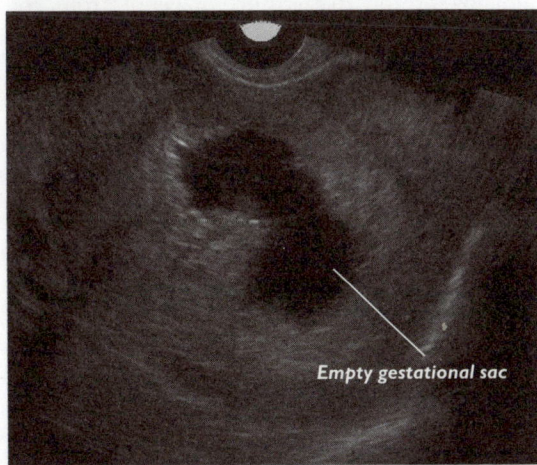

The uterus showing an empty gestational sac (missed abortion)

What are the types of miscarriage?

Threatened abortion or miscarriage

In a threatened miscarriage, there may be a small amount of painless bleeding from the vagina early in the pregnancy. In a threatened abortion or miscarriage, the baby's heartbeat can be seen on the ultrasound and there is a good chance that the pregnancy will continue. Your obstetrician may advise rest in bed for 2 to 3 days. The bed rest may stop the bleeding and the pregnancy may continue normally. Special precautions such as stopping exercise, staying off your feet as much as possible and avoiding sex may be necessary for one or two weeks.

> Over the years, medical research has clearly proven that there is no need for hormonal tablets or injections in case of a threatened abortion (miscarriage).

Inevitable abortion or miscarriage

Miscarriage becomes inevitable if the bleeding and cramping continue and the cervix begins to open. An inevitable miscarriage means that nothing can be done to prevent the miscarriage. When the uterus expels its contents entirely, it is called a **complete abortion (miscarriage).**

Incomplete abortion or miscarriage

The miscarriage is incomplete if only a part of the contents of the uterus is expelled. A dilatation and curettage (D&C) or suction procedure may be required to remove the remains of the foetus and placenta from the uterus. If the bleeding is not heavy, tablets of **misoprostol** may be inserted in the vagina or given orally to complete the miscarriage.

Missed abortion or miscarriage

If a missed abortion (miscarriage) is diagnosed (the foetus has died but there is no bleeding), the doctor may perform a D&C or induce labour to remove the foetus and placenta. In recent times, **misoprostol** tablets are more often used instead of a D&C in early miscarriage.

> In any pregnancy it is important to know your blood group and Rh type. If you are Rh negative your doctor will give you an injection after the abortion to prevent future problems.

When can you try for another pregnancy?

Give yourself time to heal both physically and emotionally before you try for another pregnancy. Apart from the physical reasons to avoid a pregnancy, it is also important to wait until you have dealt emotionally with the loss. If you have just had one miscarriage, no tests are needed before you try for another pregnancy. If you have had two or more miscarriages, you and your husband need to be tested before attempting another pregnancy.

Your obstetrician may advise you to avoid sexual intercourse for 2 to 4 weeks after a miscarriage Depending on your age, you can wait three to six months before trying for another pregnancy. Use some form of birth control till then. Your obstetrician will advise what is best for you.

> **Do not blame yourself for the miscarriage**
> Most miscarriages are spontaneous and not precipitated by anything you did.
> For example, miscarriages are not caused by strenuous exercise, emotional stress or sexual intercourse.
> Grief, anger and feelings of guilt are common and completely normal reactions to a miscarriage. Allow yourself to grieve over the loss of the baby. Seek support from relatives and friends. You may find it helpful to talk to others who have had miscarriages. You may be afraid that your miscarriage means that you won't be able to have a baby. Remember, however, that for most women, the next pregnancy is normal.

Some women do have repeated miscarriages. (A series of three or more consecutive miscarriages is called **recurrent or habitual miscarriage.**) These miscarriages may be caused by conditions that can be treated. If you have three or more miscarriages, it is important to be tested to determine and treat the cause.

What happens after a miscarriage?

- Your recovery will take 4 to 6 weeks.
- You may have some spotting and discomfort for a few days.

- If you were pregnant for more than four months before the miscarriage, you may still look pregnant and your breasts may leak milk.
- Low-impact exercises, such as walking or swimming, will not hurt you. Gradually exercise more as you feel better.
- Usually your doctor will give you an appointment for a check-up in 2 to 4 weeks.

> When you get pregnant again, there is no need for bed rest or restricted activity in the first three months. If the pregnancy is normal, nothing can dislodge it. If the pregnancy is abnormal, even lying in bed without moving will not prevent a miscarriage.

When should you call your doctor?

If you are pregnant and have bleeding from your vagina, with or without pain, call your doctor. If the bleeding is heavy or you have severe pain, see your doctor immediately.

If you are recovering from a miscarriage, call your obstetrician immediately if you have any of these symptoms:

- heavy bleeding
- fever
- chills
- severe abdominal pain

Recurrent pregnancy loss

When there have been 3 or more miscarriages, it is called **recurrent** or **habitual miscarriage**. If a woman loses her pregnancies repeatedly, she and her husband need to undergo a few tests to find out the cause.

Known causes of recurrent pregnancy loss

Sometimes a miscarriage can be linked to chromosomal problems in the foetus, medical conditions in the woman, or problems with the woman's uterus. There are tests to help your obstetrician determine what caused the miscarriage and, in some cases, treatment is available to avoid problems in future pregnancies.

Chromosomal abnormalities

In a small number of cases, problems with the couple's chromosomes can cause repeated miscarriage. **Karyotyping** is a test to check the chromosomes of the couple. It is a blood test and may pick up a cause for recurrent miscarriage.

Problems of the uterus

Several problems of the uterus are linked to repeated miscarriage. Most are not common. They include:

- **Uterine defects** present from birth, such as a uterus that is divided into two sections by a wall of tissue (septate uterus).
- **Cervical incompetence** (also called **cervical insufficiency**) sometimes causes miscarriage, usually after the 4th month. The cervix is the lower part or mouth of the uterus. During

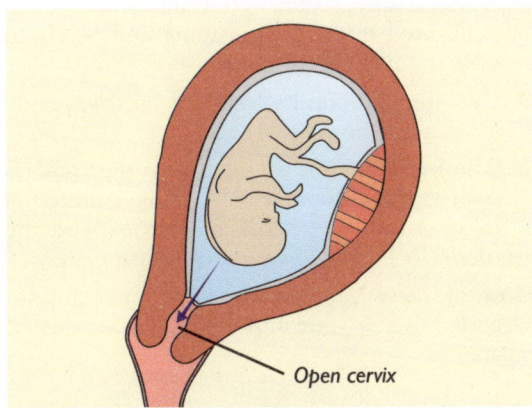

Cervical incompetence (insufficiency)

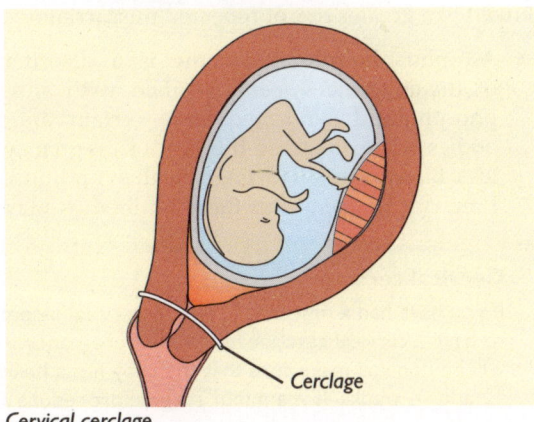

Cervical cerclage

labour, the cervix widens to allow the baby to leave the uterus and pass through the vagina. A cervix that starts widening and opening too early in the pregnancy may result in miscarriage. Often, if the problem is caught early, it can be treated and the pregnancy can continue.

Miscarriages that result from cervical incompetence (or insufficiency) generally occur after the 4th month of pregnancy. About 25 per cent of miscarriages that occur after the 14th week of pregnancy are due to cervical incompetence.

Uterine abnormalities (other than cervical incompetence) can be diagnosed with tests to locate any defects in the uterus:

- **Hysterosalpingography:** An X-ray of the uterus and fallopian tubes is taken after the organs are injected with a small amount of dye.
- **Hysteroscopy:** A thin, light-transmitting device is inserted through the vagina and cervix to view the inside of the uterus.
- **Ultrasound:** Sound waves are used to create an image of the internal organs.
- **Sonohysterogram:** A vaginal ultrasound is used to view the uterus. A saline solution is injected into the uterus to help expand the uterus for better viewing of the uterine cavity.

Most of these problems can be treated with surgery. Discuss your options with your obstetrician.

Medical conditions

Certain conditions in the mother have been linked to a greater risk of repeated miscarriage.

- **Antiphospholipid syndrome** is a disorder of the immune system. Women with antiphospholipid syndrome have certain antibodies which increase the risk of pregnancy loss. Blood is tested to diagnose this condition. Pregnant women with these antibodies may be prescribed blood thinners like low dose aspirin and heparin.
- **Thrombophilia** is a type of disorder that can make blood clot more than it should. There are several types of genetic disorders that can lead to thrombophilia. One type of disorder, Factor V Leiden mutation, may allow clots to form in the blood vessels to the placenta and lead to miscarriage. Pregnant women with this disorder may be prescribed blood thinners like low dose aspirin and heparin.
- **Diabetes** and **thyroid disease** when untreated, can cause recurrent pregnancy loss.
- **Systemic lupus erythematosus** is a chronic inflammatory disease that occurs when your body's immune system attacks your own tissues and organs.
- **Heart disease.**
- **Severe kidney disease,** mainly when linked with high blood pressure.
- Women who have undergone treatment for **polycystic ovarian syndrome** have an increased risk of miscarriage.

Sometimes, it is impossible to pinpoint the exact reason for recurrent pregnancy loss. Many times, it is the presence of a **single abnormal gene** in either the husband or the wife which causes the formation of an abnormal foetus. Unfortunately, a single gene disorder is difficult to confirm or treat.

> The loss of a pregnancy, no matter how early or late, can cause feelings of intense grief and despair. Many women feel they are somehow defective and unable to have a baby. You may feel discouraged. You and your husband may be troubled and even overwhelmed by these feelings. Remember it is not your fault. Most women can expect to have a normal pregnancy even after having more than one miscarriage.

Cervical cerclage

If you have had a miscarriage due to cervical incompetence (insufficiency), your obstetrician will advise you to have a cervical cerclage in the next pregnancy. Once you reach 12 weeks of pregnancy, an ultrasound will be done to make sure that the baby has a healthy heartbeat. A cerclage will then be done between 12 and 14 weeks. It is a minor surgical procedure and will require hospitalisation for a few days.

Miscarriage: myths and misconceptions

Having a miscarriage is a sad event in any couple's life. It is almost impossible for you to believe that you did not do something which caused the miscarriage. To add to this, friends and relatives try to come up with some explanation for the miscarriage.

Remember, all the usual reasons given for causing a miscarriage are only myths and misconceptions.

The following are usually blamed but **do not cause a miscarriage:**

- Climbing stairs
- Strenuous activity
- Travelling by autorickshaw
- Travelling in a bus
- Travelling on a bumpy road
- Travelling by air
- Having a fall
- Drinking something hot or cold
- Eating fruits like papaya, pineapple and mango
- Eating sesame seeds (til seeds)
- Going out during a solar or lunar eclipse
- Having sexual intercourse
- Being emotionally upset

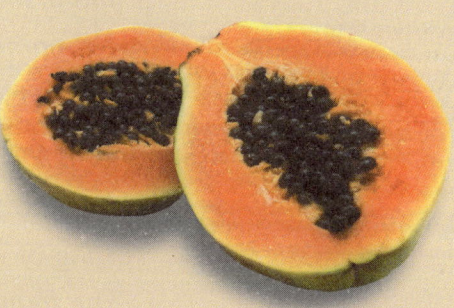

One of the commonest questions asked after a miscarriage is, "Do I have a weak uterus?" **There is nothing known as a 'weak' uterus.** There is no medicine which 'strengthens' the uterus. There is no need for injections and tablets in the next pregnancy. Remember, miscarriages happen because the pregnancy is abnormal to begin with. A miscarriage is Nature's way of getting rid of an abnormal or defective foetus.

CHAPTER 28

Bleeding in pregnancy

Shanthi is frightened. She is two months pregnant. She woke up this morning to find a small amount of blood on her underclothes. She is extremely concerned.

Samhita is 20 weeks pregnant. She was working in her office when she had a feeling of wetness. On checking, she found she was bleeding. She rushed to her obstetrician.

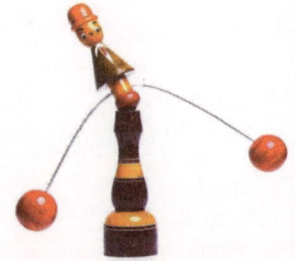

28 Bleeding in pregnancy

One of the more frightening yet common experiences in pregnancy is vaginal bleeding. This may vary from a small amount of spotting to heavy bleeding with clots and cramps. In pregnancy, even a small amount of vaginal bleeding can be alarming. Though bleeding may be a warning sign of an abnormality, it is not always a serious complication. Many pregnant women experience light vaginal bleeding at some point during pregnancy, particularly during the first three months.

Though you need not panic, it is important to seek medical help if you have bleeding anytime during pregnancy.

Vaginal bleeding in pregnancy has many causes. Though it is not an uncommon occurrence, not all bleeding is due to a serious problem. Bleeding can occur early in pregnancy, in the second or the third trimester. Slight bleeding may often stop by itself. Sometimes, though, bleeding may be serious enough to be a risk to you or your foetus. You should call your doctor or seek medical advice if bleeding occurs.

Bleeding in the first trimester (1-13 weeks)

Is it normal to have bleeding in the first trimester?

Though it is not normal to bleed early in pregnancy, it certainly is a common occurrence. Many women will experience spotting or bleeding in the first trimester of pregnancy. In most cases, women who experience slight bleeding in the first trimester go on to have a normal pregnancy. There are some signs and symptoms which may indicate that the bleeding is of serious concern.

Common causes of early pregnancy bleeding

- **Implantation bleeding:** There might be a small amount of spotting or bleeding very early in pregnancy, about 10 to 14 days after fertilisation. When the fertilised egg attaches to the lining of the uterus and starts burrowing into the lining, there can be slight spotting. Some women actually mistake this light bleeding for a period and may not realise they are pregnant.

- **Cervical changes:** In pregnancy, there is an increase in the blood supply and blood flow to the cervix. The cervix becomes soft and congested. There may be light spotting or bleeding after contact to this area, such as after sexual intercourse or a pelvic exam. This type of light bleeding in pregnancy is usually normal and will stop by itself.

- **Miscarriage:** Bleeding in the first trimester can be a sign of miscarriage. Miscarriage occurs in 15-20 per cent of pregnancies, most often during the first 12 weeks. Bleeding in the first trimester is always considered to indicate a possible miscarriage. It is called a threatened abortion. Once you are examined and an ultrasound scan shows a good heartbeat in the foetus, it indicates that the pregnancy will continue normally. **(See Chapter 27: Miscarriage (abortion).**

- **Ectopic pregnancy:** In some women, the pregnancy will not implant inside the uterine cavity but will start growing in an abnormal place, most often the Fallopian tube. This is called a tubal pregnancy. A foetus implanted outside the uterus cannot develop into a normal baby. An ectopic pregnancy can cause serious internal bleeding. Ectopic pregnancies must be treated to save the life of the mother. Symptoms of ectopic pregnancy include vaginal spotting or bleeding, abdominal pain (which is usually worse on one side) and fainting.

- **Molar pregnancy** (also called **gestational trophoblastic disease**): In this rare condition, the foetus does not form. Instead, the uterus is filled up with an abnormal mass made up of clusters of cysts. Bleeding is the most common symptom of a molar pregnancy. By itself, molar pregnancy is an uncommon cause of bleeding in the first trimester. A molar pregnancy may require treatment with suction curettage and drugs.

- **Other reasons not related to pregnancy:** Spotting or vaginal bleeding can be caused by small polyps on the cervix. Occasionally, the bleeding can be due to a small cut or tear in the vagina.

When should you seek immediate medical attention?

More than half of the women who have some bleeding in early pregnancy go on to carry the pregnancy to term. It is urgent to call your obstetrician if the bleeding is:

- heavier than a period
- accompanied by severe cramps
- accompanied by lower abdominal pain
- associated with fainting or giddiness
- associated with fever

Management of bleeding in the first trimester

When you have bleeding in the first trimester, your obstetrician will try to determine the cause of the bleeding. She will do a pelvic examination, may inspect the cervix and also may ask for an ultrasound examination. A blood test may be done to measure **human chorionic gonadotropin (hCG)**. It is a substance produced during pregnancy. You may be asked to repeat the test to see if hCG levels increase normally as the pregnancy progresses.

> **Information from an ultrasound scan (1st trimester):**
>
> An ultrasound scan can immediately rule out an abnormal pregnancy like a molar pregnancy and will also tell us if the pregnancy is viable (healthy) or destined for loss. When a heartbeat is identified, the chances are high that the pregnancy will continue normally. If a heartbeat is absent, then you may be going in for a miscarriage. There might also be a small clot adjacent to the placenta which can cause the bleeding. The ultrasound may need to be repeated periodically to track the course of the clot and to see when it disappears.

Bed rest

If the bleeding is slight, you may be advised bed rest and limited activity at home. If the bleeding is moderate or heavy, you might be admitted to the hospital for a few days till the bleeding stops. You will be asked to gradually increase your level of activity and if there is no further bleeding for 1 to 2 weeks, you will be asked to resume your routine activity. It is best to avoid intercourse for two weeks following any vaginal bleeding.

> **Can hormones stop the bleeding?**
>
> Over the years, medical research has clearly proven that there is **no need for hormonal tablets or injections** in case of a threatened abortion (miscarriage).

Bleeding in the second trimester (14-27 weeks)

Bleeding in the second trimester may be due to a growth (polyp) on the cervix. This can be diagnosed by the obstetrician when she inspects the cervix. Bleeding can also follow intercourse since the cervix is soft and congested.

The conditions which need to be watched out for are:

- **Miscarriage:** Although miscarriage is less common in the second trimester than the first, a risk still exists.
- **Cervical incompetence or insufficiency:** Occasionally, light bleeding from the cervix, along with profuse white discharge, may be a sign of cervical incompetence, a condition in which the cervix opens painlessly, leading to preterm delivery. This condition occurs most frequently between 18 and 24 weeks of pregnancy and requires prompt medical attention.
- **Circumvallate placenta:** This is an abnormal placenta which can occasionally cause bleeding in the second trimester. This kind of placenta may also be associated with preterm labour and decreased growth of the foetus.
- **Preterm labour:** Preterm labour can start off with vaginal bleeding and will then progress to cramping. If the obstetrician thinks that you are going in for preterm labour, she will advise bed rest and may also start you on tablets or injections which will arrest labour.

Management of bleeding in the second trimester:

Your obstetrician will examine you to make sure there is no polyp causing the bleeding. She will also check the cervix to determine whether you are in labour or not. After that, she will ask for an ultrasound scan.

> **Information from an ultrasound scan (2nd trimester):**
>
> An ultrasound in the 2nd trimester can help identify an incompetent cervix. It may also identify if there is any bleeding from the placenta. If there is any abnormality in the foetus, it will be picked up.

Bed rest

If the bleeding is slight, you may be advised bed rest and limited activity at home. If the bleeding is moderate or heavy, you might be admitted to the hospital for a few days till the bleeding stops. You will be asked to gradually increase your level of activity and if there is no further bleeding for 1-2 weeks, you will be asked to resume your routine activity. It is best to avoid intercourse for two weeks following any vaginal bleeding.

Cervical cerclage

If there is evidence of cervical incompetence (also called cervical insufficiency), an attempt will be made to suture the cervix shut. **(See Chapter 27: Miscarriage (abortion))**. The suture will be left in place till term and then it will be removed to allow for labour. Sometimes, the cervix may have dilated too much and the cerclage procedure may not be feasible.

Bleeding in the third trimester (28- 40 weeks)

Bleeding late in pregnancy may threaten the health of the woman or the foetus. Bleeding in late pregnancy will usually require hospitalisation. **Preterm labour** can also cause vaginal bleeding and may be associated with abdominal cramping or intermittent pain.

The two most common causes of heavy vaginal bleeding in late pregnancy are due to a problem with the placenta. They are **placental abruption** and **placenta praevia**.

Placental abruption

One of the emergencies that can occur before or during labour is placental abruption. This problem occurs only in 1 out of a 100 pregnancies. In this condition, the placenta separates or detaches from the uterine wall, either before or during labour. This may cause vaginal bleeding. This can also be associated with severe abdominal pain. It usually occurs during the last 12 weeks of pregnancy. When the placenta becomes detached, the blood flow to the foetus can get reduced or cut off. This endangers the oxygen supply to the foetus and can jeopardise its health.

Who is at high risk for placental abruption?

Women who have had pregnancies before, are over 35, have had an abruption before or who have high blood pressure in pregnancy are at high risk for developing placental abruption.

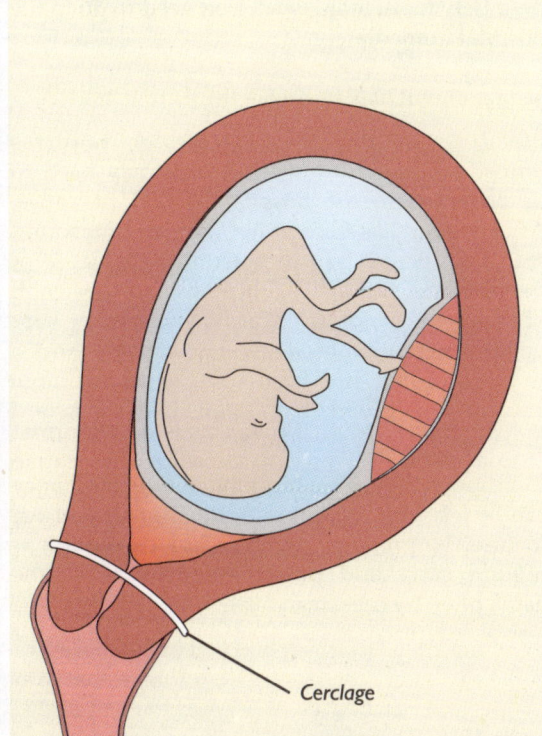

Cervical cerclage for cervical incompetence

Very rarely, blows or other injuries to the stomach can cause an abruption.

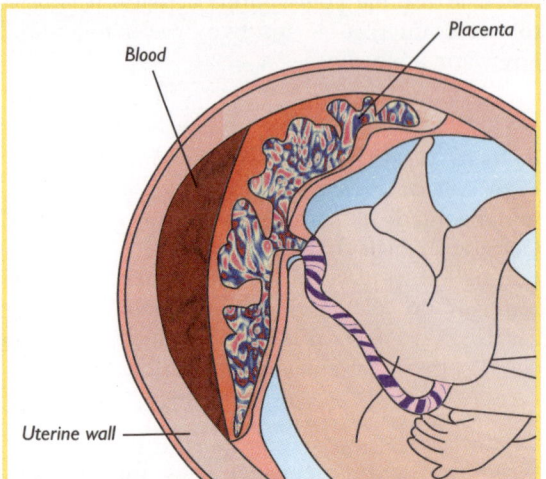

Placental abruption: the placenta has separated from the uterine wall

Placenta praevia

Placenta praevia occurs in 1 woman in 200. When the placenta lies low in the uterus, it is called placenta praevia. It may partly cover the cervix **(partial placenta praevia)** or completely cover the cervix **(total placenta praevia).**

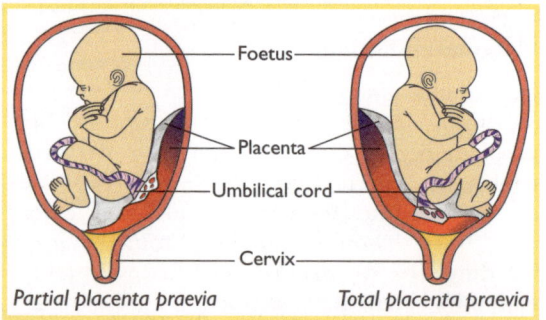

Placenta praevia can cause painless vaginal bleeding. Most of the time, this is managed conservatively. You might be admitted to the hospital for observation. If the bleeding stops, you might be allowed to go home. An elective caesarean section will be done when your baby is mature enough to be delivered. If the bleeding is profuse and uncontrollable, then an emergency caesarean section will be done, whatever the age of the foetus.

Who is at high risk for placental praevia?

Placenta praevia is more common in women who have had more than one child, who have had a previous caesarean section, or who are carrying twins or triplets.

Bleeding due to labour

Late in pregnancy, vaginal bleeding may be a sign of labour. A mucous 'plug' that covers the opening of the uterus during pregnancy is passed just before or at the start of labour. This results in a small amount of mucous and blood passing from the cervix. This is called **bloody show.** It is a common occurrence and usually happens close to your due date. Sometimes this can be more than usual and can cause concern. If you have to use a pad, the bleeding is definitely more than usual. You need to go to the hospital immediately.

Management of bleeding in the third trimester

Bleeding in the third trimester requires immediate medical attention. You may need to be admitted to the hospital to find its cause. After labour has been ruled out, an ultrasound scan may be advised to determine the cause of the bleeding. If the bleeding stops and the health of the foetus is not in jeopardy, you may be kept under observation for a few days or even weeks. If the bleeding has been profuse and a large amount of blood has been lost, a blood transfusion may be required.

Conditions that cause bleeding in late pregnancy can be a health risk for both the mother and the foetus. The problem might be serious enough to require early and immediate delivery of the baby, often by caesarean birth.

What happens when you have bleeding in pregnancy?

Shanthi is frightened. She is two months pregnant. She woke up this morning to find a small amount of blood on her underclothes. She has no abdominal cramping or pain. She is extremely concerned.

Shanthi and her husband went to see her obstetrician. She had an internal examination. The mouth of the uterus was still closed. There was only slight bleeding present. Her doctor explained to them that this, along with the fact that she was not having any pains, was a good sign but only an ultrasound scan could confirm whether the pregnancy was healthy.

An ultrasound was done and she was delighted to see that the baby's heartbeat was seen clearly. Shanthi was having a 'threatened' abortion. Since there was very slight bleeding, Shanthi was asked to go home. She was advised to stay in bed for the next three days though she could get up to eat and to go to the bathroom. After three days, she had no further bleeding. She was asked to resume normal activity at home over the next week. She was also asked to avoid sexual intercourse for the next two weeks.

After a week at home, Shanthi had no bleeding. She resumed all her activities and started going out as usual. She had no further bleeding and had a normal delivery at term.

Samhita is 20 weeks pregnant. She was working in her office when she had a feeling of wetness. On checking, she found she was bleeding. She phoned her husband and told him to meet her at the obstetrician's clinic.

Samhita is rightfully worried. Bleeding in the second trimester is less common than in the first trimester.

Her obstetrician asked her whether she had had intercourse over the past 48 hours. Since the mouth of the uterus is very soft at this stage, sometimes there can be slight bleeding following intercourse. This is not harmful to the baby.

On examination, the mouth of the uterus was closed and showed no signs of premature labour. An ultrasound was done. The baby's heartbeat was normal. The placenta was lying a little low in the uterus. There was a small clot near the lower edge of the placenta.

Samhita was advised to get admitted to the hospital. Over the next two days, the bleeding changed from bright red to dark brown. Her obstetrician explained to her that this was a good sign. It meant that there was no fresh bleeding. She was discharged on the third day. She was advised to take it easy and avoid intercourse for the next two weeks.

Since she had no further bleeding, she went back to office after two weeks. She had two further episodes of slight brownish discharge. Her obstetrician explained that this was common. As the uterus enlarged, the placenta would keep moving away from the lower end of the uterus. The danger of bleeding would become less as the pregnancy progressed.

Samhita went into labour at 38 weeks and had a normal vaginal delivery.

CHAPTER 29

Premature or preterm labour

Susan is worried. Should she be hitting the panic button? She is only 8 months pregnant but since this morning, she has been having lower abdominal pain. In the beginning, it felt like menstrual cramping but now there is squeezing pain which comes every 10 minutes. Could Susan be in premature labour?

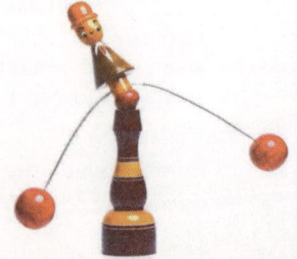

29 Premature or preterm labour

What is premature labour?

When labour begins before 37 weeks, it is considered **preterm** or **premature**. It is not known for certain what causes labour to start. Hormones produced by the woman, placenta and the foetus play a role. Changes in the uterus, which may be caused by these hormones, may cause labour to start. The exact causes of preterm labour are not known. About 10 per cent of pregnant women will have a premature delivery.

What are the problems of prematurity?

The earlier in pregnancy the baby is born, the greater the risk of serious problems for the baby. Many of the organs, especially the heart and lungs, are not fully grown or mature. Premature infants born after 32 weeks of pregnancy tend to have less chance of problems than those born earlier.

In India, a baby which is less than 1000 grams at birth or is born before 30-32 weeks of pregnancy has fewer chances for survival. These babies require a specially equipped **neonatal intensive care unit** to survive.

For infants born before 28 weeks of pregnancy, the chances of survival are slim. Many who do survive have long-term health problems. These babies may end up with chronic lung problems, and may have developmental delay both in their ability to move (motor skills) and the ability to learn (cognitive skills). Extremely premature babies may also have problems with sight and hearing.

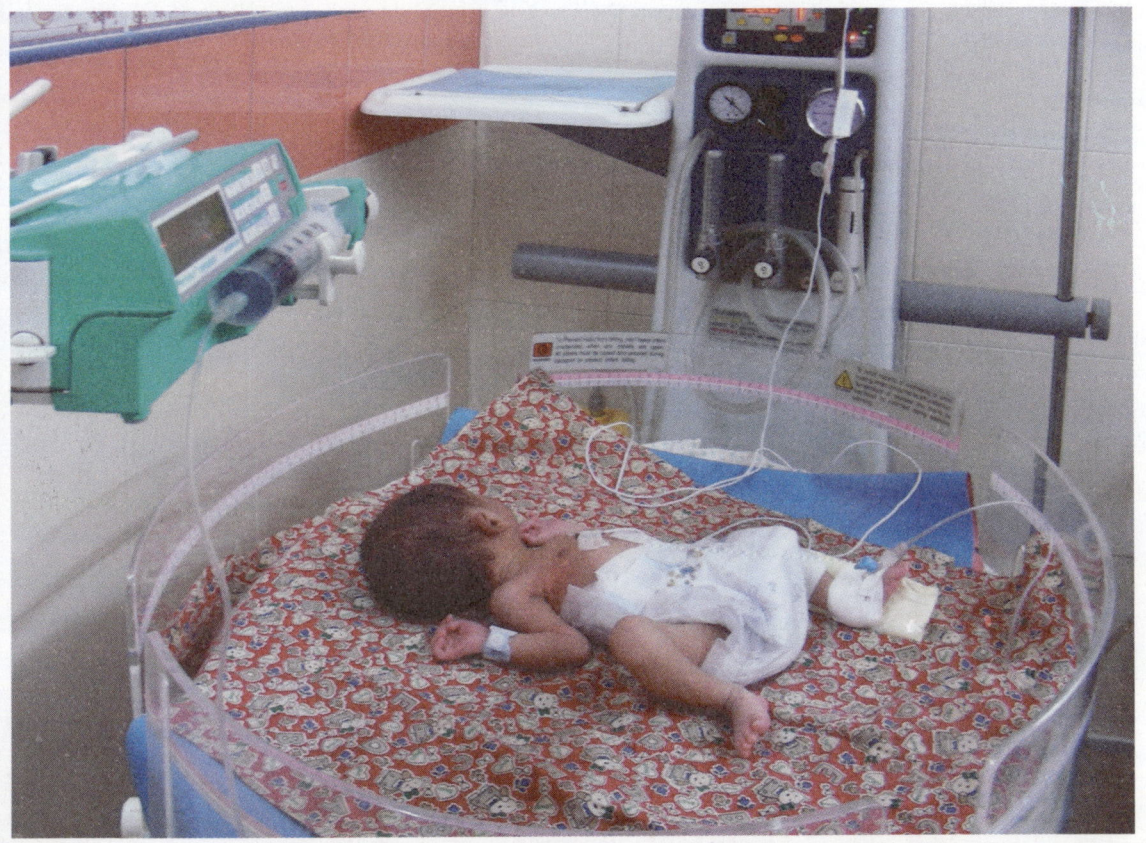

What can cause premature labour?

Some pregnancies are at a greater risk for the occurrence of preterm labour. Preterm labour can occur with:

- A previous pregnancy with preterm labour
- Infections of the urinary tract or cervix
- Cervical incompetence where the muscle fibres of the cervix are weak
- Prolonged bleeding in early pregnancy
- Twins or higher number of foetuses
- An abnormal foetus
- A growth restricted foetus (IUGR)
- Excess amniotic fluid (polyhydramnios)
- Diabetes or high blood pressure
- Malformations of the uterus
- Poor nutrition during pregnancy

Warning signs of premature labour

If preterm labour is recognised early enough, delivery may be prevented or postponed in some cases. This will give the baby extra time to grow and mature. Even a few more days may mean a healthier baby. It is important to call your doctor or go to the hospital right away if you notice any of these symptoms:

- Watery, mucoid or bloody vaginal discharge
- Sudden increase in amount of vaginal discharge
- Pelvic or lower abdominal pressure
- Constant, dull, low backache
- Mild abdominal cramps like menstrual cramps
- Regular or frequent contractions or uterine tightening, sometimes painless
- A trickle or gush of fluid from the vagina

Am I in premature labour?

It is common to have **Braxton-Hicks contractions**. These are caused by painless tightening of the abdomen in the last three months of pregnancy. They usually subside with rest.

When should you worry?

You need immediate medical attention if there are **frequent contractions**:

- at least 4 times every 20 minutes or if there have been eight contractions in an hour
- the contractions have been persisting for more than an hour

Sometimes, preterm labour can start with the **rupture of membranes.** This is called preterm premature rupture of membranes or **PPROM.**

There is a trickle or gush of fluid from the vagina which continues without stopping. This indicates that the membranes have ruptured even though pains have not started.

How is premature labour confirmed?

When you go to the hospital, your doctor will feel your abdomen to see if you are having contractions. You might also have an internal examination to assess the condition of the cervix. Preterm labour can be confirmed by finding out if **thinning and dilatation of the cervix** (mouth of the uterus) have occurred.

You might be monitored with a foetal monitor to see if you are having contractions.

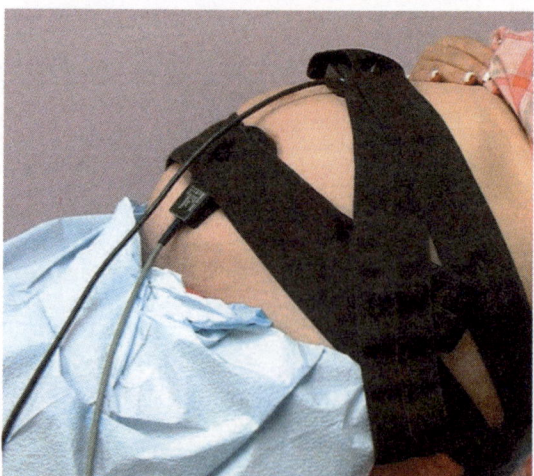

Monitoring for contractions

If you have ruptured membranes prematurely i.e. before pains have started, your doctor may do a speculum examination to see if there is **fluid leaking from the cervix** (mouth of the uterus). If there is leaking of fluid, an internal examination may be postponed till the obstetrician decides when and how she is going to deliver your baby.

Preventing premature labour

Though it is not always possible to prevent premature labour, some precautions can be taken.

Initiating regular antenatal check-ups early in your pregnancy and continuing regular check-ups with your obstetrician can help prevent premature labour.

Women who have had a previous premature delivery may be given injectable **progesterone,** a hormone to help prevent another premature delivery. This is usually started from the 16th-20th week of pregnancy.

In most cases, women at risk for premature labour do not have to be at bed rest and many of them can continue to work. You may be advised to avoid overexerting yourself and lifting heavy objects. Having intercourse during pregnancy may sometimes cause contractions so you may be advised to avoid intercourse.

Treatment of premature labour

Once premature labour is suspected, your obstetrician will admit you to the hospital for observation. The objectives of treating premature labour are twofold:

- to try and stop labour, as long as it does not jeopardise the mother's health.
- to ensure that if the baby is born in spite of preventive measures, then its lungs are mature enough for it to survive.

Tocolytics are medicines which can stop contractions. The commonest and most effective medicines used are **nifedipine, terbutaline** and **ritodrine. Magnesium sulphate** is a less commonly used medicine for stopping contractions.

Steroids are administered if it appears that the chances of the baby being born early are high. Steroids cross the placenta and help the baby's lungs mature and also prevent bleeding into the brain. Steroids increase the baby's chance of survival. Steroids are most likely to help the baby when used between 24 and 34 weeks of pregnancy.

> Steroids are very safe in pregnancy. In addition to be being used to improve foetal lung maturity, steroids may be used in asthmatics in pregnancy and also to relieve the itching which occurs in the last few weeks of pregnancy.

Delivery and care of a premature baby

A vaginal delivery will be attempted if the premature labour is progressing well and does not seem to be presenting any risk to the foetus. It may also be preferred if the chances of the baby surviving are very slim.

If there is reason to believe that the premature baby may not be able to tolerate the stresses of labour, or if there are any maternal complications, then a caesarean section may be advised.

Care of the premature baby

Many preterm babies are very small and require special care. They are kept in an incubator to keep them warm. **Surfactant** is a medication which, when administered, can prevent breathing difficulties in the baby and save the baby's life. You or your baby may be moved to a different hospital that can provide this type of care.

Today, with special care in a neonatal intensive care unit (NICU), even babies born between 28-30 weeks have a reasonable chance of survival. Babies born between 31-36 weeks have a better chance of survival.

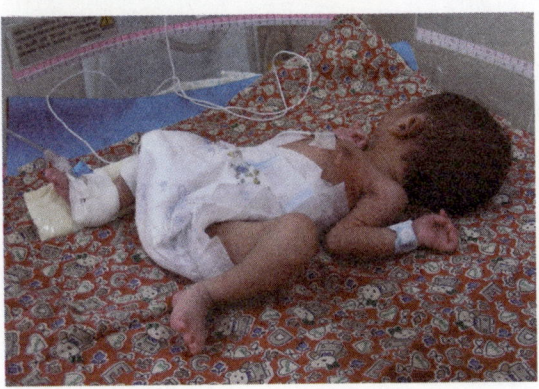

CHAPTER 30

Postdated pregnancy

Seetha is getting impatient. Everyday she gets calls from friends and relatives asking if she has delivered yet. The due date was three days ago and her baby seems to quite comfortable inside the womb. The baby is showing no signs of wanting to come out! Seetha's husband is anxious and wants the obstetrician to deliver the baby immediately. Is this necessary?

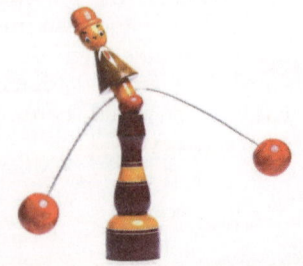

30 Postdated pregnancy

Waiting for the birth of a child is an exciting and anxious time. Most women give birth between 37 and 41 weeks of pregnancy. Very few babies are born exactly on their due date. It is quite normal to give birth as much as three weeks before or 10 days after the due date. It is important to remember that problems occur in only a small number of post-term pregnancies. Most women who give birth after the due date have no problems with the delivery and the newborn baby will do well.

The due date

The average length of pregnancy is 280 days or 40 weeks from the first day of a woman's last menstrual period. It can be hard to predict the exact date of delivery. **Only 5 per cent of babies are born on the exact due date!**

Calculating the due date helps the obstetrician know which month of pregnancy you are in and to monitor the progress of the baby, particularly its growth.

Women with irregular periods may require an ultrasound in early pregnancy to establish the actual due date. Even women with very regular periods may be asked to have an ultrasound scan in early pregnancy to confirm the age of a foetus and thereby, the due date. The due date should be confirmed as early in pregnancy as possible. Later, it becomes harder to set the due date accurately.

What is postdated or post-term pregnancy?

By definition, a postdated pregnancy is one that lasts 41 weeks or longer.

A pregnancy often lasts longer than expected because the exact time when the woman became pregnant is not known. Usually obstetricians will wait for a week beyond the calculated due date, as long as the baby's and the mother's health

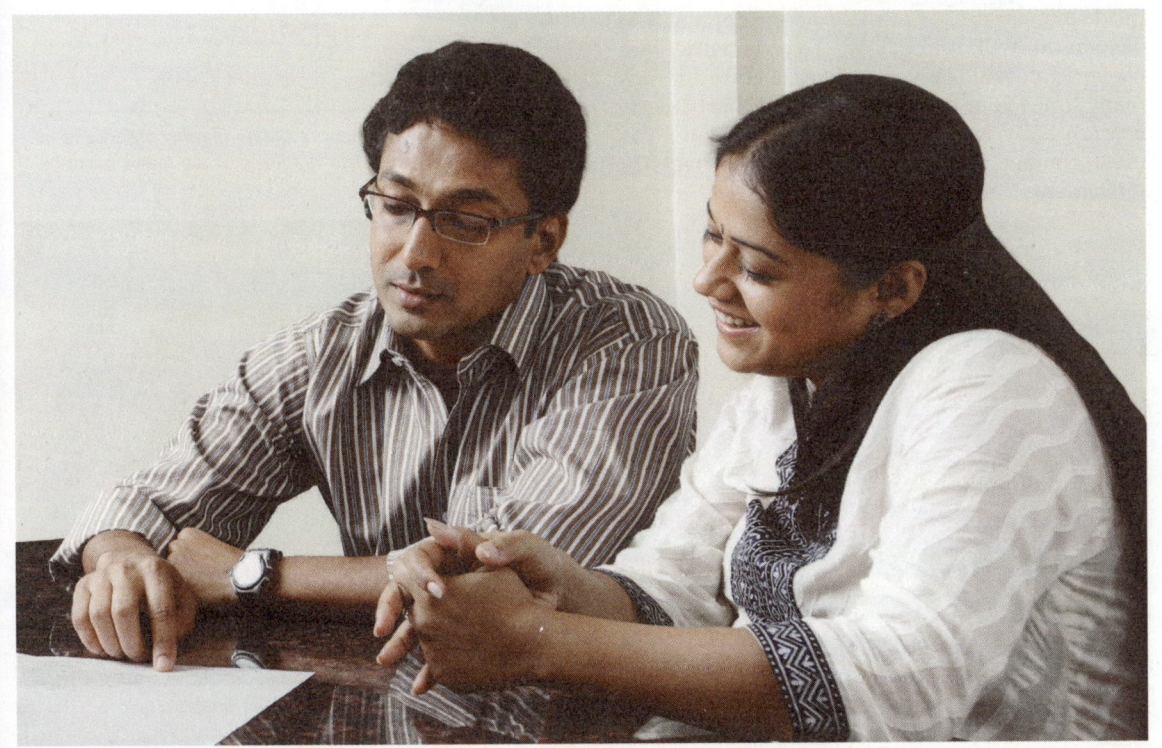

remain normal. If a pregnancy goes beyond the due date and tests show that the foetus is being affected, labour may need to be induced. Sometimes, the obstetrician may decide on a caesarean section if tests show that the baby may not be able to tolerate labour. The most common reason is a decrease in the amniotic fluid.

What are the risks of postdated pregnancy?

As the pregnancy proceeds beyond 40 weeks, the placenta may not function as well as it did earlier in pregnancy and the baby receives less blood supply. This might cause the amount of amniotic fluid around the baby to decrease. Less fluid may cause the umbilical cord to become compressed as the baby moves or as the uterus contracts. When the pregnancy goes beyond the due date, the baby also tends to pass meconium (motion) into the amniotic fluid. This meconium can be aspirated into the lungs of the baby and can cause a problem called **meconium aspiration**.

How do we know the baby is healthy?

Foetal movement count

When the baby is healthy, it will move regularly inside the uterus. When it starts receiving less oxygen, it will move less. That is why your obstetrician will ask you to keep a count of how many times your baby moves inside, particularly when a baby is not born by the due date. You must contact your obstetrician if you feel the movements have become less.

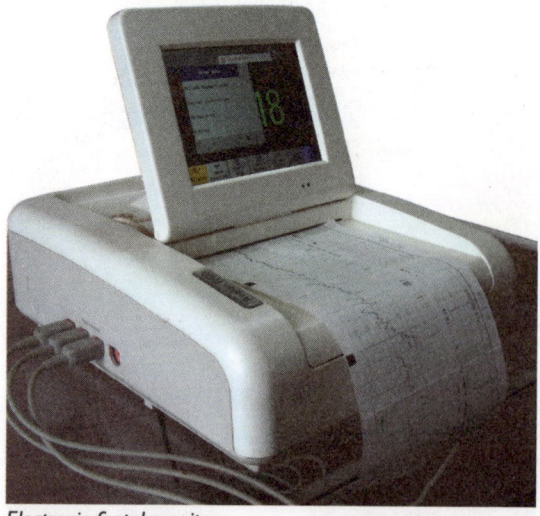

Electronic foetal monitor

Electronic foetal monitoring

This is used to record the baby's heartbeat. Looking at the recording, the obstetrician will be able to predict the baby's health.

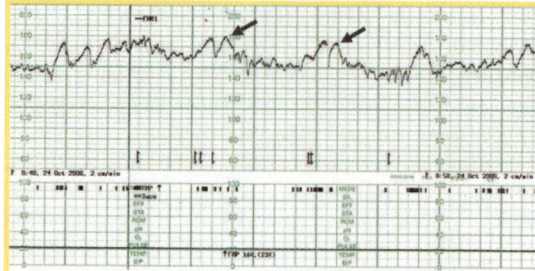

Electronic foetal monitor recording of a healthy foetus - arrows indicate accelerations which means the foetus is getting adequate oxygen from the placenta.

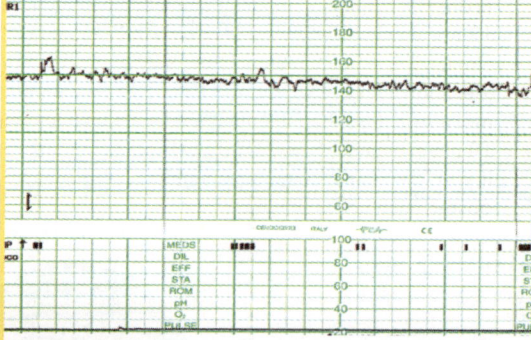

Electronic foetal monitor recording showing absence of accelerations which is a warning that the foetus might be getting less oxygen.

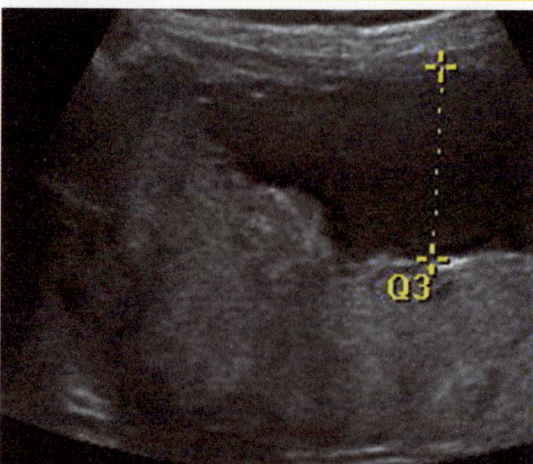

Ultrasound scan showing amount of amniotic fluid surrounding the foetus

Amniotic fluid index uses ultrasound to measure the amount of fluid around the foetus. If the fluid level remains normal, it is reassuring.

Labour induction

Most doctors wait 7 days after the due date to induce labour, as long as the mother and the foetus are healthy. Medication or other methods are used to bring on labour. The labour pains will be monitored carefully and the baby's heartbeat will also be monitored throughout the process. The incidence of caesarean section increases with labour induction for postdated pregnancy. **(See Chapter 18: Augmentation and induction of labour).**

Counting the baby's movements

There are many ways of ensuring that your baby is healthy. One of them is to count the movements of the baby. Your obstetrician may recommend a particular method for you.

One of the ways of counting the baby's movements is given below:

From the time you wake up in the morning till 12 noon, you should feel at least 10 movements. Similarly, from noon to 6 in the evening, you should feel another 10 movements. You may feel many more movements but it is essential to feel at least 10 movements. If you feel that the movements are less than 10, then lie on your side and count for 1 hour. If you have felt at least 3 movements in that hour, then the baby is doing fine. If not, you need to see your obstetrician immediately.

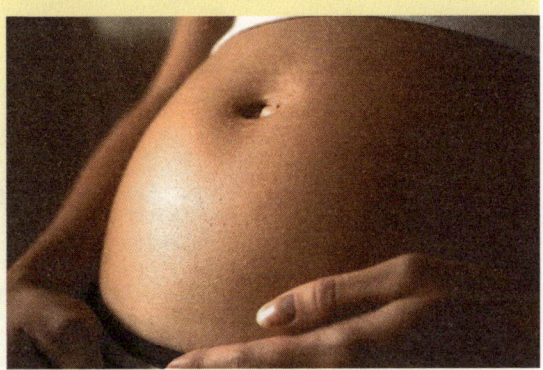

Electronic foetal monitoring or cardiotocography (CTG)

Just as the adult heart activity is recorded using an ECG, foetal heart activity is recorded using an electronic foetal monitor. This is also called cardiotocography (CTG). When the baby is receiving adequate oxygenation, the heart rate will be between 110 and 150 beats per minute.

When the pregnancy is going beyond the due date, electronic foetal monitoring is used to perform a test called a **non-stress test** (because the baby is not placed under any stress during this test). The heart rate recording will be checked to see if the heart rate is normal. The recording should also show what are known as **accelerations.** These are periodic, sharp increases in the heart rate as a response to the baby's movements. It is an excellent sign of foetal well-being.

If the baby is not receiving enough oxygen, the heart rate recording may be flat and may not show any accelerations. If the placenta is not functioning well because of being postdated, or if the cord is getting compressed because of a decrease in amniotic fluid, the baby may have **decelerations** which are periodic sharp drops in the heart rate. If there are decelerations, a decision may be made to deliver the baby immediately by a caesarean section.

CHAPTER 31

Breech delivery

Suvarna has just visited her obstetrician. She still has three weeks to go before her due date. Her obstetrician has told her that the baby is in breech position. Suvarna is a little concerned. Is being in the breech position harmful for the baby? What kind of delivery will she have?

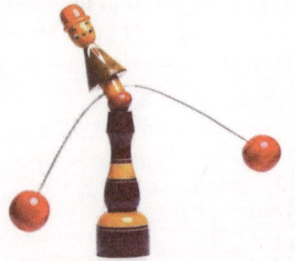

31 Breech delivery

A foetus is said to be in a **breech presentation** when the buttocks or feet of the baby are presenting first at the lowermost part of the uterus, and the head is in the upper part (fundus) of the uterus.

The baby usually reaches a stable position in the uterus by 36-37 weeks and will not move into a different position after that. By this time in pregnancy, most babies move into a head-down position. In some pregnancies, the baby's buttocks, feet or both are in the lowest position in the uterus. Most breech babies are born healthy.

Breech presentation

During the first 36 weeks, the baby is constantly changing positions - this is what is perceived as movements by the mother. In the last few weeks, the baby has less place to move around and, therefore, will not shift positions so often.

Breech presentation happens in 3-4 per cent of full-term births and requires special planning on how the baby will be born. If the baby is in a breech position, a caesarean delivery might be advised, especially if this is your first baby.

Types of breech presentation

There can be three types of breech presentations: **complete, incomplete** and **frank**. With a complete breech presentation, the buttocks are down, with the legs folded at the knees and the feet near the buttocks. If the baby is in the incomplete breech position one or both

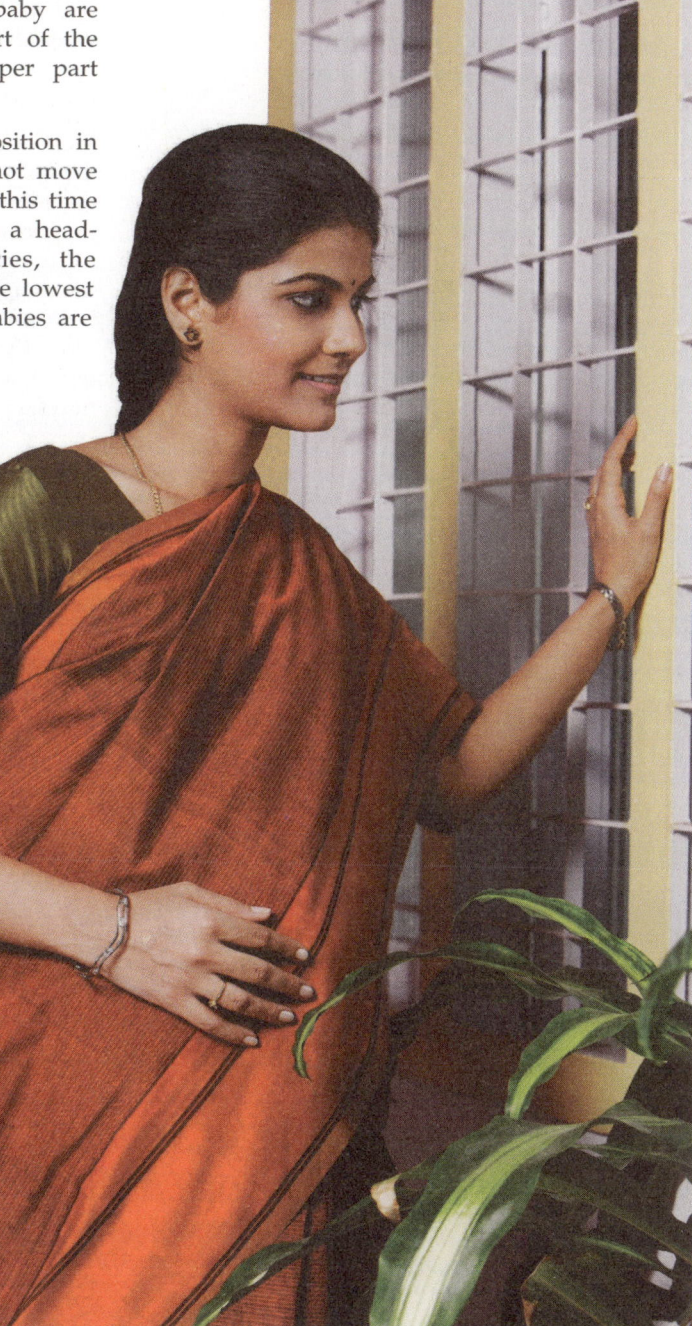

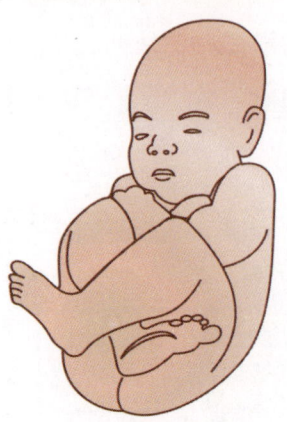
Complete breech

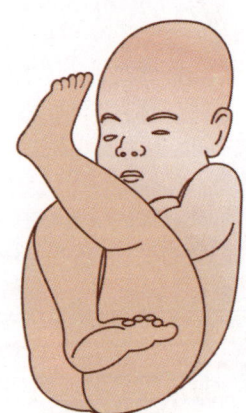
Incomplete breech

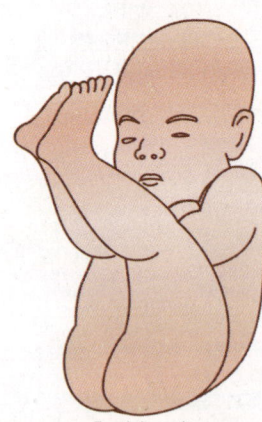
Frank breech

hips are not flexed and the feet are often below the buttocks. With a frank breech the legs are flexed at the hips and extended at the knees so the feet are up by the head. The frank breech presentation is the most common of the three and the safest position for a baby to be in if a vaginal delivery is to be attempted.

Why does breech occur?

Most of the time, there is no specific reason why the baby is in a breech position. It can be more common if the woman has had more than one pregnancy, there are twins or triplets, there is too much or too little fluid around the foetus, the uterus is not normally shaped, if the placenta is in an abnormal position or the baby is pre-term. Occasionally, the baby might have a birth defect which prevents it from getting into the normal position.

Confirming breech presentation

Every time a pregnant woman has a physical examination, the obstetrician tries to feel the position of the baby. If a breech presentation is suspected, an ultrasound exam may be done to confirm the position. Sometimes, a breech presentation is first found during a pelvic exam when the woman is in labour.

The baby's position can change till the end of pregnancy. In first pregnancies, the chances of the position changing on its own are less. If this is the second or third pregnancy, the baby will usually get into the normal head-down position spontaneously.

Changing the baby's position

If the baby is breech, your doctor may suggest **external version** which is a procedure to manipulate the baby's position into the normal

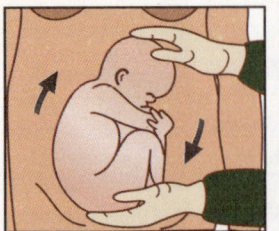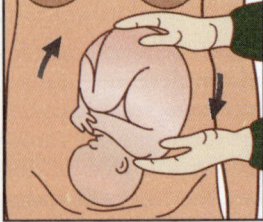

External version - turning the baby from breech to head-down position

head-down position. This increases the chance of having a vaginal birth and therefore, is highly recommended. Version is not tried until 36-37 weeks of pregnancy. If it is done before then, the baby may still go back to being a breech.

Usually medication is given to the mother which helps to relax the uterus. This may make it easier to turn the baby.

> **External version**
> The obstetrician performs a version by placing her hands on the mother's abdomen, feeling the baby's parts, and gently manipulating the baby's body into the right position. Before trying to turn the baby, an ultrasound exam is done to check the position of the baby, the position of the placenta and the amount of fluid around the baby. Scanning is done throughout the procedure to follow the position of the baby as the procedure is being done. The baby's heart rate is checked with foetal monitoring before and after version. If any problems arise with the mother or the baby, version will be stopped right away. External version succeeds in more than half the cases.

Delivery of breech

Vaginal delivery

Vaginal birth can be more difficult when a baby is breech. The risk of harm to the baby may increase in a vaginal breech birth. Particularly in a first pregnancy, the obstetrician might not recommend a vaginal delivery. If you have had a

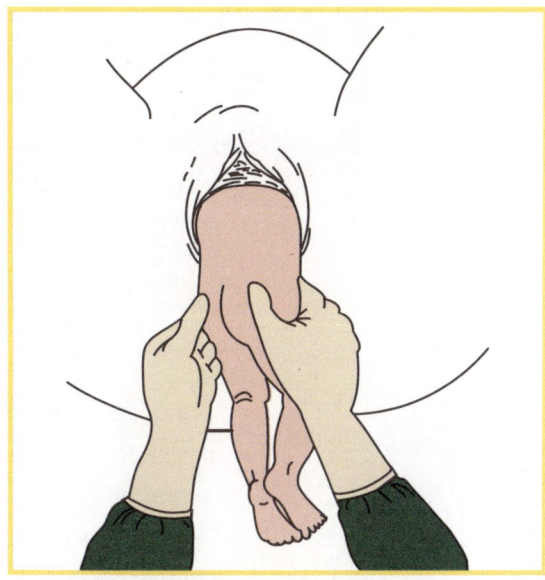
Vaginal delivery of breech

previous delivery, if the baby's position is very favourable for a vaginal delivery, and if the baby is not very large, your obstetrician might try to deliver you vaginally.

Caesarean section

If it is known that the baby is in a breech position, an elective caesarean section may be planned. If the breech presentation is discovered during labour, a decision for caesarean may depend on how far labour has progressed. Particularly in first pregnancies, a caesarean section might be the better option.

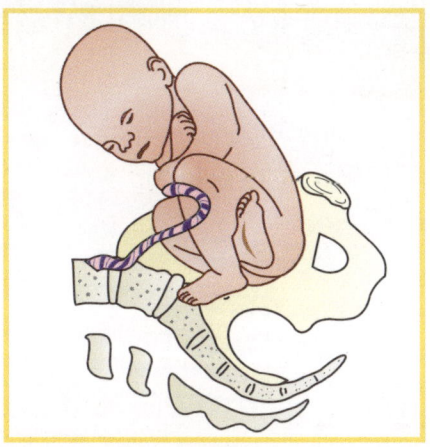
Baby in breech position

CHAPTER 32

Twin pregnancy: double trouble?

Sunanda is exhilarated and at the same time nervous. She has had an ultrasound scan and discovered she is having twins! When she saw the two little babies inside her, her heart skipped a beat and then started racing. Her husband too is thrilled at this unexpected bonus!

Sheela and her husband have been trying for a pregnancy for a few years. They had undergone treatment with medications and have now conceived after a fertility procedure. She had her pregnancy confirmed after an ultrasound scan. She too is having twins.

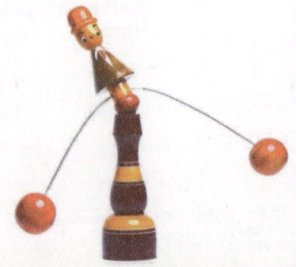

32

Twin pregnancy: double trouble?

How common is a twin pregnancy?

The chance of having **identical twins** i.e. twins from a single egg, has remained fairly constant throughout the world. One out of 250 women will have identical twins. However, the rate of having **non-identical twins or fraternal twins** i.e. twins formed from two different eggs is increasing everywhere. The chance of having fraternal twins is greater in some families.

As women are waiting longer to have babies, the increase in age triggers the increase in twinning. There is also an increase in the use of fertility drugs which boost the chance of having twins.

The advent of **IVF (in vitro fertilisation or 'test tube baby')** has also contributed to the increased rate of twins. This procedure typically involves implanting more than one embryo in the uterus and, therefore, is more likely to result in twins, triplets, quadruplets or more.

How are twins formed?

There are two different kinds of twins:

- **Identical twins** are rarer and are derived from a single fertilised egg. Identical twins may share a placenta, but each baby usually has its own **amniotic sac**. The twins will have identical genes and be of the same sex, have the same blood type, hair colour and eye colour, and are difficult to differentiate in appearance.
- **Non-identical twins or fraternal twins** are derived from two fertilised eggs released during the same menstrual cycle. These twins will have genetic differences in the same way as normal brothers and sisters. Fraternal twins have their own **placenta** and **amniotic sac**. They may or may not be of the same sex.

If a woman has triplets or more foetuses, they can be identical, fraternal or a combination of both.

Rarely, identical twins fail to completely separate into two individuals. These babies are known as **conjoined twins**.

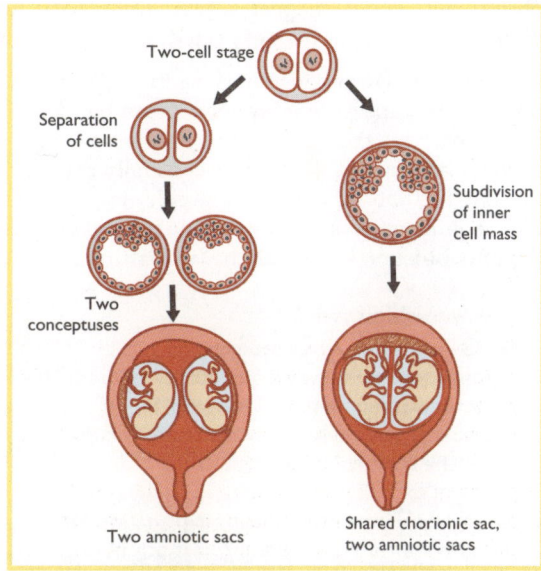

Formation of identical twins

Diagnosing a twin pregnancy

There are certain situations when your obstetrician may suspect twins:

- if there is a history of twins in your family
- if you have had twins in an earlier pregnancy
- if you have had treatment for infertility
- if your uterus appears unusually large

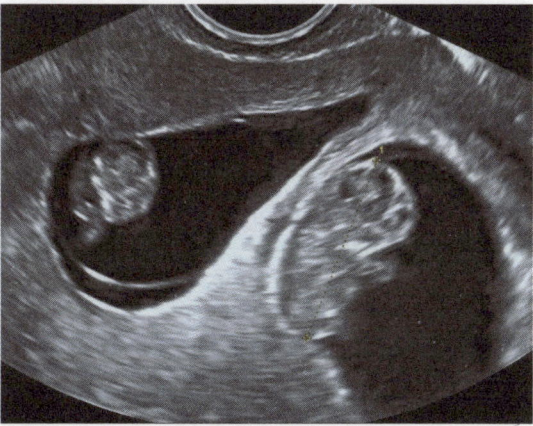

Twins at 8 weeks - two foetuses in two sacs

A twin pregnancy is almost always diagnosed before delivery. Usually it is difficult to diagnose twins in early pregnancy just from a physical examination. As the pregnancy grows, your obstetrician might suspect a twin pregnancy if your uterus is larger than expected.

A suspected twin pregnancy is confirmed with an ultrasound scan. A twin pregnancy can be identified as early as the 5th week of pregnancy. Your obstetrician may tell you that it is usually prudent to wait for one or two more weeks to confirm that it is actually a twin pregnancy because of the phenomenon known as the **'vanishing twin'**.

> **The 'vanishing twin'**
> Sometimes when an early ultrasound examination has shown the presence of twins, a repeat ultrasound done a little later in pregnancy, may reveal that there is only baby left in the uterus. The woman might or might not have experienced bleeding in early pregnancy. There is no known explanation for this phenomenon but certainly it is not because of anything you did or did not do.

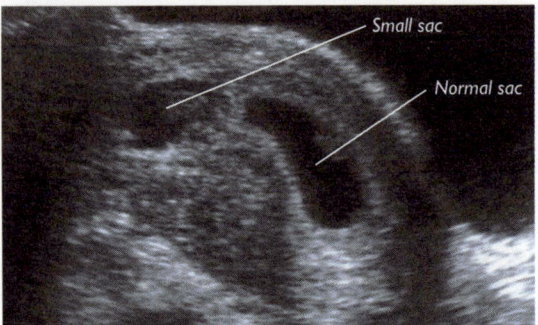

Ultrasound scan of twins in early pregnancy: the small sac on the left subsequently disappeared ('vanishing twin')

What to expect with a twin pregnancy

Having twins means that you need to take good care of yourself thus ensuring that your babies grow well and are born with the least amount of complications. Having more than one baby also means that you may have more of everything!

- **More side effects:** Due to the increased amount of hormones produced, a twin pregnancy may result in an increase in the usual pregnancy complaints, such as nausea, vomiting, heartburn, sleeplessness and tiredness. As the babies grow, the physical discomfort due to the large abdomen may result in abdominal pain, shortness of breath and pressure on the bladder. As the pregnancy progresses, you might find it difficult to find a comfortable position to sleep in.

- **More frequent check-ups:** Your obstetrician may schedule more frequent check-ups after the seventh month of pregnancy. This is to monitor the growth and development of the babies, monitor your health and watch out for signs of preterm labour.

- **More frequent ultrasound examinations** may also be advised to monitor the growth of the babies. Some twins may have a problem with growth and in some twin pregnancies one baby may grow more than the other. There are some complications which can occur specifically in twin pregnancies and these need to be carefully looked for.

- **More nutrition:** It is important for you to gain the optimal amount of weight. Eating a nutritious diet will ensure that the twins gain the right weight and are healthy at birth. When pregnant with twins, you will need to eat more than if you were carrying one baby. In addition to nurturing the babies, your diet must provide enough calories to meet your energy needs.

- **More rest:** Your obstetrician might recommend that you have more rest, particularly as you reach the seventh month of pregnancy and beyond. Due to the increased volume of the uterus, you might find it uncomfortable to move around. It is nevertheless important to be active and keep up a gentle exercise regimen. You might be asked to exert yourself less as you reach the last two months of pregnancy so that there is a lesser chance of preterm labour.

- **Anaemia** (a low blood count) is more common in women who are pregnant with twins, so it is especially important to take your prenatal vitamins and iron as prescribed. Folic acid also is important for twins. It is hard to get all the folic acid you need just from your diet, so you need to take a prenatal vitamin that contains folic acid.

The complications of a twin pregnancy

Though most twin pregnancies will progress smoothly, the risk of certain complications for both mother and child are higher. As far as the mother is concerned, there is a greater likelihood of anaemia, premature labour, high blood pressure and gestational diabetes. The babies tend to be smaller than in a pregnancy with a single foetus. There are some foetal complications which are exclusive to a twin pregnancy.

Complications for the mother

- **Premature or preterm labour:** Premature labour refers to contractions that cause the cervix to open before the 37th week of pregnancy. Most pregnancies with a single baby last 37 to 41 weeks. In a twin pregnancy, it is not unusual to go into labour between 36 and 38 weeks. You might be asked to be at rest and decrease excessive exertion from the 36th

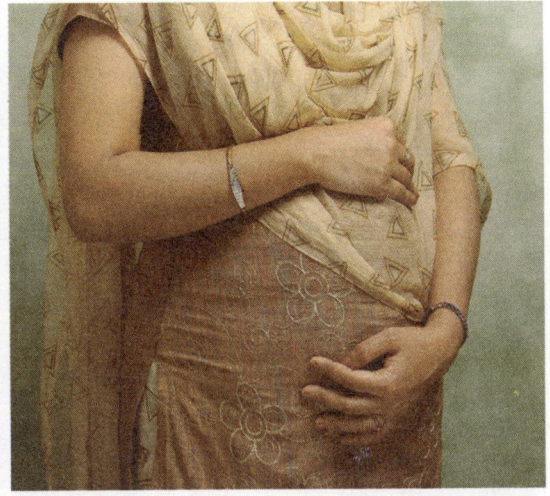

week of pregnancy. If premature labour is diagnosed early enough, delivery can sometimes be delayed with the use of medications. Postponing the birth for even a few more days can make a big difference to the babies. If you go into labour before 34 weeks, you might be given steroid injections which can help the babies' lungs mature faster so that they can breathe better after birth.

- **Premature birth:** If preterm labour cannot be prevented or stopped once it has started, the babies may be born too early. Premature or preterm birth is one of the commonest risks for twins. Twins born too early may face the same problems that any premature baby will face. **(See Chapter 29: Premature or preterm labour).**

- **High blood pressure:** A woman carrying twins has a greater risk of developing high blood pressure or preeclampsia. Preeclampsia is a condition of pregnancy in which there is

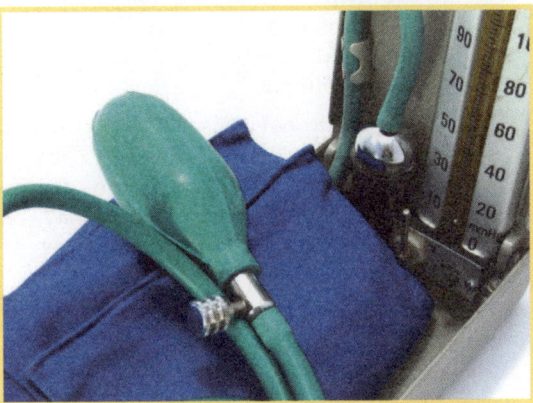

high blood pressure and protein (albumin) in the urine. Preeclampsia can be mild or severe. **(See Chapter 33: High blood pressure in pregnancy).** Preeclampsia complicating pregnancy can have harmful effects on the babies. The blood flow to the babies is reduced and this results in less oxygen and nutrients reaching the babies. Foetal growth may be affected. Preeclampsia also has deleterious effects on the mother's health. The babies may need to be delivered early if the blood pressure becomes too high.

- **Gestational diabetes:** Mothers of twins are more likely to develop gestational diabetes, a

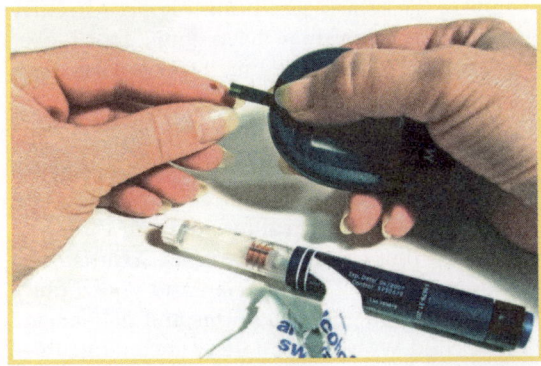

- type of diabetes that occurs only during pregnancy. Gestational diabetes may damage the placenta and increase the risk of the babies developing breathing problems at birth. **(See Chapter 34: Diabetes in pregnancy).**
- **Growth problems:** Twins are more likely to be smaller than average. Ultrasound scans are done more often in a twin pregnancy mainly to monitor the growth of the babies. The amount of amniotic fluid surrounding each baby also needs to be monitored.

  Twins are said to have **discordant growth** if one is much smaller than the other. Discordant twins are more likely to have problems during pregnancy and after birth. Twins may be discordant because of poor functioning of the placenta.
- **Twin-to-twin transfusion:** This is a rare complication and occurs only in identical twins. In this condition, a blood vessel in the placenta connects the circulatory system of one baby to the other. This causes one baby to receive too much blood and the other, too little. The twin that gives the blood ('donor twin') will be very small and have very little amniotic fluid. The other twin ('recipient twin') can have excess blood and amniotic fluid. Some of the extra fluid may need to be removed. Often, babies in this situation are delivered as soon as the benefits of early birth outweigh the potential problems of prematurity. If the condition starts early in pregnancy, there are some procedures which may be attempted to correct the condition. If the condition is severe, one or both the twins may die.
- **Loss of one twin:** In some twin pregnancies, one of the babies dies. If this happens in early pregnancy, you may have some spotting or bleeding from your vagina. This does not harm you or the other baby.

  When there is a foetal demise of one of the babies later in pregnancy, it is a more serious situation. With careful monitoring, you can often still have one healthy child. This situation is rare but can be difficult to handle. The support of your obstetrician and your family can help you go through this and deliver one live child, without any danger to your health.
- **An abnormal twin:** In some cases, an ultrasound may reveal that one of the twins is abnormal. You may still choose to carry the pregnancy to term, knowing that you can expect one normal baby. Your obstetrician will be able to guide you and counsel you about the pregnancy.

Delivery of twins

Most twins can be delivered vaginally, if the lower baby is coming down head first. A vaginal birth may be possible even when the lower twin is in the head-down position but the second twin is not. Once the first twin is born, the other twin can sometimes be turned or delivered with feet or buttocks first. When the first twin is not in the head-down position, both twins are delivered by caesarean birth.

Your obstetrician will make the decision about the type of delivery depending on the position of each baby, the weight and health of the babies. The decision will also depend on whether you are having any complications such as pre-eclampsia or gestational diabetes. Rarely, complications after the vaginal delivery of the first twin may require a caesarean section for the second twin.

Labour, especially the pushing stage, can last longer with twins. Babies usually are born several minutes apart in a vaginal delivery, but it can take longer.

Caring for newborn twins

Delivering twins is the easy part! Once you take them home, you may feel a little overwhelmed by the constant demands of two infants. You may feel exhausted and sleep deprived. Make sure you have family members to help you in the first few weeks. Get as much rest as possible. Sleep when the babies are sleeping. Also take turns with family members to handle and care for the babies.

Most twins do well at birth and can be cared for like any other healthy babies. If the babies are born prematurely, they may be kept in the nursery in the hospital after birth. Some twins may need admission to a neonatal intensive care unit.

Breastfeeding twins

Breastfeeding twins can be a challenge. You may be concerned that you may not be able to breastfeed more than one baby. Remember that mother's milk is the best food for any infant. It has the right amount of all the nutrients the baby needs. When you breastfeed, your milk supply will increase to meet the amount needed by your babies. You will need to eat healthy foods and drink plenty of liquids. If you are exhausted and feel that you are not be able to breast feed both babies despite your best efforts, your paediatrician may prescribe a milk supplement so that you can alternate between breast feeding and supplement.

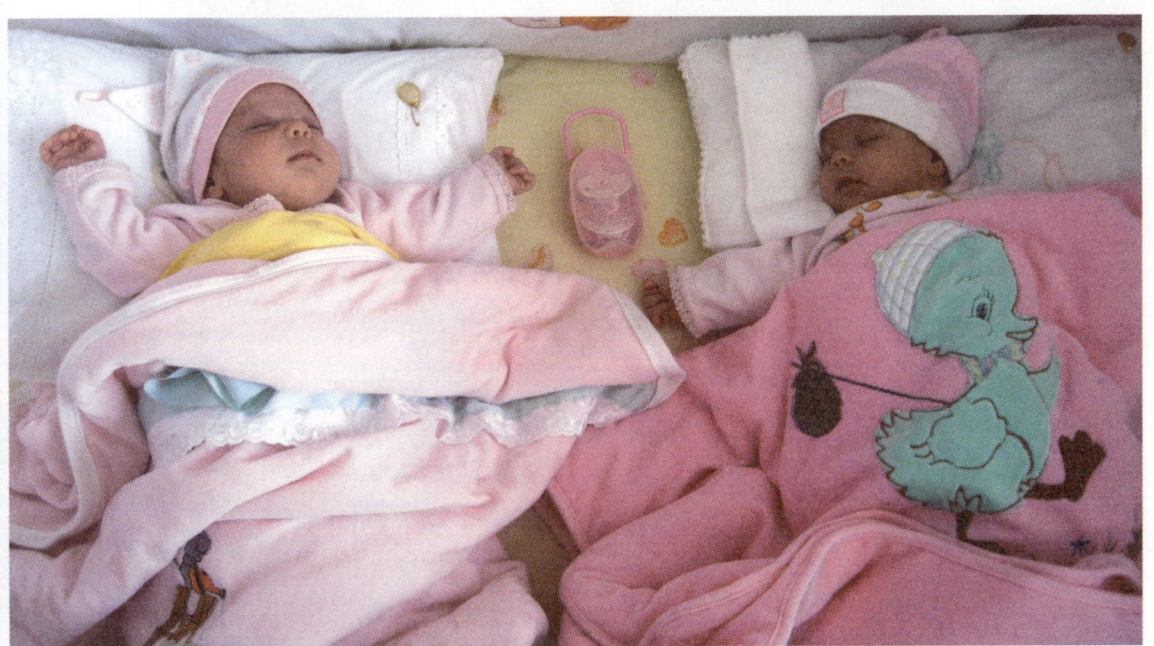

Names for twins

If you are having twins, use your imagination and name the babies with something unique! Some parents choose to name the twins with rhyming or interlinked names.

Some examples for a boy and girl combination are Maya and Mayank, Michael and Michelle, Neel and Neelanjana.

Two girls could be called Archita and Rachita, Manasa and Madhuri, or Devyani and Devanshi.

Two boys could be called Vinay and Vijay, Tarun and Varun or Manav and Pranav.

What a great opportunity to come up with something appealing and attention-grabbing!

CHAPTER 33

High blood pressure in pregnancy

Sabrina has just come back from a check-up with her doctor. She is 34 weeks pregnant and her blood pressure was 140/90. Her doctor has told her to rest and come back after two days to check her blood pressure again. Sabrina is naturally concerned. How will the high blood pressure affect her and her baby?

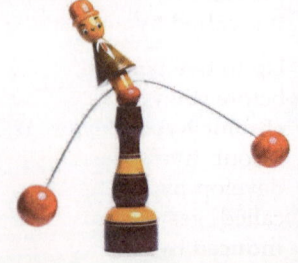

High blood pressure in pregnancy

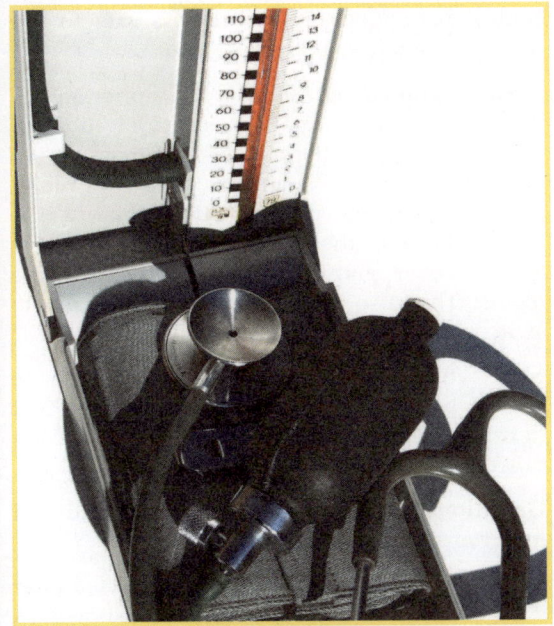

One of the important steps in every antenatal check-up is the measurement of your blood pressure. Why is this done? Having a normal blood pressure is an important component of good health at any time of life. In pregnancy too, a normal blood pressure through the course of the pregnancy will ensure good health for you and the baby.

What is blood pressure?

Blood pressure is the force of the blood pushing against the walls of the arteries. Arteries are blood vessels that carry oxygen-rich blood from the heart to all parts of the body. **When the pressure in the arteries goes beyond a set limit, it is called hypertension.**

Up to five per cent of women have hypertension before they become pregnant. This is called **chronic hypertension** or **essential hypertension**. About five to eight per cent of women will develop hypertension during pregnancy. This is called **gestational hypertension** or **pregnancy induced hypertension (PIH)**.

Hypertension during pregnancy can cause complications for mother and baby. Fortunately, serious problems usually can be prevented with proper prenatal care.

Your blood pressure reading

Blood pressure varies from person to person. It may even change with the time of day. It can increase if you are excited or if you exercise. It decreases when you are resting. These short-term changes in blood pressure are normal. When your blood pressure stays persistently high, even after being checked two or three times, you are said to have **high blood pressure** or **hypertension**.

In most pregnant women, readings of 120/80 or less are normal. If you are pregnant and your systolic pressure is 140 or the diastolic pressure is 90 on two or more readings, you are considered to have high blood pressure.

If you have one high reading, another reading will be taken at least six hours later. If your diastolic blood pressure is persistently over 90, then you will be considered to have hypertension in pregnancy.

A blood pressure reading has two numbers, separated by a slash: for example, 110/80 (referred to as "110 by 80.") The first number is the pressure in the arteries when the heart contracts. This is called the **systolic pressure.** The second number is the pressure in the arteries when the heart relaxes between contractions. This is the **diastolic pressure.**

110	Systolic	Pressure in arteries when heart contracts
80	Diastolic	Pressure in arteries when heart relaxes

How does hypertension affect pregnancy?

When the mother has a normal blood pressure, the blood flow through the placenta remains normal. This enables the growing foetus to get all the necessary nutrients and oxygen from the mother.

High blood pressure in pregnancy can cause:

- **Intrauterine growth restriction (IUGR):** When high blood pressure occurs in pregnancy, the placenta is often abnormal and the blood flow through the placenta is affected. This effectively means that the baby is receiving less nutrients and oxygen. This in turn causes growth restriction in the foetus, sometimes resulting in **low birth weight.** This effect is seen most severely in women who develop hypertension before 32 weeks of pregnancy or those who have uncontrolled chronic hypertension.
- **Premature or preterm delivery:** Hypertension also increases the risk of premature delivery (before 37 weeks of pregnancy).
- **Premature and low birth weight babies** face an increased risk of health problems during the newborn period and may have lasting disabilities, such as learning problems and cerebral palsy. (See Chapter 29: Premature or preterm labour).

Types of high blood pressure in pregnancy

Chronic hypertension

Chronic hypertension is high blood pressure that has been present for some time before pregnancy or that is diagnosed before the 20th week of pregnancy. It is also called **essential hypertension.** This form of hypertension will persist even after the delivery. The causes of chronic hypertension are not clearly understood, although heredity, obesity, diet and lifestyle may play a role.

During pregnancy, chronic hypertension may also affect the growth of the foetus. If you have been taking medications before pregnancy to control your blood pressure, ask your doctor if it is safe to use them during pregnancy. Some women with chronic hypertension can stop taking medication during pregnancy because their blood pressure returns to normal. Other women need to continue treatment during their pregnancies. In some cases, a woman may need to switch to a different medication that still helps control her blood pressure but is safe to use during pregnancy.

Preconceptional counselling: It is important for women who have hypertension prior to pregnancy to see their physician before attempting to conceive. This will ensure that the blood pressure is well under control before the pregnancy and therefore, will have the least amount of negative impact on the growing foetus. This also will allow your physician to switch you to a drug that is safe in pregnancy.

Most women with chronic hypertension have healthy pregnancies. However, about 25 per cent develop a form of gestational hypertension called **preeclampsia,** which poses special risks.

Gestational hypertension or pregnancy induced hypertension (PIH)

When high blood pressure is first detected after the 20th week of pregnancy, it is known as gestational hypertension. This kind of blood pressure usually returns to normal once the baby is born. In fact, in severe gestational hypertension, delivering the baby (even if it is premature) may be the only way of treating the condition.

Once high blood pressure is detected in pregnancy, you will be required to see your obstetrician more often to monitor the blood pressure. When gestational hypertension is associated with certain other signs, it is called **preeclampsia.** Gestational hypertension may lead to preeclampsia and can jeopardise the health of the mother and the baby.

Preeclampsia

To this day, it is not clear why some women develop preeclampsia. Earlier, preeclampsia was also referred to as **toxaemia of pregnancy.** Preeclampsia can occur anytime after the 20th week of pregnancy and up to six weeks after the baby is born.

When gestational hypertension is associated with one or more of the following signs, then the condition is called preeclampsia:

- Protein (albumin) in the urine
- Persistent headache
- Visual problems like blurring, double vision
- Rapid weight gain
- Swelling (oedema) of the hands and face
- Pain in the upper right part of the abdomen

Who is at risk for developing preeclampsia?

Women are at risk of developing preeclampsia if they:

- Are pregnant for the first time
- Have had preeclampsia in a previous pregnancy
- Have a history of chronic hypertension
- Have twins or triplets
- Are 35 years or older
- Are diabetic
- Have kidney disease
- Are overweight
- Have antiphospholipid antibody syndrome

Eclampsia

When preeclampsia becomes severe, the woman's organs can be damaged, including the kidneys, liver, brain, heart and eyes. In some cases, seizures (fits) will occur. This is called **eclampsia**. This is a severe and dangerous situation for both the mother and the baby. Immediate delivery is sometimes the only way of saving the mother. Fortunately, eclampsia is rare in women who receive regular antenatal care.

Management of hypertension in pregnancy

Antenatal care

Women who already have blood pressure before pregnancy should bring their blood pressure to normal levels before proceeding with a pregnancy. They should have blood tests to make sure that their kidneys are functioning well.

At each antenatal visit, a woman's weight, blood pressure and a urine sample (to check for protein) are taken. This helps in catching the earliest changes that might occur. Once high blood pressure is detected in pregnancy, you will be required to see your obstetrician more often to monitor the blood pressure. If the blood pressure does not come down to normal levels, you might even be admitted to the hospital for a few days for blood pressure control with medications.

Treatment

Bed rest

If there is only a mild increase in blood pressure, and you are not close to your due date, you might be advised rest at home. The best is to lie on your side for an hour after breakfast, two hours after lunch and to lie mostly on your sides in the night. Of course, this may not be possible if you are a working woman, so you might need to take a week or two off.

> There will be no change prescribed in the diet. Salt restriction is only advised for women with chronic hypertension. Women who have developed hypertension in pregnancy need not cut down on their salt, except avoiding very salty food like pickles and chips.

Blood pressure medications

If the blood pressure does not get under control with these measures, you might be prescribed blood pressure medications. There are medications which are safe for both you and your baby.

If the blood pressure is abnormally high, you might be admitted to the hospital and your

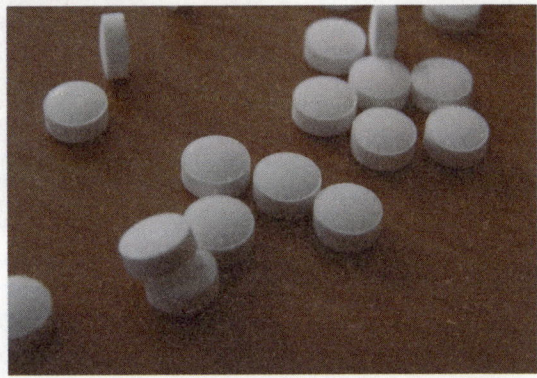

medications will be monitored till the optimal dose is reached. If the blood pressure does not increase to dangerous levels, and if you do not develop preeclampsia, pregnancy may be allowed to continue until labour begins naturally.

HELLP syndrome

About 10 per cent of women with severe preeclampsia also develop a disorder called HELLP (Haemolysis, Elevated Liver enzymes, and Low Platelet count) syndrome, which is characterised by blood and liver abnormalities. Symptoms may include nausea and vomiting, headache, upper abdominal pain and general malaise. HELLP syndrome is a life threatening condition. Women who develop HELLP syndrome during pregnancy require intensive monitoring. They almost always require immediate delivery to prevent serious complications.

Monitoring the foetus

Your baby's well-being will be closely monitored with tests such as ultrasound and foetal heart rate monitoring. The ultrasound scans will show how well your baby is growing and if the high blood pressure is having any adverse effects on it. The amount of amniotic fluid around the baby will also be monitored.

Delivery

The decision on when to deliver depends on the severity of the condition and the duration of the pregnancy. If a woman is at term (37 to 40 weeks), the preeclampsia is mild and her cervix has begun to thin and dilate (signs that she is ready for delivery), her obstetrician will consider inducing labour. If the cervix is not yet ready for labour, medication may be used to ripen the cervix before inducing labour.

Sometimes, despite treatment, the blood pressure will continue to rise. If you have **severe preeclampsia,** you will be hospitalised, whatever the week of pregnancy you are in. If there is persistent protein (albumin) in the urine, the blood pressure is very high or if the foetus shows signs of being affected by the condition, a decision will be taken to deliver the baby. The risk of prematurity is outweighed by the risk of progression to eclampsia. **Eclampsia is a life threatening condition and is best avoided.**

If you are between 28 and 34 weeks of pregnancy and your obstetrician has made a decision to go ahead with the delivery, you will be given steroid injections which will help increase the

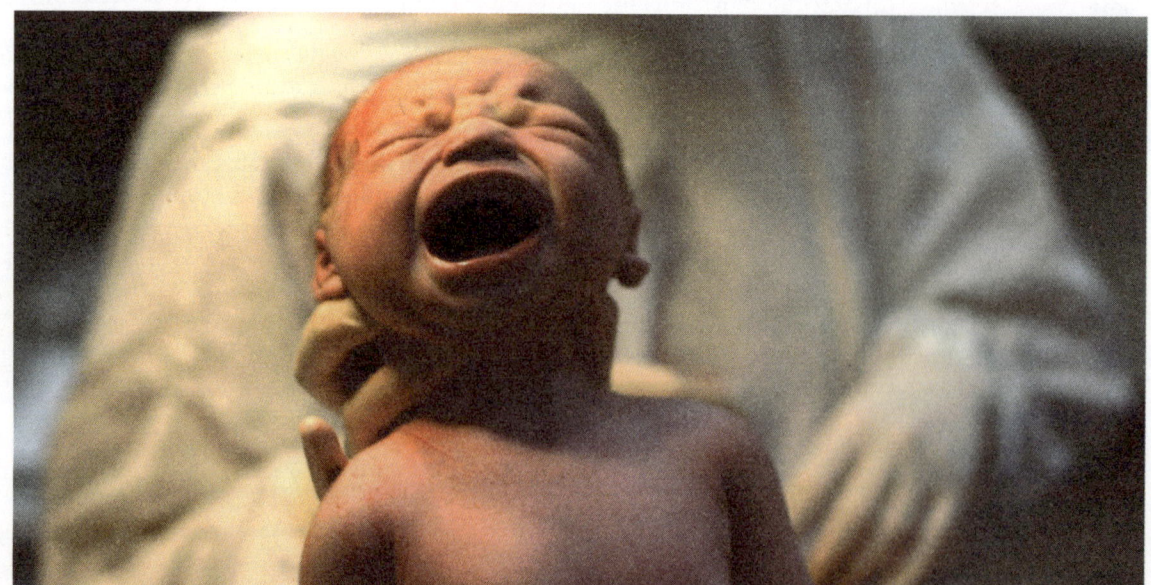

maturity of the lungs of the foetus. This will make it easier for the baby to breathe once it is born. Most premature babies have to be monitored carefully in a newborn nursery.

Since in most cases, delivery of the baby is the "cure" for preeclampsia, either labour will be induced or a caesarean section will be done (if the conditions are not favourable or the foetus cannot tolerate labour).

Is preeclampsia likely to recur in another pregnancy?

Only about 20 per cent of women who have developed preeclampsia after the 37th week of pregnancy develop it again. The risk of recurrence appears to be highest when preeclampsia has occurred before the 30th week of gestation and, in some cases, may be as high as 65 per cent in another pregnancy.

Can preeclampsia and gestational hypertension be prevented?

Since nobody really knows why high blood pressure occurs in pregnancy, currently, there is no way to prevent gestational hypertension or preeclampsia. However, the complications arising from high blood pressure in pregnancy can be minimised with regular antenatal check-ups and appropriate intervention.

Women who had developed high blood pressure before 34 weeks of pregnancy in an earlier pregnancy may be started on **low dose aspirin (50-80 mg per day)** in the first trimester to prevent recurrence of high blood pressure in the present pregnancy. Women who already have high blood pressure before they become pregnant may also be started on low dose aspirin in early pregnancy to prevent the development of preeclampsia.

CHAPTER 34

Diabetes and pregnancy

Sunanda is in her 28th week of pregnancy and has just been told that she has developed diabetes in pregnancy. Diabetes that develops or is first detected in pregnancy is known as gestational diabetes.

Sunetra, on the other hand, has been a diabetic for the past three years. She is 29 and pregnant for the first time.

Both of them may expect some problems in pregnancy if the sugar levels are not kept under good control. However, if they follow instructions and the appropriate treatment, they both have a good chance of delivering a healthy baby.

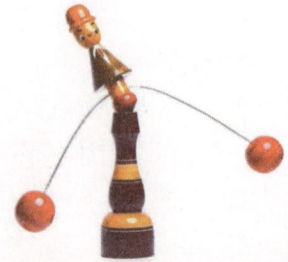

34 Diabetes and pregnancy

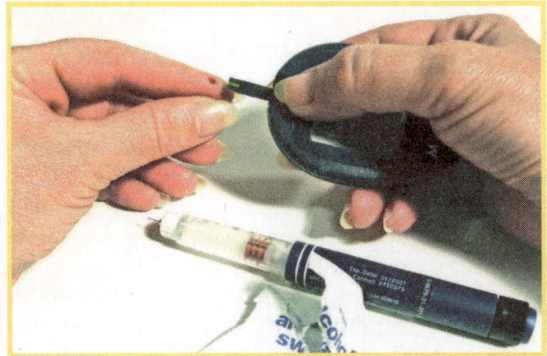

Gestational diabetes

Diabetes caused by pregnancy is known as **gestational diabetes.** Gestational diabetes can develop during pregnancy in a woman who has not previously had the condition. It is becoming more common in Indian women and may affect more than 10 per cent of pregnant women. Unless properly controlled, it can lead to problems for both the mother and her baby.

Insulin is the hormone which normally controls blood sugars. It enables the body to break down sugar (glucose) to be used as energy. Without sufficient insulin, the level of sugar in the blood rises. During pregnancy, the placenta produces certain hormones that prevent insulin from working well. They cause what is known as **insulin resistance.** Insulin resistance can lead to diabetes during pregnancy.

> Developing diabetes in pregnancy is a warning that you might develop diabetes in later life. It is important not to take this lightly. If you stick to a healthy diet, walk daily and maintain the appropriate weight for your height, you can prevent the development of full blown diabetes.

Gestational diabetes usually begins in the second half of pregnancy. The blood sugar levels, as a rule, return to normal after the baby is born. Nevertheless, it is important to remember that developing gestational diabetes is a warning that a woman may develop full-blown diabetes later on in life. To avoid this, she must make definite lifestyle modifications.

What increases the chances of developing diabetes in pregnancy?

Indians, as a race, are at high risk for developing diabetes in pregnancy. The risk of developing gestational diabetes increases with

- age over 25
- being overweight prior to pregnancy
- a family history of diabetes
- a history of diabetes in a previous pregnancy
- a big baby in a previous pregnancy
- a history of a stillbirth late in pregnancy
- high cholesterol
- polycystic ovarian syndrome

Will you know if you have gestational diabetes?

Unfortunately, in most women, gestational diabetes causes no symptoms. It is a silent disease and is usually discovered only following a blood test. All women should be tested for diabetes in pregnancy.

How is gestational diabetes diagnosed?

At every antenatal check-up, urine is routinely tested for sugar. If there is sugar detected in the urine, you will be tested to see if your blood sugar levels are abnormal.

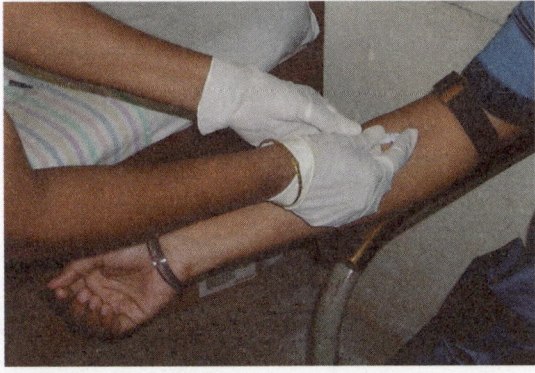

Blood tests (glucose tolerance tests):

Your obstetrician will administer the glucose tolerance test between **24 and 28 weeks of pregnancy.** You do not have to be on an empty stomach for this test. The **50 gm oral glucose tolerance test** involves drinking a glucose solution. After waiting one hour, blood is taken from a vein in the arm and the glucose level is checked. If your glucose level is **less than 140 mg/dl,** you are considered not to have gestational diabetes and no further testing is done.

If the glucose level is **above 140 mg/dl,** there is a chance that you might have gestational diabetes. To confirm this, a **three-hour 100 gm glucose tolerance test** will be performed. You are advised not to eat or drink anything except water for about 12 hours before the test. A fasting blood sample is first taken. This blood sample is used to determine the fasting glucose level. You are given a 100 gm glucose solution to drink. Blood will be drawn every hour for three hours after the drink has been consumed. If two or more of the glucose levels are higher than the normal values, a diagnosis of gestational diabetes can be made.

If your obstetrician believes that you are at high risk for developing gestational diabetes, this test may be carried out earlier than 24-28 weeks.

If you have had gestational diabetes in an earlier pregnancy, your blood sugars will be checked at your first antenatal check up and if normal, will be repeated at frequent intervals during your pregnancy.

Why you should be concerned

Diabetes in pregnancy can have a deleterious effect both on the growing foetus and the mother unless the blood sugar levels are kept well under control.

Diabetes before pregnancy

If you have diabetes before pregnancy, you must be particularly careful about keeping your blood sugar levels well under control before you try for a pregnancy. Despite medical advances, babies born to women with diabetes, especially women with poor control of diabetes, are still at greater risk for **birth defects.**

A growing foetus is particularly vulnerable in the first few weeks of pregnancy, when its organs are forming. Since most women will not know they are pregnant until the baby has been growing for two to four weeks, high blood sugars at this stage can be harmful to the baby. For this reason, good blood glucose control before you get pregnant is very important.

Pre-pregnancy counselling: If you are a diabetic, it is essential for you to have pre-pregnancy counselling. Your pregnancy must be planned and your blood sugar levels must be made optimal. If your blood sugar levels are not under good control, work to bring your diabetes under control before getting pregnant. It is a good idea to be in good blood glucose control three to six months before you plan to get pregnant. You might be switched from oral medication to insulin when you start planning a pregnancy.

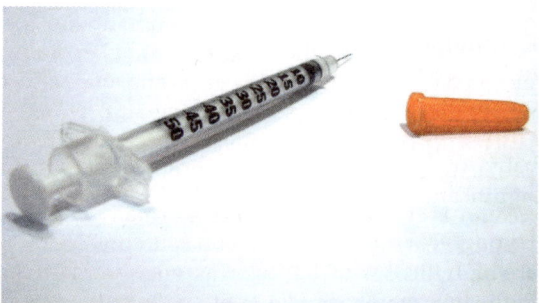

Some oral medications for diabetes are not considered safe in pregnancy. You might be advised to start insulin injections, or switched to another medication.

Effect of diabetes on the baby

Macrosomia: When the mother's blood sugars are high, the baby's weight and growth may be excessive, leading to an **overweight** or **big baby.** How do high blood glucose levels cause problems? The extra sugar circulating in your blood is absorbed by the baby. All this excess sugar can make the baby excessively big and fat. This in turn may cause complications during labour. The chance of caesarean section increases because the baby may be too big to be born through the normal birth passage.

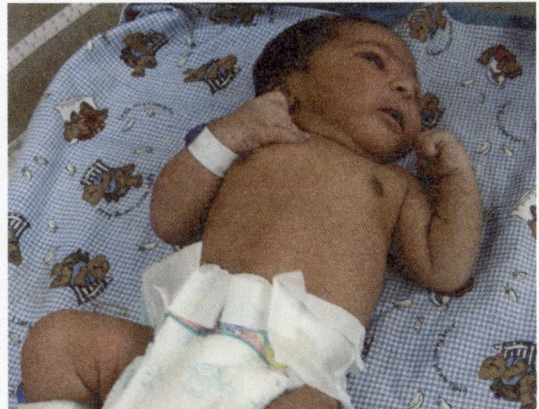

Large baby born to a diabetic mother.

Polyhydramnios: The water surrounding the baby (amniotic fluid) may also increase significantly due to the diabetes and this can lead to premature labour and premature delivery.

Respiratory distress after birth: There is an increased chance of the baby developing breathing difficulties (respiratory distress) after birth. The lungs do not mature on time in the baby of a diabetic mother. This may cause significant difficulty in breathing.

Hypoglycaemia: When your blood sugar levels are high, the foetus also gets extra sugar. To deal with this, the foetus produces extra insulin. Immediately after birth, the baby continues to produce extra insulin. This extra circulating insulin can cause low blood sugars or hypoglycaemia. The baby must be monitored, and treated if the blood glucose level drops too low.

Hyperbilirubinaemia (newborn jaundice): For some reason, newborn jaundice occurs more often in babies of women with diabetes. Jaundice is a build-up of old red blood cells that the body is unable to process in the normal manner. This problem can be treated by placing the baby under special lights which help the jaundice pigments get absorbed faster. This is called 'phototherapy'. (See page 254).

Stillbirth (delivery of a baby that has died before birth) occurs more often in babies of women whose diabetes was not well controlled before and during pregnancy.

It is important to remember that having gestational diabetes does not mean that the baby will have diabetes at birth.

Effect of diabetes on the mother

Gestational diabetes is not an immediate threat to your health. Most women with gestational diabetes, whose blood sugar levels stay within the safe range, deliver their babies without complications.

Women who develop diabetes in pregnancy also have a greater risk of developing high blood pressure. This is called **pregnancy induced hypertension or PIH. (See Chapter 33: High blood pressure in pregnancy).**

As mentioned earlier, if you get gestational diabetes, you are more likely to develop gestational diabetes in future pregnancies. You are also at a higher risk of developing **type II diabetes** (non-insulin dependent diabetes) later in life.

Managing diabetes in pregnancy

Controlling sugar levels

In gestational diabetes, the key to a good pregnancy outcome is maintaining blood sugars in the normal range. This reduces the risk of complications. Your sugar levels must be maintained at less than 100 mg/dl in the fasting state and less than 140 mg/dl 1 hour after a meal (or 120 mg/dl 2 hours after a meal). Dietary modification and exercise will help to control blood sugars initially. If this alone is not enough, then insulin injections may be needed.

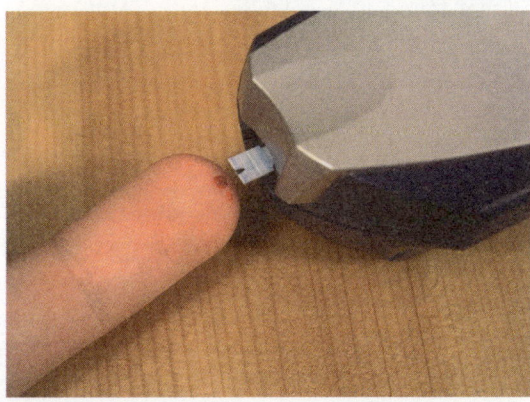

Doctors usually advise blood glucose testing once a week, although for some women this may need to be done more often. Glucose needs to be measured in the morning before breakfast and again one or two hours after breakfast. Some women, especially those on insulin, may need to test levels before and after each meal till the dose of insulin is stabilised.

> **Home glucose testing kits (glucometers)** are available now. These usually involve taking a tiny blood sample with a pinprick device. The blood is put on to a strip and inserted into the glucometer, which gives the blood glucose level.

Diet

Remember, a diabetic diet is an extremely healthy diet. Everyone can follow this diet. The basic principles you have to follow are:

- Avoid sugar and sweets completely. This includes the sugar in your tea or coffee. Honey and jaggery should also be avoided.

- The carbohydrate content in your meals should be reduced. This means that you will have to reduce the quantity of rice, wheat and other cereals. Wheat or ragi can be substituted for rice at one or two meals. It is the total calorie restriction which is important.

- Increasing fibre is also helpful. Fibre includes that found in vegetables, and also in carbohydrates like wheat, oats, ragi, soya and barley.

- You are allowed to eat only certain fruits. These have to be restricted to a small apple, guava or orange or 1/3 cup pomegranate.

- A low fat diet is helpful as it prevents excess weight gain. This means avoiding deep fried food, ghee, butter and coconut.

- You do need a certain minimum number of calories, so an appropriate diet chart will be given to you by the dietitian. Eating too little is also not good for the baby.

Exercise

Any activity that keeps you moving, and gets your heart rate up (what is referred to as aerobic activity), is helpful as it makes your insulin work better. Walking for a minimum of 30-45 minutes daily is necessary. This can be done at any time, morning or night, or can be split up. If you are on insulin, have a discussion with your doctor before you start a vigorous exercise programme.

Insulin

Despite making the above lifestyle changes, blood sugar levels may remain high. In such a situation, you may need daily injections of **insulin.** You might need to be admitted for a few days to the hospital initially to adjust the dose of insulin. Your obstetrician will usually refer you to a physician or endocrinologist who deals with diabetic patients on a regular basis.

The amount of insulin needed to control glucose levels throughout the day varies from woman to woman and depends on many factors. Your doctor will tell you how to use insulin and how many daily injections you will need. The number of injections and dose of insulin you need may change as the baby grows. When insulin is needed to control diabetes during pregnancy, the diet and the insulin dose must be balanced at all times to prevent harmful levels of glucose. Any woman who needs to take insulin can easily be taught how to take it herself.

Sometimes, a slightly higher dose can cause low blood sugar (**hypoglycaemia**). Common symptoms of this are weakness, shaking, hunger and sweating. For women taking insulin, it is a good idea to keep a snack handy at all times in case low blood sugar develops.

> Many pregnant women are worried that insulin will affect the baby. The insulin will not cross the placenta and will not affect the baby. On the other hand, the good control of your blood sugar levels with insulin will ensure that your baby will be healthy.

Managing pregnancy with diabetes

As mentioned earlier, the baby of a diabetic mother has chances of developing problems (see page 204). To make sure the baby is doing fine, some or all of these tests will be done during the pregnancy:

- Regular monitoring of your blood sugar levels.
- Ultrasound examination of the baby at regular intervals to make sure the baby is neither too big (macrosomia) nor too small (intrauterine growth restriction). The fluid around the baby will also be monitored closely.

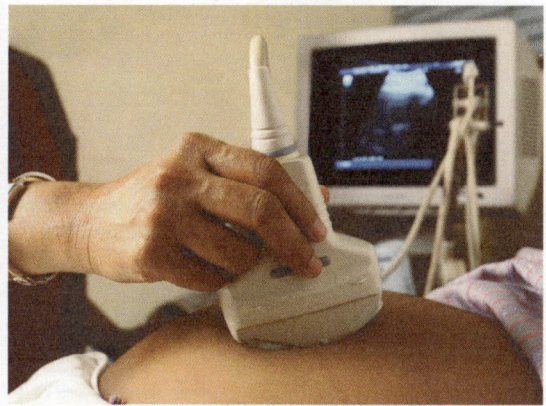

- Recording of the baby's heartbeat (electronic foetal monitoring) closer to the due date.

Delivery

If you have diabetes which has been well controlled with just a diet and exercise regimen, and the baby does not have any complications, your obstetrician will wait for you to go into labour. If you or the baby has any complications, then a caesarean may be decided upon.

If you are on insulin to control your sugar levels, then labour may be induced between 37 to 38 weeks. If there are any other complications, then a caesarean may be done between 37 to 38 weeks.

Your blood glucose levels will be monitored and kept under control during labour and delivery.

After delivery

If you are a gestational diabetic, your sugar levels will come back to normal immediately after delivery. You will be asked to check your blood sugars 6-8 weeks after the baby is born.

If you were a diabetic before you became pregnant, you may not need as much insulin as you were taking during pregnancy.

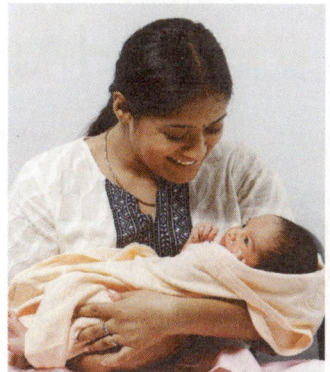

Breastfeeding

Breastfeeding is good for your baby. It is also good for you because women who breast feed use up more calories. During the first weeks at home with the baby, you are likely to be tired and stressed from lack of sleep. If you are still on insulin, it might be a little difficult to get back on schedule. Low blood glucose is a real danger.

To help prevent low blood glucose levels due to breastfeeding:

- Plan to have a snack before or during nursing
- Drink enough fluids
- Keep a snack nearby to treat low blood glucose when you nurse, so you do not have to stop feeding to treat hypoglycaemia

Contraception

Women with diabetes or those who develop gestational diabetes must plan future pregnancies with care. It is smart to begin using a form of birth control after a reasonable interval following delivery. In general, women with diabetes can use most of the available methods. At your first postnatal check-up, discuss with your obstetrician which method would be best for you.

Preventing diabetes

You can prevent diabetes by:

- Maintaining your weight close to the ideal for your height.
- Exercising regularly: this has been shown to decrease the chances of developing diabetes. Walking briskly for 30-45 minutes daily has consistently been proved to cut down the risk of diabetes.
- Staying on a healthy diet.

CHAPTER 35

Rh factor: how can it affect pregnancy?

Srinidhi is pregnant for the first time. She knew that she was Rh negative. When she went for her first antenatal check-up, her obstetrician tested her husband and found that he was Rh positive. Srinidhi and her husband had many questions. Would this difference in their Rh factor affect the baby? Would she have to take any precautions? Would this affect her next pregnancy? Srinidhi and her husband need not worry.

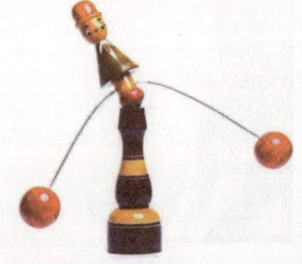

35 Rh factor: how can it affect pregnancy?

The Rh factor

There are four blood groups: **A, B, AB,** and **O.** Each of the four blood groups is additionally classified according to the presence of another protein (antigen) on the surface of red blood cells that indicates the **Rh factor.** If this antigen is present, you are classified as being **Rh positive.** If this antigen is absent, you are considered **Rh negative.**

About 85 per cent of Indians are Rh positive. This percentage varies in some ethnic communities. If a woman who is Rh negative and a man who is Rh positive conceive a baby, there is the potential for the baby to have a problem during pregnancy.

Approximately half of the children born to an Rh-negative mother and Rh-positive father will be Rh positive. The problem arises only if the baby developing inside the Rh-negative mother has Rh-positive blood, inherited from the father. This problem is called **Rh incompatibility.** Luckily, Rh incompatibility has a harmful effect in only 10 per cent of women who are affected.

Rh incompatibility usually does not lead to a problem in the first pregnancy. In the subsequent pregnancies, however, problems can arise for the foetus.

> If a pregnant woman is Rh negative, her foetus can be Rh positive only if the father is Rh positive. If both the mother and the father are Rh negative, there is no chance that the foetus will be Rh positive. The mother therefore does not run the risk of sensitisation.

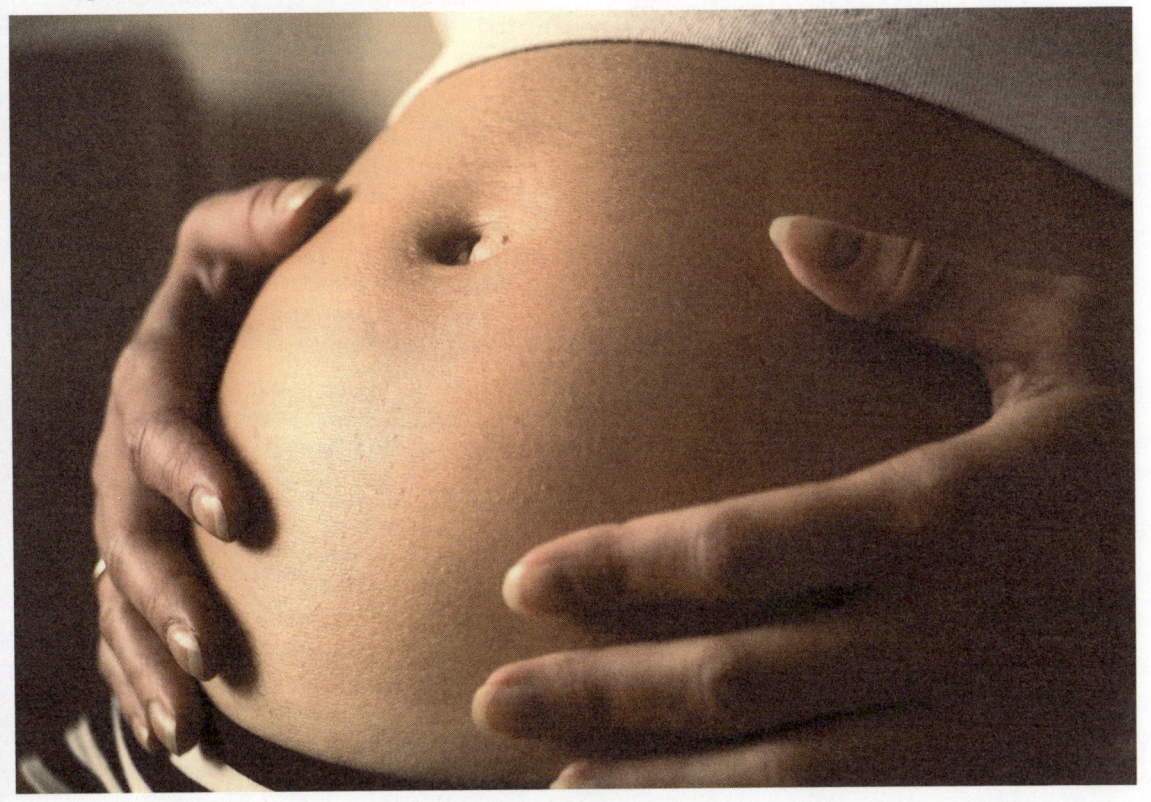

What is Rh sensitisation?

The exposure of an Rh negative woman to Rh positive blood is called **sensitisation.** During delivery, the mother's and baby's blood can get mixed. If the baby is Rh positive, the problem arises when his blood enters the mother's blood stream. The mother's body identifies the Rh protein as a harmful substance and will begin producing **antibodies.** These antibodies are protein molecules in the immune system that recognise, and later cause destruction of any Rh positive blood cells they encounter.

> Rh incompatibility will usually not affect the first pregnancy - it will only cause problems in subsequent pregnancies. These problems can be prevented by the mother taking an Rh immunoglobulin injection within 72 hours after the birth of the baby.

What is the effect of Rh sensitisation?

When the mother has become sensitised and has developed Rh antibodies, the antibodies attack the red blood cells of the baby in the subsequent pregnancy. This swelling and rupture of the red blood cells is called **haemolysis.** If this happens, the baby's blood count can get dangerously low. This can lead to severe **foetal anaemia** while the baby is still inside the uterus. If the condition is mild, the baby may survive during pregnancy but may develop anaemia and jaundice after birth. This is called **Rh disease of the newborn.**

> **What if the father is Rh negative and the mother Rh positive?**
>
> If the father is Rh negative and the mother is Rh positive, sensitisation does not occur. There is no effect on the baby.

Other conditions causing Rh sensitisation

Rh-negative pregnant women can be exposed to the Rh protein that might cause antibody production in other situations too:

- Blood transfusions with Rh-positive blood
- Miscarriage or induced abortion
- Ectopic pregnancy
- Invasive prenatal procedures like chorionic villus sampling (CVS) or amniocentesis
- Significant bleeding during pregnancy

Preventing Rh sensitisation

The most important step in preventing Rh disease is by preventing the formation of Rh antibodies. This is done by giving an injection of **Rh immunoglobulin (Anti-D)** immediately after an event where foetal blood can mix with the mother's blood e.g. delivery, abortion, ectopic pregnancy or prenatal procedures. Rh immunoglobulin is a blood product that can prevent an Rh-negative mother from being sensitised. It prevents her body from responding to Rh-positive blood cells of the foetus. Rh immunoglobulin can prevent sensitisation in almost all cases.

> If you are Rh negative, an injection of Rh immunoglobulin must be given if you have had a miscarriage, have undergone an induced abortion, have an ectopic pregnancy or have had significant bleeding in the pregnancy.

Before giving the Rh immunoglobulin, the mother is always tested for the presence of antibodies. **Rh immunoglobulin will be effective only if the mother has not developed antibodies.** This simple blood test is called an **indirect Coomb's test.** If a woman has antibodies in her blood, the test will be called positive. If she has no Rh antibodies, then the indirect Coomb's test will be negative.

Rh immunoglobulin is injected into a muscle of the arm or buttocks. Occasionally there might be swelling or pain over the site of the injection.

Timing of Rh immunoglobulin

During pregnancy and after delivery

If a woman with Rh negative blood has not been sensitised (as shown by the absence of Rh antibodies in her blood), the doctor may suggest that she receive an Anti-D injection around the 28th week of pregnancy to prevent sensitisation for the rest of the pregnancy. This prevents problems in the small number of women who can become sensitised during the last three months of pregnancy. Because of the cost of the injection, some doctors might suggest not taking the injection at the 28th week but might wait till after the delivery of the baby.

As soon as the baby is born to an Rh negative mother, the blood group and Rh status of the baby are determined. If the child has Rh positive blood, the mother should be given a dose of Anti-D within 72 hours of birth. In almost all cases, this prevents the woman from making antibodies to the Rh positive blood cells she may have received from her baby before and during delivery. **The injection is not needed if the baby is Rh negative.**

The Anti-D injection given during a particular pregnancy is only effective for that pregnancy. Any subsequent pregnancies must be treated in the same way.

Is Rh immunoglobulin required after sterilisation?

Your doctor will help you decide if you need Rh immunoglobulin if you are planning to undergo sterilisation. After sterilisation, you will not get pregnant again so it is possible to avoid the cost of the expensive Anti-D injection.

Some doctors might advise you to take the injection for the following reasons:

- You may decide later to have the sterilisation reversed
- Rarely, the sterilisation may fail and you may get pregnant again

Other reasons for taking Rh immunoglobulin

An Rh–negative woman also should receive treatment any time after the blood of the mother comes in contact with the foetus. This can occur during miscarriage, ectopic pregnancy or induced abortion. She also should receive it after certain procedures, such as amniocentesis or chorionic villus sampling. This prevents any chance of the woman developing antibodies that would attack a future Rh positive foetus.

What can happen if Rh disease is not prevented?

Rh incompatibility rarely causes complications in a first pregnancy and does not affect the health of the mother. It is the Rh antibodies that develop during subsequent pregnancies that can be potentially dangerous to mother and child. Rh disease can result in severe anaemia, jaundice, brain damage and heart failure in a newborn. In extreme cases, it can cause the death of the foetus because too many red blood cells have been destroyed.

In the past, Rh incompatibility was a very serious problem. Fortunately, significant medical advances have been made to help prevent complications from Rh incompatibility and to treat any newborn affected by Rh disease.

Managing an Rh sensitised pregnancy

A mother who is Rh sensitised will be monitored regularly during the pregnancy. A Doppler ultrasound is used to determine if the foetus is developing anaemia. The Doppler test is done frequently, usually after the fifth month of pregnancy. If the Doppler ultrasound shows that the foetus may be developing severe anaemia, a foetal blood sampling is done. A fine needle is inserted into the baby's umbilical cord and a blood sample is obtained. When the anaemia is confirmed, blood transfusions are given to the foetus. This is successful in 90 per cent of cases. This is a specialised procedure and can only be done in some centres equipped to handle these cases.

Newborns with Rh disease

If the foetus is near term and tests show that the baby is developing anaemia, your labour may be induced early before too many foetal blood cells are destroyed. After delivery, some cases of Rh disease are so mild that the baby does not need any treatment. If the baby has jaundice, he may be placed under special blue lights (phototherapy). In some cases, the baby may need an exchange blood transfusion.

CHAPTER 36

Pregnancy after thirty-five

Sanjana and her husband were married late. She is 36 years old and is planning to go ahead with a pregnancy.

Smriti and her husband, on the other hand, have been married for the past seven years. She has conceived now after treatment for infertility. She is 37 years old.

Shyamala is 35 and pregnant for the second time. Her first child is 13 years old. Will being 35 or older cause a problem in a pregnancy?

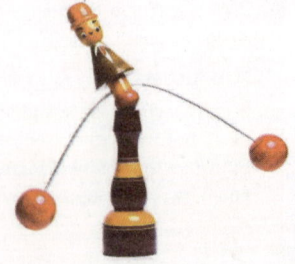

36 Pregnancy after thirty-five

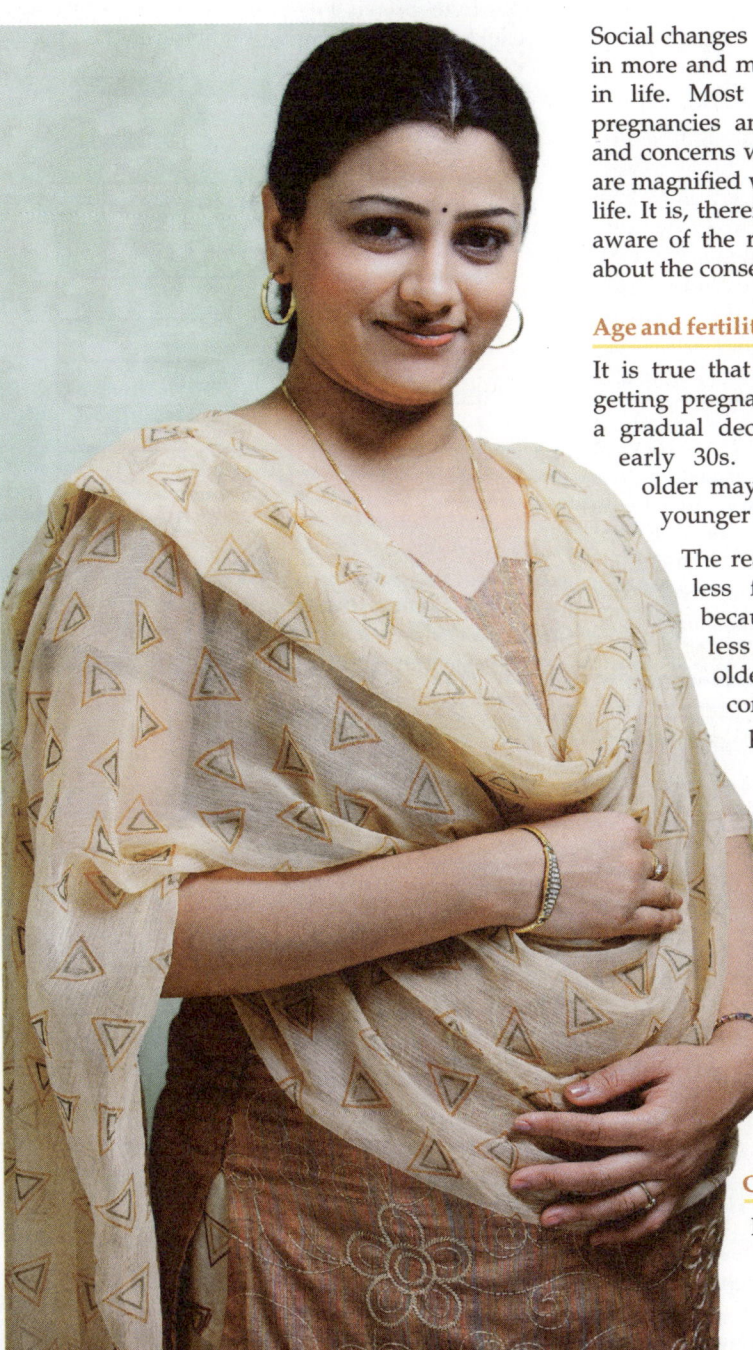

Social changes and career pressures are resulting in more and more women having children later in life. Most women over 35 have healthy pregnancies and healthy babies. The anxieties and concerns which plague all pregnant women are magnified when a woman has a child later in life. It is, therefore, important for a couple to be aware of the risks involved and stay informed about the consequences of a late pregnancy.

Age and fertility

It is true that women have more difficulty in getting pregnant as they grow older. There is a gradual decrease of fertility starting in the early 30s. A woman in her mid-30s or older may take longer to conceive than a younger woman.

The reason that women over 35 may be less fertile than younger women is because they produce an egg (ovulate) less frequently. As women grow older, they may also develop medical conditions which may interfere with pregnancy. For example, women over 35 are more likely to have endometriosis, which may contribute to decreased fertility.

If you are over 35, you should consult your gynae-cologist if you have not conceived after six months of trying. About one-third of women between 35 and 39 and about half of those over 40 have problems conceiving. Many fertility problems can be treated successfully.

Chances of twins

Paradoxically, women over 35 may have difficulty in conceiving but have a greater chance of having twins. The chance of having twins increases naturally with age. The other contributing factor is that women over 35 are more likely to undergo fertility treatment, and this may increase the chance of twins and triplets.

Risk of miscarriage

At any age, most miscarriages occur in the first three months of pregnancy. The rate of miscarriage in older women is significantly greater than in younger women. This is mainly because of the increasing risk of chromosomal abnormalities. Approximately 10 to 15 per cent of recognised pregnancies for women in their 20s end in miscarriage The risk rises to about 20 per cent at ages 35 to 39, and about 50 per cent by ages 40 to 44.

Preexisting health problems and pregnancy

At any age, when planning a pregnancy, a woman should consult her obstetrician before trying to conceive. A preconception visit helps ensure she is in the best possible physical condition before conception. Diabetes and high blood pressure are two conditions which are common in Indians and much more common in women in their late 30s and early 40s. Moreover, women over 35 are twice as likely as women in their 20s to develop high blood pressure and diabetes for the first time during pregnancy.

Careful medical monitoring is required and the appropriate medications must be started before conception and continued throughout pregnancy. This can reduce the risks associated with these conditions and, in most cases, result in a healthy pregnancy.

Risk of birth defects in women over 35

As a woman ages, the risk of bearing a child with chromosomal disorders increases. The most common of these disorders is Down syndrome, a combination of mental retardation and physical abnormalities caused by the presence of an extra chromosome 21.

Women who are 35 or older at the time of delivery should undergo prenatal testing to rule out Down syndrome and other chromosomal problems. Ask your obstetrician if the facilities are available to have the testing done. Usually a blood test along with an ultrasound will be done as a preliminary to assess the risk of your having a baby with Down syndrome. **(See Chapter 11: Tests during pregnancy).** If the test comes back positive, prenatal tests like amniocentesis and chorionic villus sampling (CVS) may be offered. **(See Chapter 13: Special tests during pregnancy).** Most women who have these tests will find that their baby does not have a chromosomal problem.

Age related risk of Down syndrome	
Age 25	1 in 1,250
Age 30	1 in 1,000
Age 35	1 in 400
Age 40	1 in 100
Age 45	1 in 30
Age 49	1 in 10

Risk of pregnancy complications

While women in their late 30s and early 40s are likely to have a healthy baby, they do face more complications along the way. It is important to keep in mind that many of these risks can be managed effectively with good prenatal care and most women will have a happy outcome.

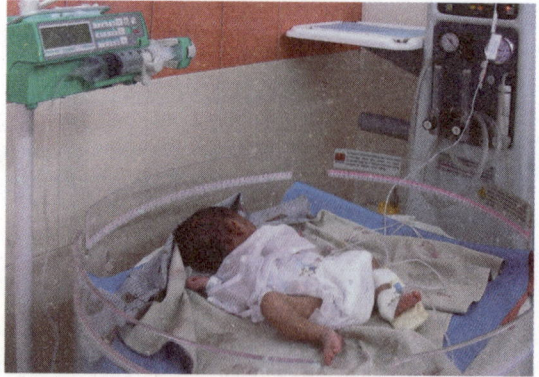

Women having their first baby at 35 or older are at an increased risk of having a baby who has a **low birth weight** or is **premature** (born at less than 37 full weeks of pregnancy). Women over 35 are 20 to 40 per cent more likely than younger women to have a baby who has a low birth weight and 20 per cent more likely to have a premature delivery. Women over 40 are

40 per cent more likely than younger women to deliver prematurely. Premature babies are at an increased risk for health problems in the newborn period. **(See Chapter 29: Premature or preterm labour).** Women in their 40s may also have a greater chance of having a low-birth weight baby.

Women over 35 have an increased risk of having **placental problems.** The placenta may not function well and may result in poor growth of the foetus. Foetal growth has to be monitored carefully both with regular check-ups and ultrasound scans. Women over 35 also have a greater chance of developing placenta praevia as compared to younger women. This risk triples in women in the 40s.

Gestational diabetes (diabetes developing for the first time during pregnancy) develops twice as often in women over age 35 as compared to younger women. **(See Chapter 34: Diabetes in pregnancy).**

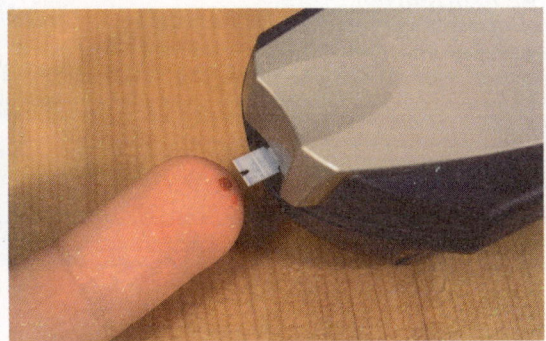

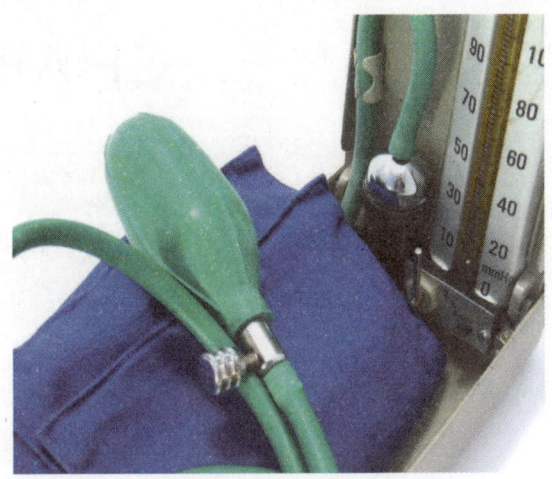

Pregnancy-induced **hypertension** and **pre-eclampsia** are more common in women over 35. **(See Chapter 33: High blood pressure in pregnancy).**

The rate of **stillbirth** (delivering a dead baby) doubles in women over 40 but the reasons for this unfortunate event in the over-40 age group are not known.

Problems in labour and delivery

First-time mothers over 35 are more likely than women in their 20s to have difficulties in labour. This may account, in part, for the increased rate of caesarean sections among women over 35. First-time mothers over 40 have the highest chance of having a caesarean section.

Reducing the risks

Most women in their late 30s and early 40s can look forward to having a healthy pregnancy and a healthy baby. However, given the special concerns about pregnancy past 35, it is especially important for older couples to seek preconceptional counselling from their obstetrician before embarking on this very important step in their lives.

CHAPTER 37

Handling pregnancy loss

Shravanthi was 32 weeks pregnant when her obstetrician told her the baby's heartbeat had stopped and she had suffered an **intrauterine foetal demise**. She and her husband are heartbroken.

Sheela was 11 weeks pregnant when she suffered a miscarriage. Having shared the happy news with everybody she knew, Sheela was upset about the miscarriage.

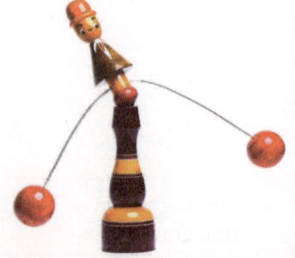

37 Handling pregnancy loss

Sunita is 24 weeks pregnant. An ultrasound has revealed that her baby has a major **birth defect** because of which the baby may not survive if born. Her obstetrician has suggested termination of the pregnancy.

Sabira had gone to the hospital in labour. Unfortunately, the labour ended with a **stillbirth**.

It is well known that 12 to 15 per cent of confirmed pregnancies do not progress to term. In older women, this rate may be even higher. Early pregnancy loss i.e. less than 20 weeks is experienced by one in five women. **(See Chapter 27: Miscarriage).**

Most women go on to have successful subsequent pregnancies. Nevertheless, the feeling of loss and grief may be difficult for some couples to handle.

The grieving is often complicated by feelings of self-blame, particularly when there is no medical explanation for the loss. This is compounded by well meaning relatives or even strangers asking if she had done something to cause the pregnancy loss. **It is important to remember that there is not much a woman can do to prevent a miscarriage, intrauterine demise, stillbirth or a birth defect.** Blaming oneself is a useless exercise and will only prolong the grief.

It is normal to experience grief and go through a grieving process after a miscarriage or stillbirth. Emotional healing after a pregnancy loss can take some time. For some, the grieving process may only last a few days, while for others, it can take a few weeks or months. Although it can be difficult, it is important to deal with your loss rather than ignore the emotions you may be feeling.

Factors which influence the grieving process:

- Having previously experienced one or more miscarriages
- Miscarrying later in gestation (especially if the woman has felt the foetus move and formed an emotional attachment to it)
- Having conceived the pregnancy at an older age
- Having conceived the pregnancy with great difficulty after undergoing treatment for infertility

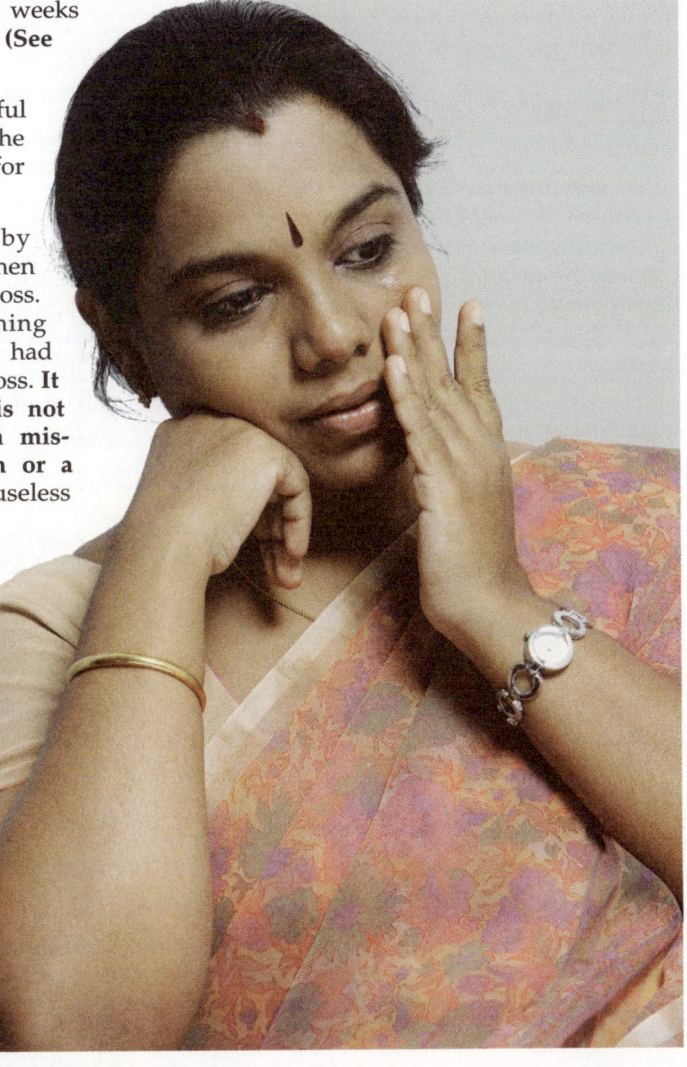

- The family and social implications of having lost the pregnancy

How does grief and healing evolve?

Immediately after the event, your emotions may range from anger to despair. **Remember that grief is not a sign of weakness.** It is a natural human emotion experienced by everyone after a significant loss. Do give yourself the time you need to mourn and accept what has happened. Sometimes, it may take weeks or months to recover.

Grief, in all individuals, follows a few well described stages. You may or may not pass through each stage but the last stage is the most important one to reach.

Common stages of grief

Denial

Faced with the news, you may refuse to believe it. You may seek opinions from another obstetrician or ask for another ultrasound scan to confirm the diagnosis. You may bargain with a higher power to make the bad news go away.

Anger

You may be angry at yourself, your husband or a higher power for letting this happen.

Guilt

As a woman, you may wonder if you could have avoided the pregnancy loss by being more careful. Don't blame yourself. There is very little a woman can do to avoid an unexpected pregnancy loss.

Depression

Your pain and sorrow may lead to symptoms of depression. These feelings usually resolve in time with strong support from your husband, family and friends. About 10 per cent of women may end up with clinical depression. If your depression is prolonged, you may need to seek professional support.

Acceptance

Each step in the grieving process brings you closer to acceptance. You will always carry the memory of your baby, but acceptance may ease your pain. Slowly, time and day-to-day living will help you overcome the acute pain.

There will be certain days and occasions when the memories will come flooding back and overwhelm you. You may surprise yourself by the anger and jealousy you might feel towards other women who are happily pregnant. Seeing a newborn baby or another mother with a baby may trigger feelings of sadness. Again, these are not unusual emotions to experience; after all, you are only human. Just don't let these feelings consume you – you will only hurt yourself more. Remember that eventually these feelings will pass. Let your mind heal and learn acceptance even if it is a tough lesson to imbibe.

You do not have to be alone

There is no need for you to keep your feelings bottled up. Your husband and you should be able to talk it over with each other. You have to be the most important support system for each other because no one else can feel the intensity of loss as much as the two of you. Your relationship with your husband might be particularly strained during this time. Remember, he is also grieving. However, he may not be able to express what he is feeling, which can make you feel he is not sharing your grief.

At the same time, do not exclude your parents from the grieving process. They also have lost a grandchild. The older people in the family have experienced life and may be able to provide you with wisdom and support in dealing with this sorrowful life event.

Discuss the loss with your obstetrician. Try to find out what are the causes, if any, for the loss. Find out how soon you can plan the next pregnancy. Taking positive steps like this will help you resolve your feelings of loss.

If you have friends or relatives who keep bringing up stories about other women who have lost a pregnancy or tell you what you should have done to avoid this loss, stay away from them. You do not need the aggravation of people who are insensitive or thoughtless at this time. Be direct and let them know when you don't want to discuss your pregnancy loss with them.

Planning your next pregnancy

Even though it seems good sense to plan another pregnancy immediately so that you can 'forget' the pregnancy loss, it may not be such a good idea. Give yourself time to recover physically. More important, you need to heal emotionally. This emotional healing may take a few months. Only when you are fully recovered can you go through the next pregnancy with confidence. If you get pregnant immediately, your pregnancy may be overshadowed with anxiety and fear.

Talk to your obstetrician about the best form of birth control till you decide on your next pregnancy.

When grief overwhelms us

Be on the lookout for signs which will warn you that you are not moving towards acceptance and healing. You may:

- Work hard to the point of complete exhaustion to avoid being overwhelmed by your emotions
- Suppress your emotions and resent those who try to help you
- Remain depressed well past the normal healing period and be unable to function normally

One of the commonsense pieces of advice given to those who are grieving is, "Running away from grief postpones sorrow; clinging to grief prolongs pain; neither leads to healing."

The healthy path to healing

Be compassionate with yourself and accept support from family, friends or a spiritual advisor. Loss can also affect you physically. It is not unusual for someone who is grieving to have shortness of breath, palpitations, stomach pain, and sleep irregularities. Sometimes, it may be difficult to see that the physical pain is tied to the emotional, but they often go hand in hand.

Reaching equanimity and acceptance

Although you will not forget your loss, and there will always be a tender spot in your heart, the intensity of the pain will diminish over the years. Time really is a great healer.

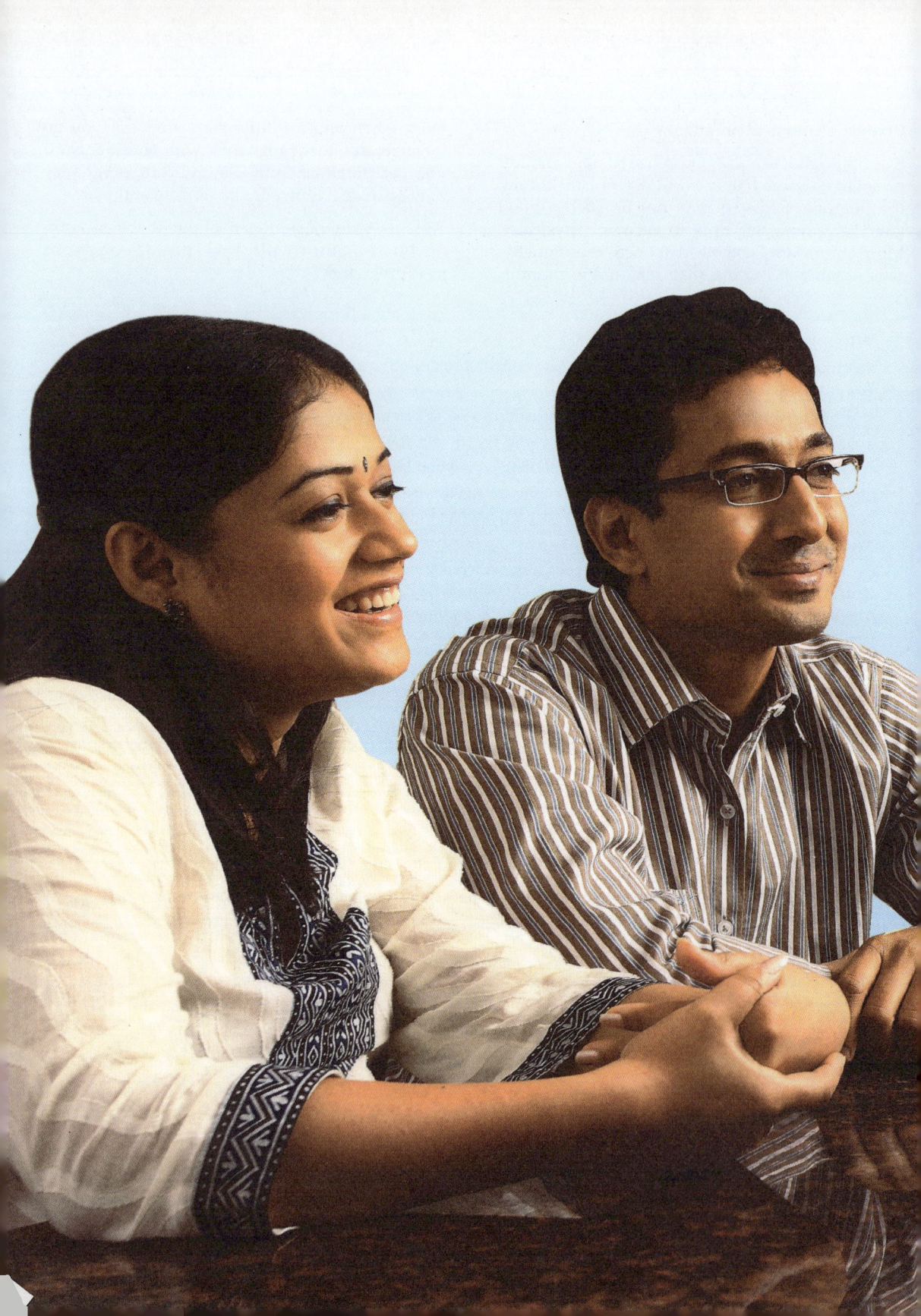

Common illnesses in pregnancy

CHAPTER 38

Fever in pregnancy

Shamini is running a high temperature. She is six months pregnant. Her husband is anxious. Will the fever affect the baby? Will the tablets she needs to take have any harmful effect on the growing foetus?

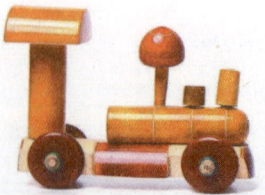

38 Fever in pregnancy

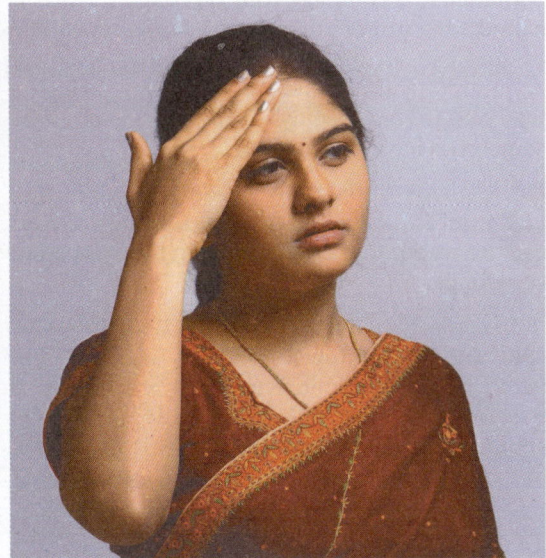

The common causes of fever in pregnancy are

- Cold and cough
- Influenza ('the flu')
- Malaria
- Typhoid
- Chickenpox
- Measles and German measles
- Urinary tract infection **(See Chapter 39: Urinary tract infection and vaginitis).**

Cold and cough in pregnancy

Colds are so common that it would be unusual for you to go through your pregnancy without catching a cold at least once. Colds, coughs and most fevers are usually due to a viral infection. Most of the time, there is no need for antibiotics. They can be treated with medications which are safe in pregnancy and relieve the symptoms.

Coughs, colds and viral fevers may make you feel tired and miserable but do not have any effect on the baby. Even when you have a severe cough, the coughing will not in any way disturb or harm the baby.

If the cough persists for more than a few days or is accompanied by a large amount of phlegm, you might want to see your doctor to rule out a severe infection. Do not take an antibiotic unless it is prescribed by a physician. Women who have had sinusitis earlier may need to take specific medication to relieve the symptoms.

Immediate home remedies

- Drink plenty of fluids, as this will help to thin secretions. Water, juices and warm tea are good for you
- Steam inhalation will help clear a stuffy nose and also help relieve coughs
- Sleep in a reclining position with plenty of pillows under your head so that breathing is easier
- Hot water gargles are soothing for a sore throat
- Use mentholated lozenges which help to relieve throat pain

Medications to relieve symptoms

Decongestants: This group of medications is used to treat colds or allergies. They relieve stuffiness of the nose.

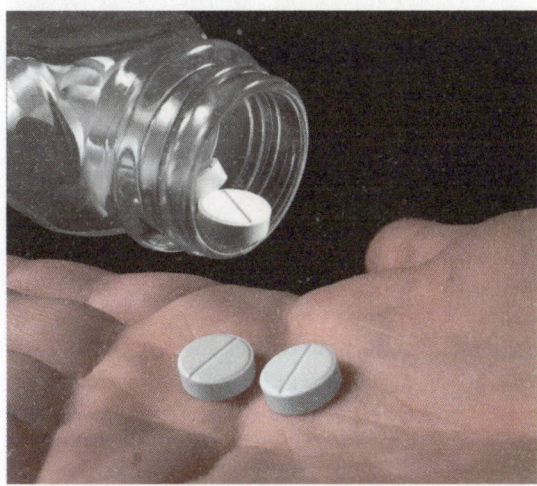

Cough suppressants and expectorants: Dextromethorphan, a common ingredient found in cough and cold medications, suppresses cough and is effective for a dry cough. Guaifenesin is an expectorant in many cough and cold medicines.

Antihistamines: Cough syrups and cold remedies may also contain an antihistamine.

Headache and body ache: It is safe to take paracetamol for headache and also to bring down a fever. Body pain can be treated with ibuprofen.

Fever: It is best to avoid high fevers in pregnancy, especially in the first three months. Take paracetamol (which can be taken every 4-6 hours) to keep your temperature as near normal as possible.

Food

Having a cold, cough or fever does not mean that you cannot eat a normal diet. Make sure you drink plenty of fluids and don't get dehydrated. You do not have to avoid cold drinks, juices or curds. They do not aggravate fever or cold. If drinking something cold makes your throat hurt, then you may avoid it.

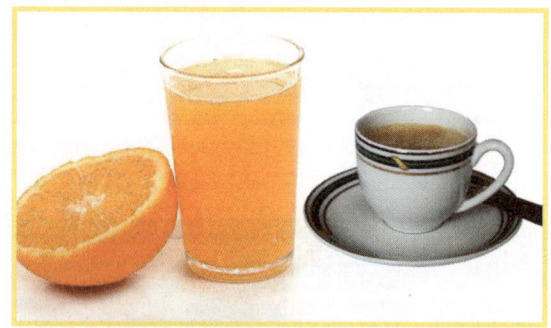

Influenza ('the flu')

Having the flu can be very tiring in pregnancy. It can cause severe body pain. The best thing to do is to drink plenty of fluids, eat a healthy diet and rest till you feel better. The body pain will respond to paracetamol and ibuprofen, both of which are safe in pregnancy. The fever can be kept under control with paracetamol. Remember that the flu is caused by a viral infection and does not require antibiotics.

Lower respiratory infection

Sometimes, a common cold or cough (which is called an upper respiratory infection) can progress to an infection in the lungs (a lower respiratory infection). You might start bringing up yellow or greenish phlegm which may sometimes have a bad odour.

Drink plenty of fluids to loosen up the phlegm. Steam inhalations will also help. Cough syrups can be used to suppress annoying, incessant coughing.

If the infection does not respond to the usual cold and cough remedies, your doctor might prescribe an antibiotic if she feels it is due to a bacterial infection. The antibiotic prescribed should be carefully chosen to make sure that it does not have any adverse effect on the baby.

Typhoid fever

Typhoid fever spreads through the consumption of contaminated food and water or through close contact with someone who is infected. Typhoid is suspected when there is persistent high fever, headache, abdominal pain, and either constipation or diarrhoea.

Once signs and symptoms do appear, you are likely to experience fever, often as high as 103^0 or 104^0 F (39^0 or 40^0 C), headache, weakness and fatigue, sore throat, abdominal pain, diarrhoea or constipation.

Cause of typhoid fever

Typhoid fever is caused by virulent bacteria called **Salmonella typhii**. The bacteria that cause typhoid fever spread through contaminated food or water and occasionally through direct contact with someone who is infected. In India, where typhoid is endemic, most cases result from contaminated drinking water and poor sanitation. S. typhii is passed in the faeces and sometimes in the urine of infected people. You can contract the infection if you eat food handled by someone with typhoid fever who has not washed carefully after using the bathroom. You can also become infected by drinking water contaminated with the bacteria.

Diagnosis of typhoid fever

Typhoid is diagnosed by a blood test. The blood test will come back as positive only after the fifth day of fever. Testing for typhoid before the fifth day of fever is not useful.

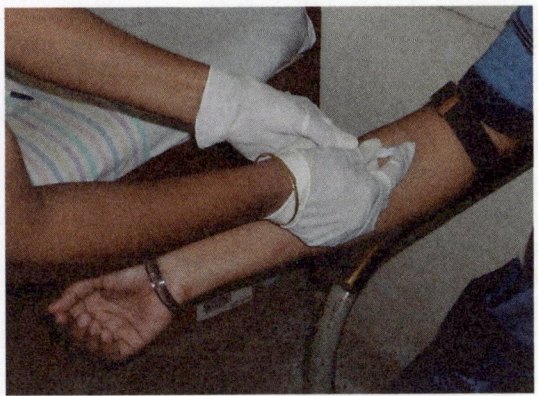

Treatment of typhoid fever

Women who are pregnant respond well to **amoxycillin** tablets or **ceftriaxone** injections. Ciprofloxacin is not recommended in pregnancy. The treatment has to be given for 7-14 days for complete cure.

Diet during typhoid fever

- Drinking fluids: This helps prevent the dehydration that results from prolonged fever and diarrhoea. If you are unable to drink enough fluids, you may be given fluids through a vein in your arm (intravenously).
- Eating a healthy diet: Low fibre, non-bulky, high-calorie meals can help replace the nutrients you lose when you are ill.

To prevent infecting others

These following measures can prevent others in your family from getting infected:

- Wash your hands often. This is the single most important thing you can do to keep from spreading the infection to others. Use plenty of hot, soapy water and scrub thoroughly for at least 30 seconds, especially before eating and after using the toilet.
- Avoid handling food. Avoid preparing food for others until your doctor says you are no longer contagious.
- Keep personal items separate. Set aside towels, bed linen and utensils for your own use and wash them frequently in hot, soapy water. Heavily soiled items can be soaked first in disinfectant.

Malaria

Malaria is an infectious disease caused by a parasite that is transmitted by the bite of a female anopheles mosquito.

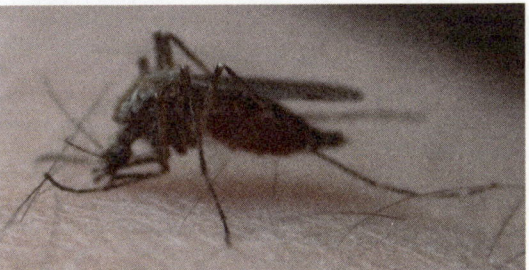

Symptoms

A malaria infection is generally characterised by recurrent attacks of high fever with moderate to severe shaking chills and profuse sweating as body temperature drops.

Tests and diagnosis

A blood sample and a blood smear can usually confirm the presence of the malaria parasite and its type.

Treatment and drugs

A malaria infection requires prompt evaluation and treatment. In most cases, doctors can treat malaria effectively in pregnancy with tablets of chloroquine.

Avoiding malaria

- Use mosquito repellant.
- Wear protective clothing.
- Use mosquito netting.

CHAPTER 39

Urinary tract infection and vaginal infection

Shabana has been running to the bathroom every five minutes. There is severe burning when she passes urine. Does she have a urinary infection?

Sameera is six months pregnant. She has developed a thick white vaginal discharge. She also has severe itching which seems to be worse at night. Does she have a vaginal infection?

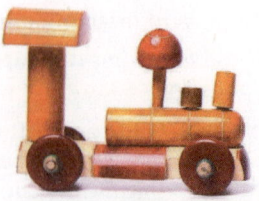

39 Urinary tract infection and vaginal infection

Urinary tract infection

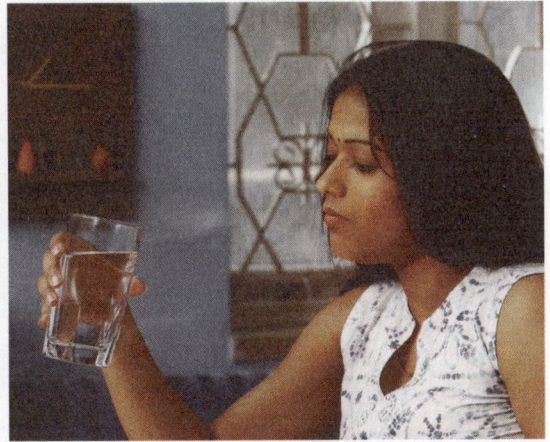

A urinary tract infection (UTI) can be very distressing. You can suspect that you have a urinary tract infection when you have an urge to pass urine very frequently but pass only small quantities or just a few drops every time. This may be accompanied by burning or pain. You may also have pain in the lower part of your abdomen. If the infection has spread to your kidneys, you might have pain over your flanks and back. Urinary tract infection can also be accompanied by fever and chills.

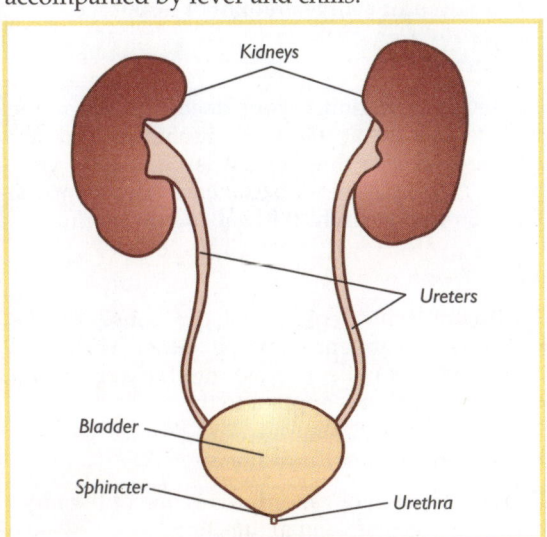

An infection involving the bladder is called **cystitis.** When it spreads upwards to the kidneys, it is called **pyelonephritis.** This can be suspected when you have pain over the kidneys when the doctor examines you. These infections are caused by bacteria.

When should you suspect a urinary tract infection?

An urge to pass urine frequently, burning or pain on urination, a feeling that you need to urinate right after you have just passed urine are all signs of a UTI. Sometimes there may be blood in the urine.

Does a urinary infection affect the baby?

An infection in the bladder will not affect the baby. If you have a UTI which is not treated promptly, it may lead to a kidney infection. Bladder and kidney infections may sometimes cause premature labour.

> It is important to confirm the urinary infection with a **culture and sensitivity test** before starting on antibiotics. This allows the appropriate antibiotic to be used and will prevent recurrence of the infection.

Diagnosis of urinary infection

When a urinary infection is suspected in pregnancy, it is absolutely essential to get the urine tested before treatment is started. When there is a UTI, a microscopic examination of the urine might show pus cells. When the **pus cells** are more than 8-10 per high power field, it is suggestive of a urinary

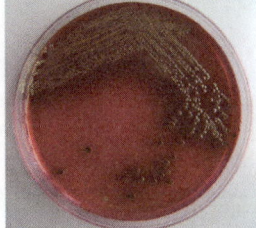

Bacteria growing in culture

infection. **Red blood cells** might also be seen. A **culture and sensitivity test** must also be performed on the urine. This will tell us which type of bacteria is responsible for the infection.

> **Collecting urine for a culture and sensitivity test**
>
> The lab will provide you with a sterile wide-mouth container. Wash your genital area well and then pass a little urine into the toilet. Collect the remaining urine in the container. Make sure the container does not touch your skin. This is called a 'mid-stream sample'.

A colony count should be reported and if the colony count of the bacteria is more than 100,000 per ml, only then is an infection confirmed. A culture and sensitivity report usually takes 48 hours.

How is a urinary infection treated?

An appropriate antibiotic will be prescribed. Usually the course of antibiotics is for 3 to 5 days. Your obstetrician will prescribe an antibiotic that is safe for you and the baby. The choice of antibiotic will depend on the report of the culture and sensitivity test. Sometimes, if the pain and other symptoms are very severe, you might be placed on an antibiotic before the report comes back and this may be continued or changed depending on the report.

You can help by increasing your fluid intake to help flush out the germs from the urinary tract. You can drink plenty of water and also juices, coconut water and buttermilk *(lassi)*.

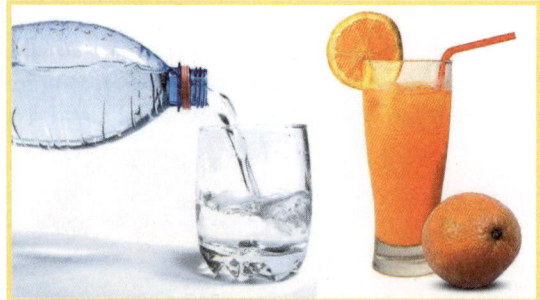

Was the treatment effective?

You should call your doctor if you have a persistent fever (over 100°F or 38°C), chills, lower abdominal pain, nausea, vomiting or flank pain. If after taking medicine for three days, you still have a burning sensation when you urinate, check again with your doctor.

Preventing a urinary tract infection

You can help prevent UTIs in several ways. First, you should always drink plenty of liquids especially in the hot summer months. Water is the best and cheapest fluid! You should urinate often and not have long intervals between urination. Always urinate after sexual intercourse.

Vaginal infection

Vaginitis is an inflammation or infection in a woman's vagina. Many pregnant women develop vaginitis in pregnancy. Sometimes, the infection may spread over the groin area and cause intense itching. When there is any abnormal discharge associated with burning or itching, it is best to contact your obstetrician.

All women have a small amount of vaginal discharge. This may become more during ovulation. In pregnancy, it is common for women to find an increase in vaginal discharge, starting even in the first few weeks of pregnancy. Closer to term the discharge may increase. This is because the cervix is soft and has started to open. Discharge without itching is a normal occurence.

The vagina has many organisms, such as bacteria and yeast. These are usually in balance and do not cause any problems. Pregnancy may upset this balance and one or other of the organisms may start to increase, resulting in an infection (also called vaginitis). **Vaginitis** may cause itching, a bad odour or a large amount of discharge.

Diagnosis

To diagnose vaginitis, your doctor will examine you to see what kind of discharge you are having and also the effect it is having on your body. A sample might be taken to check for the kind of organism which is causing the vaginitis.

Treatment

Treatment will depend on the cause of the vaginitis. Treatment may be either with oral tablets, tablets to be inserted into the vagina or a cream or gel that is applied to the vagina.

Fungal infection or candidiasis

Fungal infection or candidiasis is one of the most common types of vaginal infection.

This infection is caused by a fungus called Candida. It is found in small numbers in the normal vagina. However, when the balance of bacteria and yeast in the vagina is altered, the yeast may overgrow and cause symptoms. Women who have diabetes in pregnancy have an increased risk of developing candidiasis.

Some types of antibiotics increase the risk of a fungal infection. Overgrowth of candida also can occur if the body's immune system (which protects the body from disease) is suppressed. For example, in women infected with **human immunodeficiency virus (HIV)**, yeast infections may be severe. They may not go away, even with treatment, or may recur often.

The most common symptoms of a fungal infection are itching and burning inside the vagina and over the area outside the vagina. The area may be red and swollen. The vaginal discharge usually is white and curdy.

Treatment

In pregnancy, fungal infections are treated by placing anti-fungal tablets into the vagina, since oral antifungal agents are not safe in pregnancy. Treatment is not necessary for your husband. Ointments will also be prescribed to treat the itching outside the vagina.

Avoiding recurrence of fungal infection

Because the Indian climate usually causes sweating, it is better to wear cotton underclothes and avoid synthetics. This allows better air circulation and also helps in absorbing the sweat, thus decreasing the chances of fungal infection.

Trichomoniasis

Trichomoniasis is a condition caused by the microscopic parasite Trichomonas vaginalis. The diagnosis is confirmed by identifying the parasite under the microscope. The infection is spread through having intercourse.

Symptoms

Symptoms of trichomoniasis may include a yellow-gray or green vaginal discharge. The discharge may have a fishy odour. There may be burning, irritation, redness and swelling of the vulva. Sometimes, there is pain during urination.

Treatment

Treatment of Trichomoniasis in pregnancy usually consists of applying metronidazole gel or cream around the vagina. Oral medications which are used for Trichomoniasis are better avoided in pregnancy. Your husband will be given an oral medication since the infection may spread back and forth between the two of you if he is not treated.

CHAPTER 40

Medical disorders in pregnancy

Suzanne has had asthma from childhood. Will the asthma affect the baby?

Shabana is on medication for epilepsy for the past two years. She was married eight months ago. She is now pregnant and her doctor has told her to continue her medicines. Is this safe?

Sundari's thyroid gland does not produce enough hormone. She takes thyroxine regularly. Her thyroid function tests have been normal. Her doctor has advised her not to reduce the dosage in pregnancy.

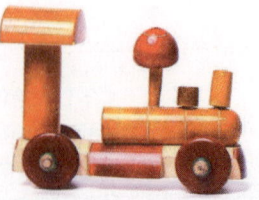

Medical disorders in pregnancy

Asthma

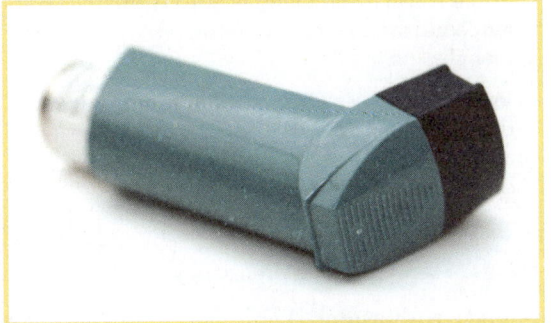

Suzanne has suffered from asthma for many years. She knows the triggers that can aggravate the wheezing and knows how to handle an attack. She is now in the second month of her pregnancy. She is concerned that her asthma may affect the baby. Can she continue her usual medications?

Asthma is the most common condition that affects the lungs during pregnancy. About eight per cent of pregnant women have asthma. Before becoming pregnant, women with asthma should discuss their condition with their physician. Women who become pregnant should continue their asthma medications. Stopping medications all of a sudden could result in a bad attack of asthma. Remember, the risk of poorly controlled asthma is much greater than the risk of taking medications to control the condition.

What causes asthma?

The basis of an asthma attack is inflammation of the bronchioles, the narrow tubes that carry air into the lungs. The inflammation leads to constriction and narrowing of the bronchioles and results in wheezing, tightness of the chest and a persistent dry cough. Substances like dust, mold, pollen and smoke trigger cell inflammation and mucous production. The basis for this is an allergic reaction. People who have a tendency to have allergies have a greater chance of developing asthma.

Asthma is not always triggered by allergies. Women can also have asthma attacks after taking drugs such as aspirin or ibuprofen. Some women develop asthma in the workplace due to exposure to certain chemicals or other substances. Sometimes, asthma is triggered by exercise. Exercise-induced asthma is caused by dry air coming into the lungs or a change in the fluid balance of cells. Within five to ten minutes after beginning exercise, individuals experience asthmatic symptoms such as chest tightness, coughing or wheezing.

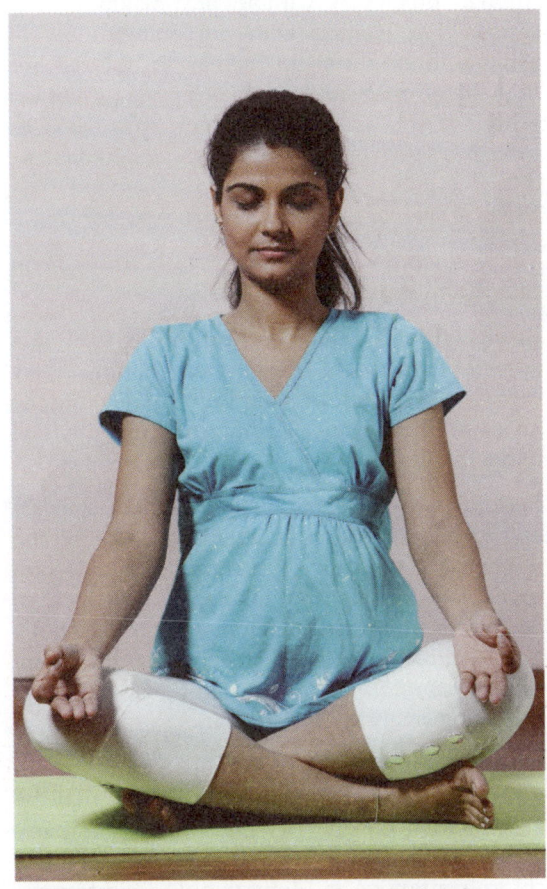

Breathing exercises like **pranayama** are excellent for asthmatics and complement medical treatment.

Effect of pregnancy on asthma

It is difficult to predict the effect of pregnancy on asthma. The severity of asthma during pregnancy varies from one woman to another. As a rule of thumb, during pregnancy, asthma worsens in about one-third of women, improves in one-third and remains stable in one-third. Women who have severe asthma are more likely to face a worsening of the disease in pregnancy.

Asthma tends to worsen in the third trimester. This may have something to do with the size of the uterus and the pressure of the diaphragm on the lungs.

Effect of asthma on pregnancy

Women who have mild asthma usually go through pregnancy without any major complications. For women with moderate to severe asthma, there is a slight increase in the risk for high blood pressure or preeclampsia. Women with severe asthma also run the risk of premature delivery and low birth weight babies.

Medications for asthma during pregnancy

The commonly used drugs which are safe in pregnancy are:

Bronchodilators: Short-acting bronchodilators appear to be safe during pregnancy. They rapidly relieve asthma symptoms by relaxing the airways. They include salbutamol, theophylline and terbutaline.

Steroids: Experience shows that the use of steroids by pregnant women is generally safe for both the mother and the baby. The steroids include oral prednisone tablets and inhaled drugs such as beclomethasone, triamcinolone, and budesonide. Budesonide is thought to be one of the safest inhaled steroids. Beclomethasone has also been used extensively during pregnancy.

Antihistamines: Although antihistamines are not used to directly treat asthma, they may be used to treat the allergies that often accompany asthma. These drugs include diphenhydramine, chlorpheniramine and cetirizine. These drugs are safe in pregnancy.

Women with mild asthma: Asthma can be managed with inhaled bronchodilators. If needed, inhaled steroids can be added. These drugs are also available as combination inhalers.

Women with moderate asthma: In addition to the above medications, women with moderate asthma may be given oral theophylline.

Women with severe asthma: In addition to the above medications, women with severe asthma may be given oral steroids, either as short courses or as a daily dose.

Drugs to be avoided in pregnancy

Women with asthma know that their condition can get aggravated by taking aspirin or ibuprofen. They should also be aware that certain drugs used in pregnancy can worsen their wheezing. The **F-series of prostaglandins, sometimes used in pregnancy to make the uterus contract and control bleeding after delivery, must be avoided in an asthmatic.**

Monitoring the baby's growth

Since women with moderate to severe asthma have a greater risk of delivering a low birth weight baby, the baby's growth must be monitored with ultrasound scans.

Labour and delivery

The medications that you are taking will be continued during labour and delivery. Epidural analgesia for pain relief is safe for a woman with asthma. If general anaesthesia has to be given for an emergency caesarean section, the anaesthetist will also give an injection to prevent wheezing.

Women who are given oral steroids for asthma may develop gestational diabetes. Therefore, their blood sugar levels must be monitored carefully.

Breastfeeding

Women with asthma are encouraged to breastfeed because there are a number of benefits for both her and her infant.

Epilepsy

Subbulakshmi has been married for two years. She is an epileptic and has been avoiding a pregnancy because she and her husband are worried the baby might be affected by the medicines she is taking. They need not worry. With good preconceptional counselling and optimal obstetric care, she can have a normal pregnancy and a healthy baby. She can also safely breastfeed her baby.

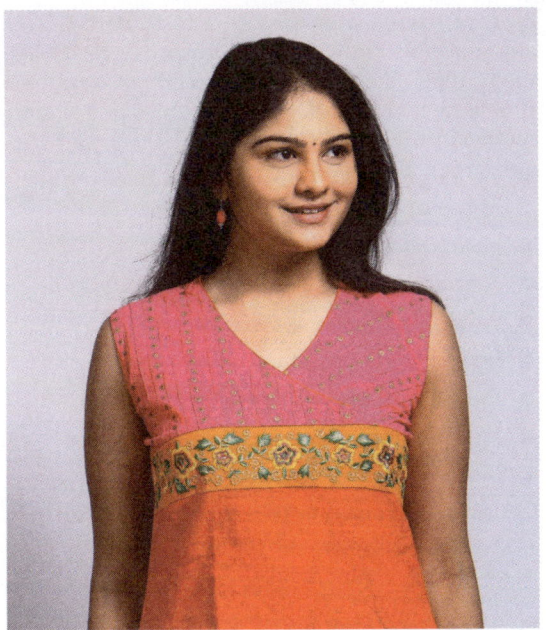

How common is epilepsy?

There are 5.5 to 7.8 million persons with epilepsy in India. Unfortunately, both in the urban and rural population, people still try to conceal the disease. Girls and women particularly delay seeking professional help. To avoid problems later in the marriage, it is best to have an informal discussion with a doctor by both parties so that all doubts can be laid to rest. There are many cases where a disclosure of epilepsy after the marriage ends up in the woman being sent back to her parents' home, even if she is pregnant.

Epilepsy and pregnancy

The chances of having a normal, healthy child are excellent and are greater than 90 per cent. Both the neurologist and the obstetrician need to be involved in reviewing the anti-epileptic drug that the woman is taking and in deciding whether there is need for a change in medication prior to conception. It is best to be on a single drug rather than a combination of drugs.

Though there is a slightly increased risk of certain abnormalities in the baby due to anti-epileptic drugs, these problems can be prevented by taking folic acid supplementation (5mg/day), particularly prior to conception and in the first three months of pregnancy. A good quality detailed ultrasound in the 5th month can ensure that the foetus does not have a birth defect. There may be a need to increase the dose of the antiepileptic drug in pregnancy.

Before conception

If you have epilepsy, it is smart to take certain precautions before you get pregnant to ensure that you stay healthy and have a healthy baby. See your doctor before getting pregnant to discuss your medication. If there has been no seizure in two or more years, it may be possible to stop the medication gradually. If the medications cannot be stopped, your doctor may suggest that you switch to a medication which is safer for the foetus. However, seizures are more harmful to you and your baby than any medication; so do not abruptly stop your medication and make sure your obstetrician and neurologist are in agreement about the medications you are taking.

Antiepileptic drugs affect the way the body uses folic acid. So make sure you take a folic acid supplement along with your medication.

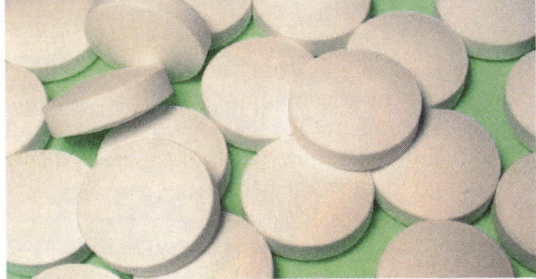

Risks for the baby

In all women, the risk of having a baby with a birth defect is 2 to 3 per cent. Women with epilepsy have a slightly higher risk (6 to 8 per cent) of having a baby with a birth defect. This risk may be related to the disorder or to the medication used to treat it. Though rare, the problems that may be seen in babies of epileptic mothers include:

- Cleft lip or palate (the lip or roof of the mouth is not completely closed)
- Heart defects
- Neural tube defects (such as spina bifida)
- Small head
- Low birth weight (small baby)
- Intrauterine growth restriction
- Mental retardation
- Bleeding problems at birth

Children of women with a seizure disorder may also run the risk of developing epilepsy later in life.

Delivery

There is no reason why a woman with epilepsy cannot have a vaginal delivery. Like any other woman, she may require a caesarean only if there is a problem during pregnancy or labour.

Postpartum care

After delivery, the medication to control the seizures may need to be adjusted. Just after birth, your baby will be given an injection of vitamin K to prevent any bleeding problems. This is because antiepileptic drugs lower the natural levels of vitamin K (the vitamin that helps with blood clotting) in the body.

Breastfeeding

Women on a single drug can safely breastfeed their babies in consultation with their paediatrician. Antiepileptic drugs are found in small amounts in breast milk, but in most cases this is not enough to affect the baby.

Birth control methods in women with epilepsy

All available birth control methods can be used by women with epilepsy. Birth control pills and intra-uterine devices are safe and reliable contraception. It is important to know that some antiepileptic drugs can make birth control pills less effective in preventing pregnancy. It is best to involve both the neurologist and the obstetrician in deciding on the best method of contraception.

Thyroid disease in pregnancy

The thyroid gland is butterfly-shaped and located at the base of the neck. The thyroid gland has an enormous impact on your health. Every aspect of your metabolism, from your heart rate to how quickly you burn calories, is regulated by thyroid hormones. You cannot live without your thyroid gland or the thyroid hormones.

Occasionally, the thyroid may not produce enough of the hormone thyroxine. This is called **hypothyroidism.** Sometimes, there is an overproduction of the hormone. This is called **hyperthyroidism.**

Diagnosis of thyroid disease

Blood tests are done to measure TSH and free T4. If the TSH is raised and the free T4 is low, then you have hypothyroidism. Decreased TSH and raised free T4 are indicative of hyperthyroidism.

Hypothyroidism and pregnancy

This is a condition in which the body lacks sufficient thyroid hormone. Since the main purpose of thyroid hormone is to regulate the body's metabolism, people with this condition will have symptoms associated with a slow metabolism.

Causes of hypothyroidism during pregnancy

The most common cause of hypothyroidism is the autoimmune disorder known as Hashimoto's thyroiditis. Inadequate treatment of a woman already known to have hypothyroidism or overtreatment of a hyperthyroid woman with antithyroid medications can also result in problems.

The risks of hypothyroidism to the mother

Most women with mild hypothyroidism may have no symptoms. Untreated, or severe hypothyroidism has been associated with anaemia, muscle pain and weakness, low birth weight infants, and postpartum haemorrhage (bleeding).

The risks of maternal hypothyroidism to the baby

The thyroid hormone is critical for brain development in the baby. Do not stop your thyroid medication when you find out you are pregnant. The effect of maternal hypothyroidism on the baby's brain development is not clear. It is important that hypothyroidism be adequately treated in pregnancy. TSH and free T4 levels must be checked regularly in pregnancy to monitor if you are getting enough hormone replacement.

Treatment of hypothyroidism during pregnancy

There must be adequate replacement of thyroid hormone in the form of synthetic **thyroxine** Thyroxine requirements frequently increase during pregnancy, often by 25 to 50 per cent. Women with known hypothyroidism should have their thyroid function tested as soon as pregnancy is detected and their dose adjusted by their physician as needed, to maintain the TSH level in the normal range.

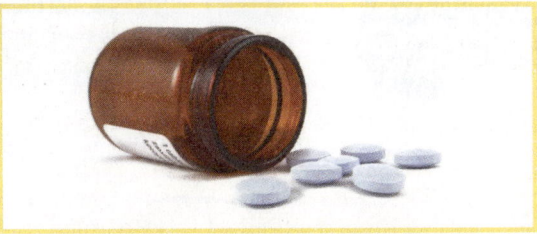

Prenatal vitamins contain iron that can impair the absorption of thyroid hormone. Consequently, thyroxine and prenatal vitamins should not be taken at the same time and should be separated by at least 2-3 hours.

Children born with **congenital hypothyroidism** (no thyroid function at birth) can have severe cognitive, neurological and developmental abnormalities if the condition is not recognised and treated promptly. It is recommended that babies of mothers with hypothyroidism be tested for thyroid function on the 3rd or 4th day of life. Ideally, for all newborns should be tested for thyroid function.

Hyperthyroidism in pregnancy

Hyperthyroidism is the medical term used to describe the signs and symptoms associated with an over production of thyroid hormone.

Causes of hyperthyroidism during pregnancy

The most common cause (80 to 85 per cent) of maternal hyperthyroidism during pregnancy is Graves' disease and occurs in 1 in 1500 pregnant patients. Diagnosis is based on a careful history, physical exam and laboratory testing.

The risks of hyperthyroidism to the mother

Graves' disease may present initially during the first trimester or may be exacerbated during this time in a woman known to have the disorder. Inadequately treated maternal hyperthyroidism can result in premature labour and pre-eclampsia. Very severe hyperthyroidism (known as 'thyroid storm') may also develop.

The risks of hyperthyroidism to the baby

If hyperthyroidism is treated adequately, the risks to the baby are very low. It is important to see your physician before you get pregnant so that the proper medication can be given in the sufficient dose.

Treatment options for a pregnant woman with hyperthyroidism

When hyperthyroidism is severe enough to require therapy, anti-thyroid medications are the treatment, with **propylthiouracil (PTU)** being the drug of choice.

After delivery

Hyperthyroidism typically worsens in the postpartum period, usually in the first 3 months after delivery. Higher doses of anti-thyroid medications are frequently required during this time. As usual, close monitoring of thyroid function is necessary.

Breastfeeding

It is safe to breastfeed the baby if you are on propylthiouracil (PTU). The baby will require periodic assessment of its thyroid function to ensure maintenance of normal thyroid status.

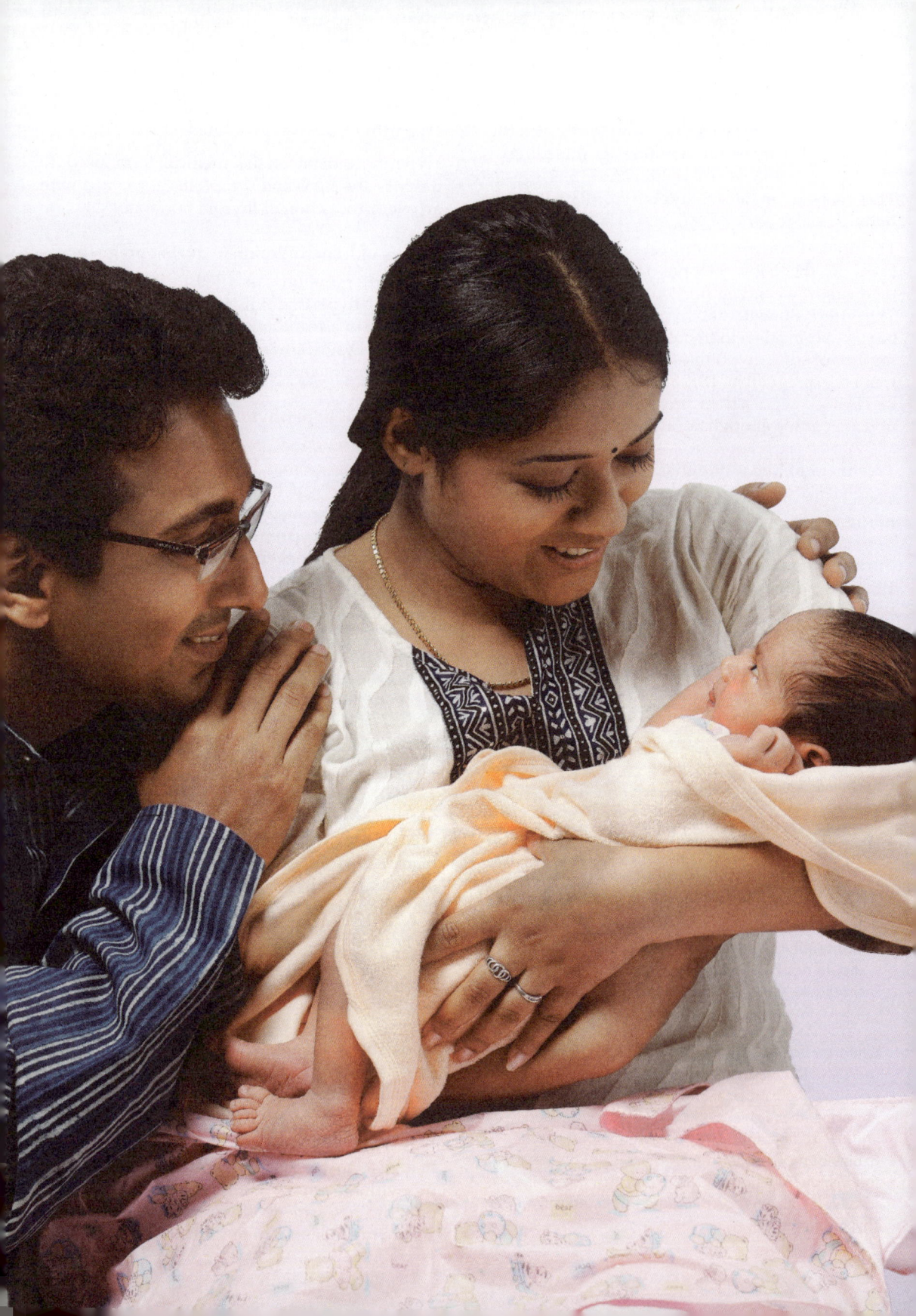

Being a parent

CHAPTER 41

Preparing your child for the arrival of the new baby

Shravanthi is the mother of a four year old toddler. She has just found out that she is pregnant for the second time. She wants her daughter to be as excited as she is about the new baby. How should she break the news to her daughter?

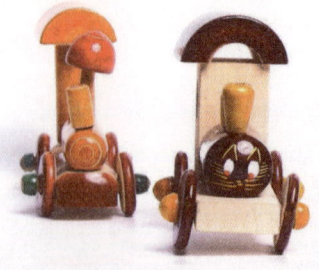

41 Preparing your child for the arrival of the new baby

However loved a child is, she will always feel a sense of displacement when she learns that a new baby is on its way. Having been the focus of attention for her parents and grandparents for three or four years, a toddler can feel threatened by the new baby and will suffer what is known as 'regression'. She may want to be fed, may want to be cuddled more often and on occasion, may even forget her potty training. The child will become difficult to handle and will throw tantrums the way only a toddler can! Getting angry with her and punishing her will only worsen the problem. Give her all the love and understanding that she deserves. After all, how would you feel if your husband suddenly asked you to share your home with another woman! That is exactly how your toddler views the new baby- as an usurper of her rightful place in the family.

Remain calm and unflustered. Do not expect your toddler to behave like an adult and display instant love for the new baby. Ease her into the fact that she is going to be the 'big sister' who will be taking care of the baby.

A good way to make your first child a part of the whole process is to discuss her own birth with her. Explain how excited you were about her coming into the world. Little children are always fascinated by stories of their childhood, especially since they are the main character in the drama that unfolds! Then involve her in the process of the arrival of the new baby. Include her by always saying "your baby", "your little one" and "the baby will expect her sister to take care of her". This will give your child a sense of ownership and she will get engrossed in the whole process of your pregnancy.

Telling your child about the new baby

There are no real rules about how you break the news to your child about the new baby. If your first child is still young, he or she might not quite understand the concept of waiting for a few months till the baby arrives. You might wake up every day to be bombarded by the same question, "Has the baby come yet?"!

If your child is going to school, you can relate the date of delivery with the school calendar. For example, you might say, "The baby will arrive just before the summer holidays."

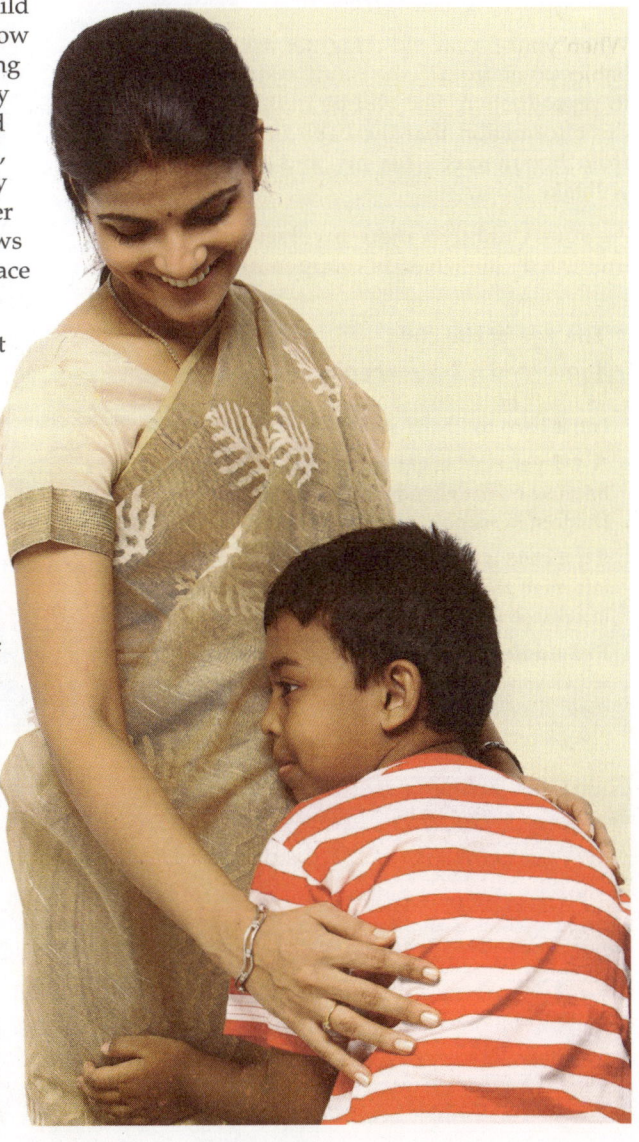

How your child handles the news also depends on the age of the child and the size of the extended family. If your child is used to being in the middle of a large family, he or she will handle the newcomer better. If the child has been the centre of attention in a small nuclear family, he may find it hard to give up his place. If there has been the birth of another child in the close family and your child has been aware of it and has participated in the fun of a new arrival, he may handle it better.

Your child is not asking for details!

When your 5 year old daughter asks, "Where do babies come from?" she is not asking for a lesson in reproduction. She will be quite satisfied with the information that the baby is going to come from her mother's tummy and that the doctor will take it out.

As your child gets more involved and is really interested in what is happening, help him understand by showing him what he looked like when he was a baby. His own baby pictures will help him realise how small the new arrival is going to be.

If your child is old enough, you can share the pictures in this book about how the baby is developing **(Chapters 5 to 7)**. You can also take him to see a friend who has had a baby. Let him give you suggestions about baby names. Don't be surprised when he wants to name the baby after his best friend in school or his favourite teacher!

> Regardless of the child's age, parents have to be realistic and need to know that each child will react differently to the arrival of a new baby. Be patient and most importantly, don't feel guilty about having another child!

Involve your child during pregnancy

If your child is small but old enough to understand the concept of another baby, tell her

> **The age of the child**
>
> If your child is **2-3 years** old, she might tend to be more possessive of your affections and might find it hard to 'share' you.
>
> A **4-5 year** old might find it easier to share because he has already learnt to deal with other children in school.
>
> If the child is **six or older,** he might want to be informed about all that is happening and might be interested in helping out with the new arrival.
>
> **Pre-adolescents** or **adolescents** could swing either way. They might resent this 'usurper' of their place in the family or they might be completely overjoyed with the new one.

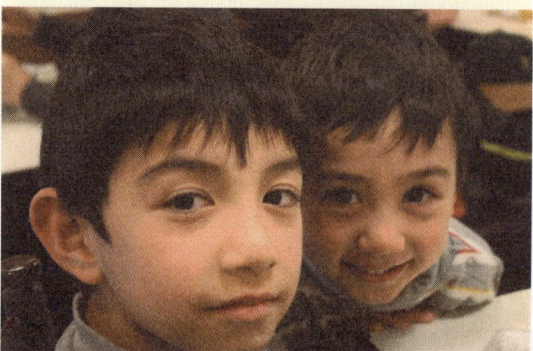

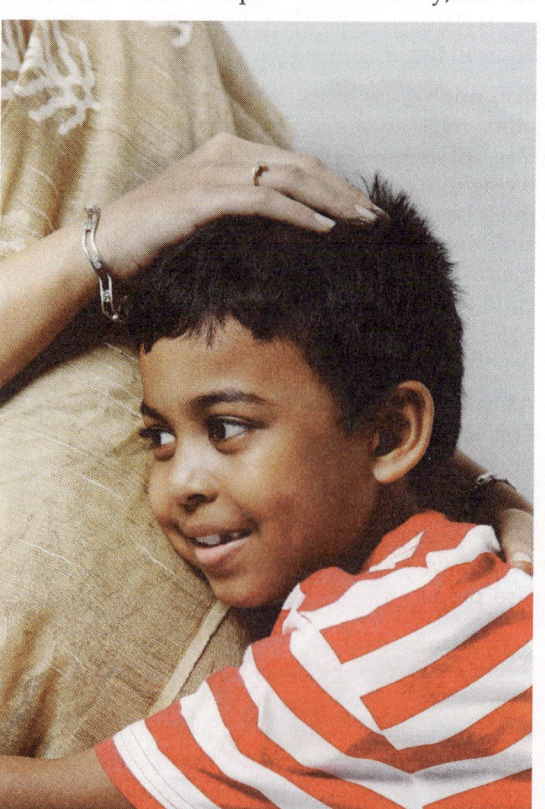

around the third month of your pregnancy. Of course, if your child is older and understands your conversations well, tell her as early as possible so that she does not feel left out.

Take your child with you to the antenatal check-ups so that he can be involved in the process right from the beginning. Ask your doctor if he can be allowed to hear the baby's heartbeat (which is possible when using a hand-held Doppler).

Let your child help in picking stuff for the new arrival.

Either directly or by suggestion, do not influence the child to say that she specifically wants a sister (or a brother). Encourage her to say that she wants a baby and it does not matter whether it is a boy or a girl. When you keep stressing that you want the baby to be of the opposite sex of your child, she might feel that you don't appreciate her or that she was a disappointment. She will then resent the new baby.

You might also want to talk to your parents or other relatives about what to say to your child. Very often, the elders in the family may keep trying to tutor the child into saying that the baby must be a boy (or a girl). This only confuses the child into believing that you can actually choose the sex of the baby. Let everybody encourage the child to ask for a healthy, normal baby.

Involve your child in the hospital

As you get closer to the due date, and if your first child is old enough, then involve him in the preparations you will be making for going to the hospital.

Make arrangements for your child to be taken care of when you are in the hospital. You must also prepare the child for the separation and let him know that he is being very helpful to you by being mature and staying at home.

Let your first child come and visit you as soon as possible. Let this be an intimate time for you, your husband, your child and the newborn. Do not let this be a big gathering of friends and relatives where your first child will feel that all the attention has been taken away from him.

Your child will want to touch and feel the baby. Do not get agitated and angry. Let him gently touch the baby while you are holding it. Calmly explain that the new baby is fragile and needs gentle handling.

Do not be surprised if your first child regresses and wants to be held and cuddled by you. Give him all the hugs and reassurances he needs.

After bringing the baby home

When you come home, reserve some special time for your first born. Have someone handle the baby for a while and give all your attention to the first one.

Visitors will have a tendency to make a big fuss over the newborn. Make sure your first child is involved in introducing "our baby" to others. Remind visitors that your older child may not really be interested in conversations which revolve only round the new baby.

Include your first one in pictures of the baby. Have her help you with the little chores involved in baby care.

If your child sulks and throws a tantrum, be patient and calm. Do not lose your temper or tell her that she is a bad sister. Be firm and allow the child to calm down. Be lavish with your hugs and cuddle her as much as she wants.

If the child continues to be aggressive, make sure that you do not leave him alone with the baby. The aggression will become less eventually - you have to be calm and firm at all times.

Don't forget that a new baby is as great a transition for your child as it is for you. It may bring on a feeling of insecurity as well as anticipation. Try to make this a positive experience for the entire family.

CHAPTER 42

Your new baby

Sheeba and her husband can't take their eyes off their new baby. How tiny and perfect she is! They want to make sure they know how to take care of their baby so that when they get home, they will feel confident enough to handle her.

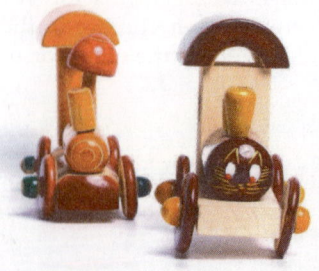

42 Your new baby

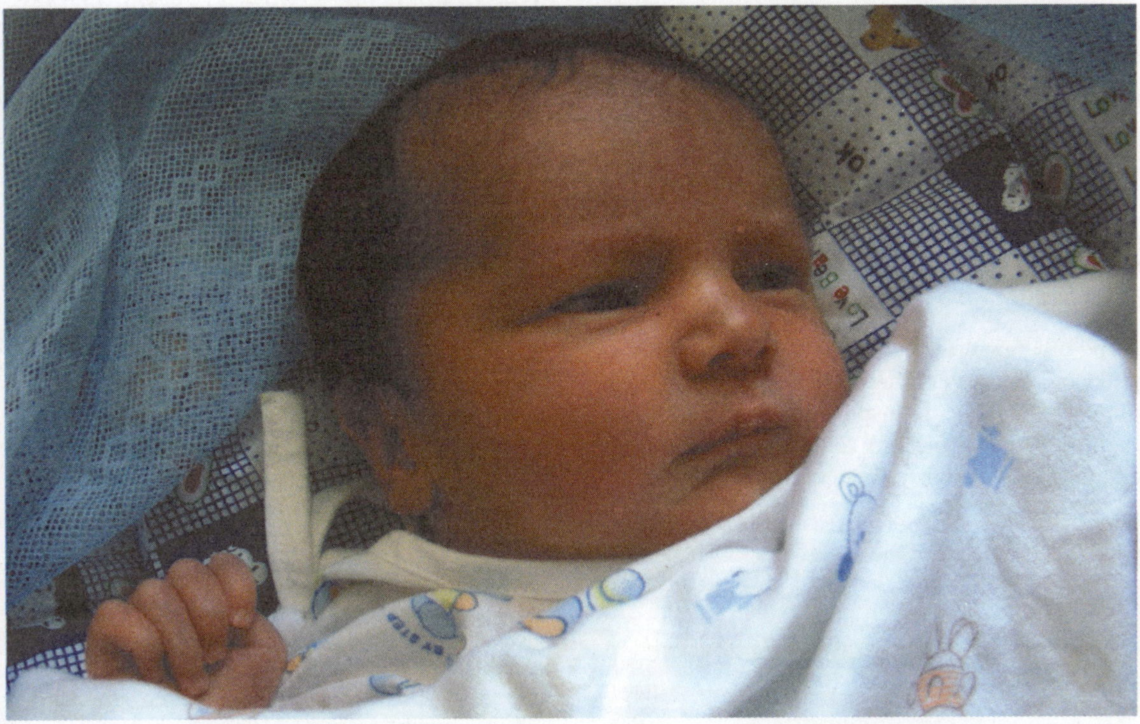

As a new parent, you might be filled with trepidation. You need not worry - you will do fine! Newborns do not come with instructions, but like all responsible parents, you will pick up the skills as you go along. Remember, parenting is an instinctive and intuitive process.

Holding your baby

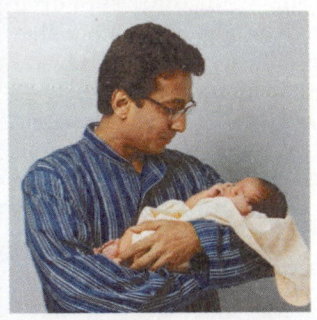

Always make sure you support the newborn baby's neck when holding her. She will feel safe and secure if you support her head and neck with one arm and her bottom and thighs with the other hand. Hold her close to your body for added security.

The baby's skin

At birth, your newborn may be covered with a thick greasy substance called **vernix caseosa** which protected her from the amniotic fluid that she was surrounded by in the uterus. This is usually wiped off when she has her first bath. You might still find traces of it in the folds of her body for a few days.

The baby's skin may be red and wrinkled at birth. After a few hours, you may notice that the skin colour is patchy - areas of pale skin alternating with pink. This is due to the blood vessels under the thin skin and will disappear as the baby matures.

The skin will also be covered with fine **lanugo hair** which may be found on the shoulders, forehead and sometimes over the legs and arms. This soft hair will disappear soon.

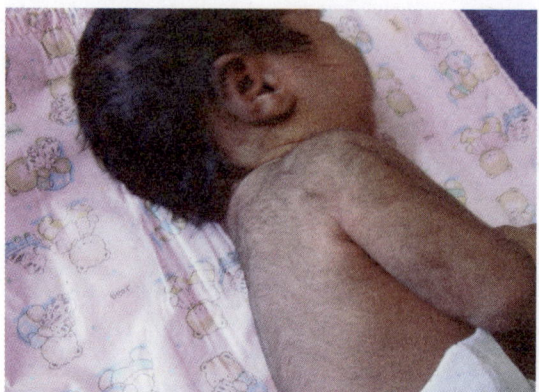
Lanugo hair

In the first few weeks, most babies will develop a pinkish rash over their cheeks, almost like **pimples.** This is in response to the mother's hormones. This does not require any treatment and may last for two to three months.

The baby may have greenish black patches over the buttocks or the lower back. These are called **Mongolian patches** and disappear in a few weeks.

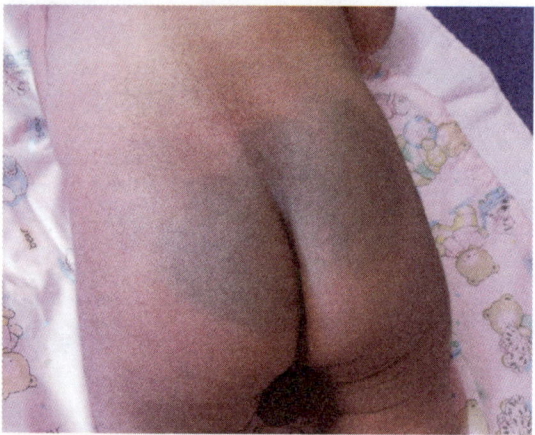
Mongolian patches

The baby may have little white bumps on the nose and face called **milia**. These are caused by blocked oil glands. When the baby's oil glands enlarge and open up in a few days or weeks, the white bumps will disappear.

Another common newborn rash looks like mosquito bites and can occur anywhere over the body, most commonly over the back. This is called **erythema toxicum.** The cause is unknown, and it resolves without treatment after a few days or weeks.

Dry, peeling skin is often due to a baby being born a few days after the due date. The underlying skin is perfectly normal and soft.

In hot weather, your baby may develop **prickly heat** or **heat rash.** It looks like tiny raised red bumps on a red patch and is most often found around the neck, on the chest, back and the scalp. This rash is more common if the baby is overdressed. A cool bath and light clothing may help the baby be comfortable.

During a baby's first few months of life, she may develop a **cradle cap,** a condition that looks like dirty, rough skin on the scalp. Washing the scalp daily with soap and water will clear it up in most cases. You can also gently brush the scalp with a soft baby brush or toothbrush. Sometimes, rubbing a little oil into the scalp before washing the head will help. If the condition persists or spreads, see your paediatrician.

A **diaper rash** is very common and usually clears up in three or four days. Diaper rashes can be prevented by frequent diaper changes, increasing air exposure by keeping the diaper off as much as possible, and using a mild soap after bowel movements. A cream containing zinc oxide can be used to protect the delicate skin and this can be applied after every diaper change or if it is not severe, after every two or three diaper changes.

The baby's eyes

The eyes may be puffy at birth. The baby will try to open her eyes but will scrunch her eyes up if the light in the room is bright. Remember that the baby will not be able to focus for several weeks. The eyes may also keep watering because the tear ducts may not have opened up. In a few weeks, this problem will resolve by itself. If there is a sticky discharge in the eyes, wipe the eyes gently with a cotton ball soaked with warm water. If the discharge persists, it is best to consult the paediatrician.

Do not be alarmed if the baby seems to have a squint and appears cross-eyed. This is a temporary condition and once the baby matures enough to focus his eyes, this condition will correct itself.

The umbilical cord

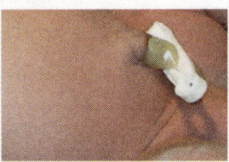
Clamped umbilical cord

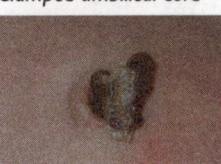
Cord drying up

When the baby is born, the umbilical cord is clamped and cut close to the baby's body. About 2-3 cm of the cord will still be attached to the baby's body. Within a day or two, the umbilical cord which was shiny and moist at birth, will shrivel up and darken in colour. This umbilical stump will dry and drop off in ten to twenty days. The stump must be kept clean and dry. Fold the baby's diaper below the stump so it is exposed to the air. This will prevent it from being constantly soaked by urine. A wet cord may smell and appear infected. Do not worry, this is normal. When the stump falls off, you may detect a little blood on the diaper, which is normal.

Do not apply any ointment, creams or home remedies to the cord or stump.

Sometimes, the cord will dry and will continue to hang from the umbilicus by just a small thread like attachment. Do not pull it off. It will fall off by itself.

Sometimes, after the stump falls off, a pink or yellowish piece of flesh may remain, which will disappear by itself. This is called an **umbilical granuloma**. At times, there is a yellowish discharge or even a small amount of bleeding from this. The paediatrician may apply medication to this to help it dry up.

Regurgitation of milk or spitting up

A common problem that worries new parents is regurgitation or spitting up. Most newborn babies will bring up a small amount of milk soon after feeding. This happens because the baby swallows air while feeding. The swallowed air comes up as a burp and part of the milk also

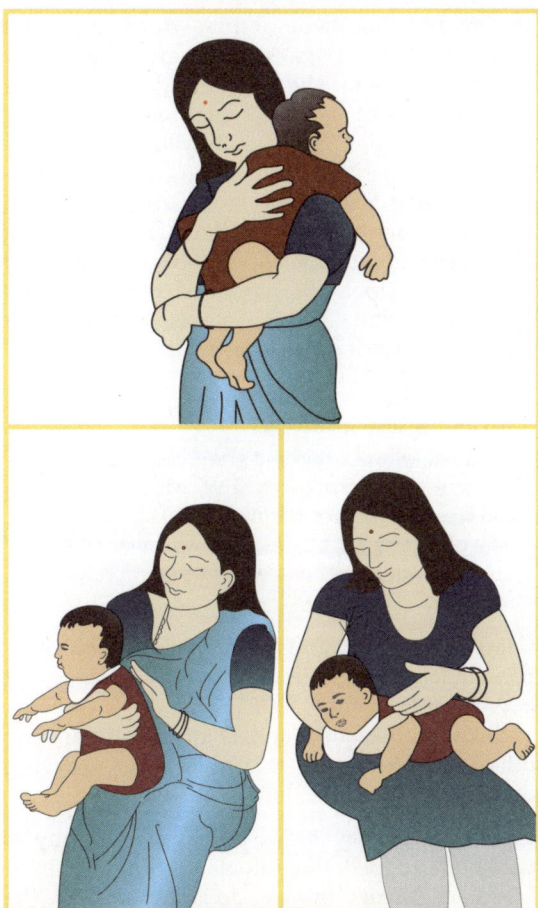

Methods of burping a baby

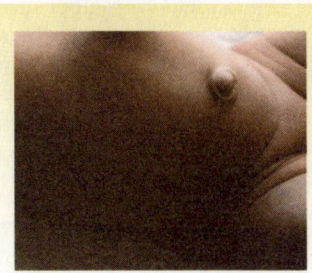

Umbilical hernia

Some babies may have a very prominent umbilicus. Every time the baby cries, the umbilicus and the area around it will bulge out, sometimes alarmingly. The swelling will become less prominent when the baby stops crying or straining. Do not worry. This is an umbilical hernia and many babies are born with it. Usually this will become smaller and may even disappear completely within a year. You need to see your doctor immediately if the swelling is hard, appears red and does not go down on gently pressing down with a finger.

comes out along with the air. Burping the baby by holding him upright on the shoulder for 5 to 10 minutes after the feed relieves the gas and regurgitation. Some babies just spit up more than usual. Make sure you burp the baby well. The problem will usually settle down in a few weeks.

Stools

During the first two to three days, the baby passes black, tarry stools which are followed by greenish stools for the next few days. With the establishment of regular breast feeds, the baby will pass regular, semisolid, yellowish stools. Most babies pass 4 to 8 stools in a day. Remember that some babies pass stools after each feed. This does not mean that the baby is having diarrhoea. Some babies pass stools once in 2 to 3 days. If the stools are hard and the baby cries excessively while passing stools, consult your doctor to rule out constipation.

> **Straining and grunting**
> Most babies will strain and grunt almost like they were severely constipated. They will go red in the face and grimace alarmingly. This is just a way of passing gas or even passing urine. This straining will usually decrease in a few weeks.

Diarrhoea is diagnosed when the baby is passing large quantities of watery, loose stools at a greater frequency. When the baby is being exclusively breastfed and is not receiving any other top feeds, it is unlikely to develop diarrhoea due to infection.

Constipation may be suspected if the baby is passing hard, pellet-like stools that cause pain or bleeding. The first thing to do is to make sure the baby is getting enough milk. If necessary, some water may be given. If this does not help, your paediatrician may prescribe a medicine.

Urine

Most newborns pass urine within 48 hours of birth. If the baby has not passed urine within 48 hours, the paediatrician will make sure the baby is not dehydrated. If the baby does not pass urine in spite of adequate feeds, tests will be done to make sure that the baby has no kidney problem. A normal baby passes urine about 5-10 times per day. Babies usually cry on passing urine. This does not mean that the baby is having pain. This just helps them push the urine out.

Sleep

During the first few days of life, most babies keep their eyes closed with occasional attempts to open their eyes. Of course, there are some babies who open their eyes immediately and seem to be quite alert and awake!

Most newborns sleep during the day and are awake and playful during the night. You might have noticed during your pregnancy that the baby is usually less active during the daytime and up and kicking when you want to rest at night! This sleep rhythm continues even after the baby is born. Babies tend to fall into a set sleep pattern in 4 to 6 weeks.

> When you put your little one down to sleep, move slowly and gently to prevent him from getting startled or even waking up. Put his head down first. Always make sure to support his neck. Then gradually lay the rest of his body down. Gently slide out your hand from under his head. Then remove the other hand. Stay by his side, stroking him and speaking or singing to him softly. He will hopefully settle down to sleep.

It is best to put the baby to sleep on his back or on his side. It is better not to place the baby on his stomach to sleep.

Babies also tend to fall asleep after taking just a few sucks at the breast. This may leave you

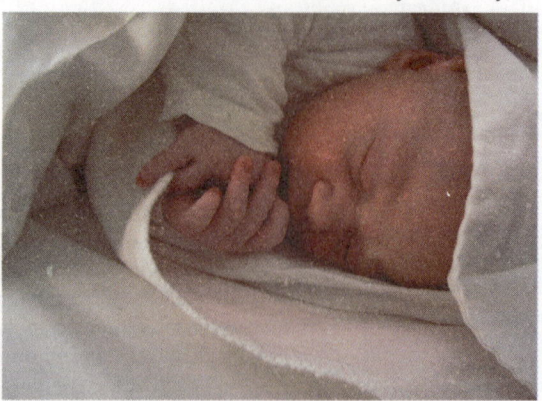

frustrated that the baby is not feeding well but soon enough the baby will get hungry and start suckling properly.

Startle reflex and other reflexes

When a newborn baby is startled by a sudden noise, he responds by arching his back, kicking his legs and jerking his arms. This is known as the Moro reflex.

When you place a finger or any object in the baby's palm, the baby will grab on tightly.

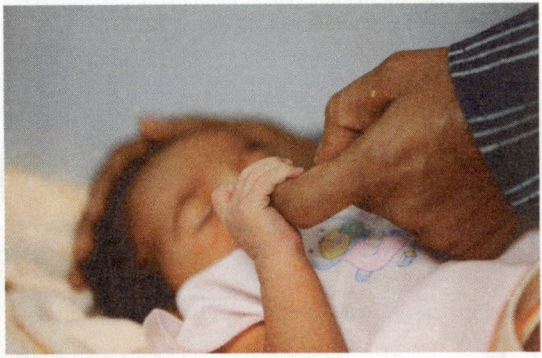

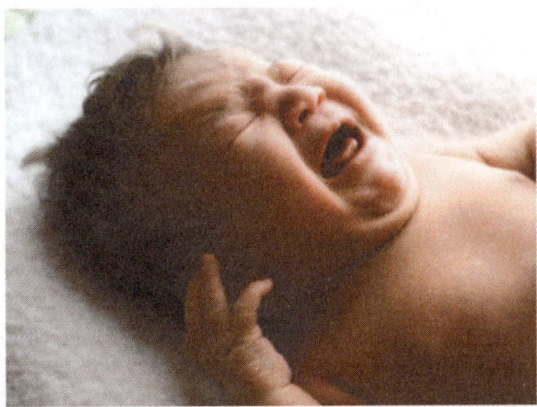

Presence of continuous crying or a high-pitched cry may suggest infection, and the baby should be taken to the doctor immediately.

Rooting reflex is when your baby is searching for food. She will open her mouth and turn her head toward your hand if you stroke her cheek.

When your baby is drowsy or sleeping, you may notice her smiling. She is in a dreamy state and this is termed **reflexive smiling.** It will be a few weeks before she will actually be smiling back in response to your smile.

Sneezing

This is very common and usually is a way for the baby to clear her nose.

Hiccups

Remember that your baby was hiccupping even inside your womb! When the baby hiccups, it does not mean anything is wrong. It will subside by itself and the baby is really not feeling any discomfort.

Excessive crying in newborns

Most babies cry when they are either hungry or having discomfort such as a wet or soiled nappy.

> Some babies suffer from **colic.** Most babies will have a particular time of the day when they will cry inconsolably for 3-4 hours. If you have fed the baby, the diaper is clean and there is no fever, you just have to walk around with the baby or rock her and hope she calms down. An infant with colic may have gaseous distension of the abdomen and usually feels comfortable when placed on her tummy which helps the baby pass gas. Colic will usually subside in a few weeks and usually does not persist after the third month.

Bleeding in baby girls

Due to the hormones passing from the mother to the baby, little girls may have a mucous like discharge or even bleeding from the vagina. This is nothing to be concerned about and will subside on its own.

Fever

It is unusual for a newborn to develop fever. The paediatrician will make sure that the fever is not due to dehydration before checking for an infection. During the summer months, some babies may develop a mild fever during the second or third day of life. If the child is active and feeds well, usually there is no cause for worry. A rise in temperature due to dehydration is easily treated by ensuring proper feeds and hydration.

Giving the baby a bath

Babies have sensitive skin that dries out easily. Till the umbilical cord falls off, it is alright to wipe the baby off with a wet cloth dipped in warm water. Once you are comfortable with giving a bath, you can use a basin to bathe the baby. The bath can be given every day but it does not matter if you skip a day as long as you keep the baby's face and bottom clean.

Ideally, a bath should be given in the morning or at the end of the day before a feeding so that the baby can then feed and fall asleep. If the baby is very hungry, feed her but wait for at least 15 minutes before you bathe her so that she does not spit up the milk.

Your newborn does not need to have a bath every day. Just wipe her face, neck and diaper area with a wet towel whenever she is dirty.

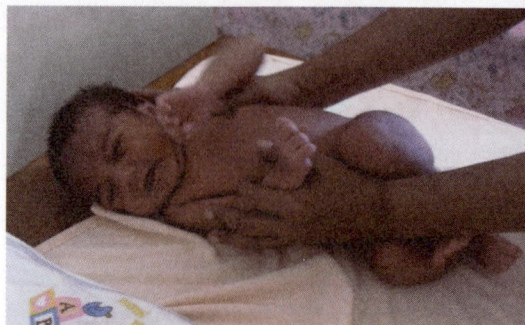

1 Take your baby's clothes off. Make sure that it is not drafty so that the baby does not feel cold.

Tips for a happy bath time

NEVER leave an infant alone near a tub or bucket of water – not even for a minute!

Make sure you have all supplies ready before you begin the bath.
- Towel
- A mild shampoo or soap
- Cotton
- A small, soft hand towel to clean the face

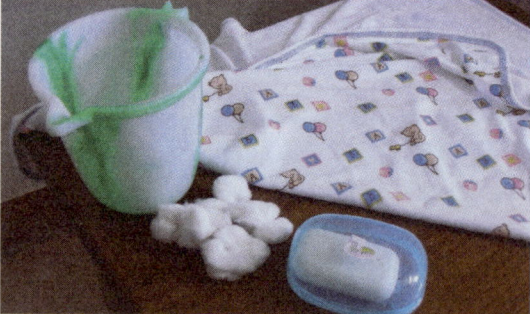

Make sure the room is warm enough and the water is not too hot or cold before putting your baby in the tub.

Use a small wet towel or your hand to gently wipe the baby's face and ears. No soap is necessary near the eyes.

Use only a mild baby shampoo and soap.

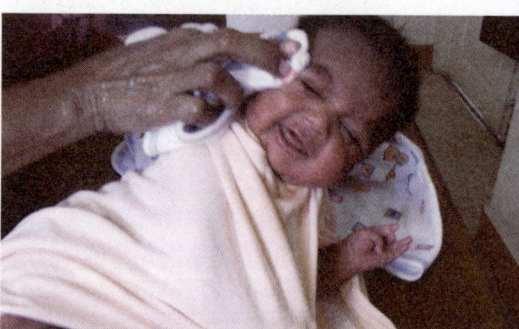

4 Use damp cotton balls to wipe your baby's eyes. Gently wipe the face with your wet hand and then dry his face with a towel.

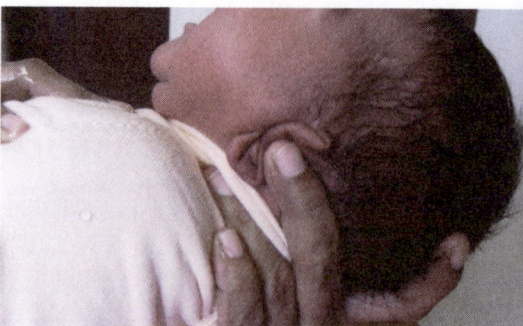

7 Wash your baby's hair and scalp very gently, using soap or a baby shampoo. You need to do this only once or twice a week.
To prevent water from entering the baby's ears, gently fold the ears and hold them in place with your thumb on one side and the middle finger on the other.

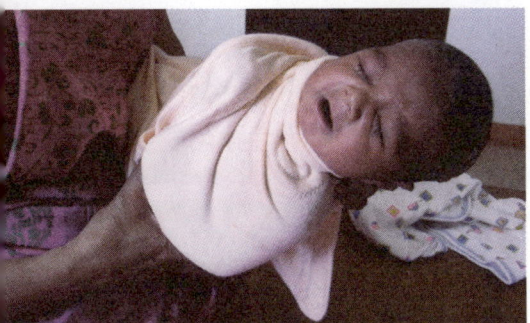

2 Keep two towels ready. Once you have undressed the baby, wrap the baby in a towel. This helps you hold your slippery baby while you wash his face and hair. Wrap the baby snugly in the towel so that his arms and legs will not dangle while you wash his hair.

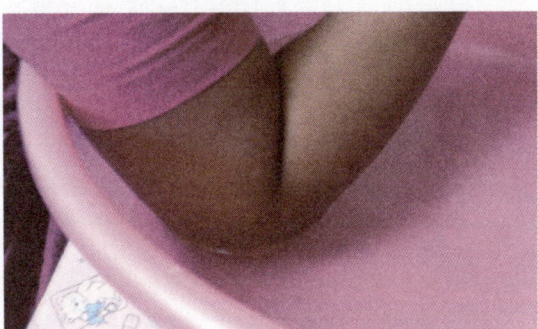

3 Fill a bowl or basin with warm water. Use your wrist or elbow to check the water to make sure it is just the right temperature. Be sure the water is not too cold or too hot. Very hot water can be dangerous.

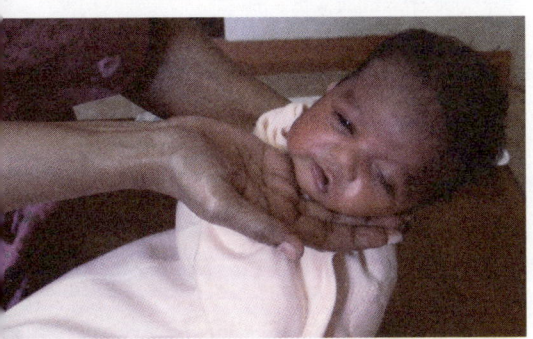

5 Wash and dry under his neck.

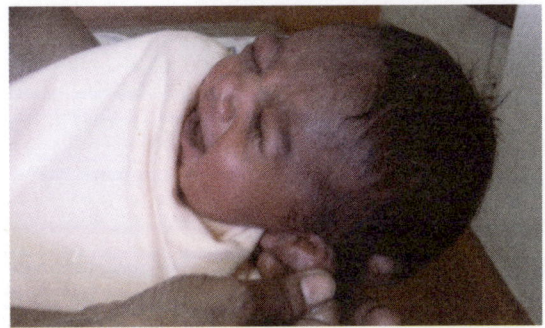

6 Gently wash the outside and back of each ear and behind his ears.

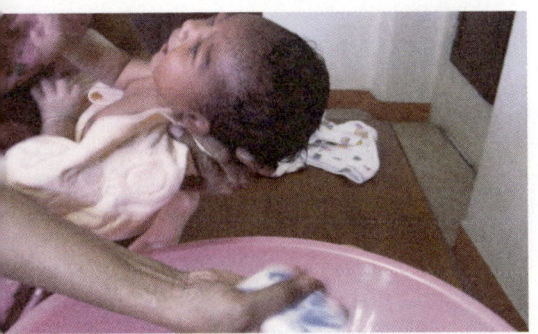

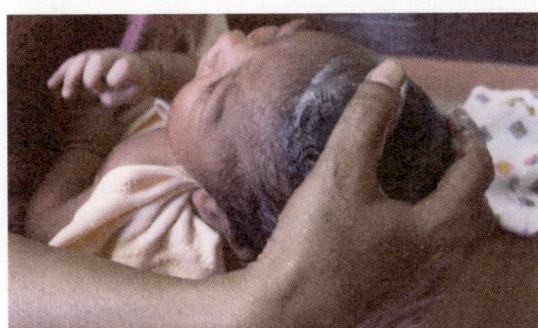

8 Hold his head over the basin and gently pour some water on his head. Hold him firmly like a bundle. Let his bottom rest on your waist, under your left elbow. Cradle his head in your left palm, with your fingers gently gripping his neck. Of course, you can use the other arm if you are left handed!

Take some baby soap or shampoo in your hand and apply it to his scalp. Rub the soap softly into the scalp till there is a lather. Remember that the baby's scalp will not be that dirty so you do not have to wash his hair every time you give him a bath. If he has a cradle cap, you can gently scrub his scalp with a soft toothbrush to loosen the flakes.

Using baby powder

You really do not need to use baby powder in the first few weeks. If you want to use powder, any baby powder may be used, but powders made with cornstarch are preferred. Make sure that you do not use powder on the face because the baby may end up inhaling too much of the powder. Shake the powder on to your hands and not directly on to the baby so that the powder does not enter the baby's lungs. A good rule of thumb is to use the powder on the body only below the baby's umbilicus.

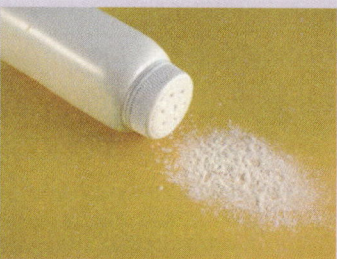

Baby oil and lotion

It is not essential to apply oil to the baby's body or head. Lotions are usually not necessary unless the skin is very dry.

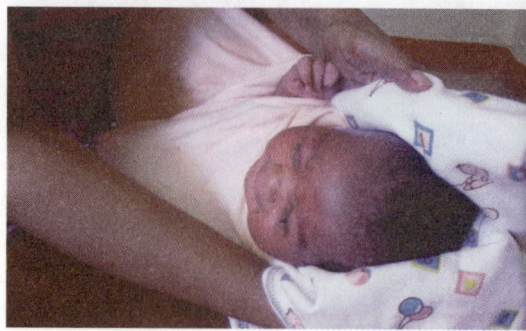

9 Wash off the soap from his hair. You can use your cupped hand to pour water over the baby's head or when you are more experienced, you can pour water using a mug. Make sure that the water does not run over his eyes or nose. Once his scalp is washed, you can wipe off his hair with a towel.

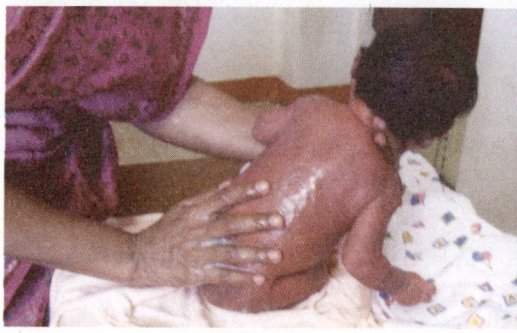

11 Supporting his chest with your palm, make sure to soap his back too.

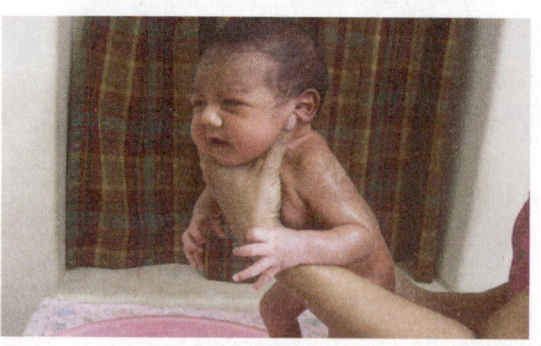

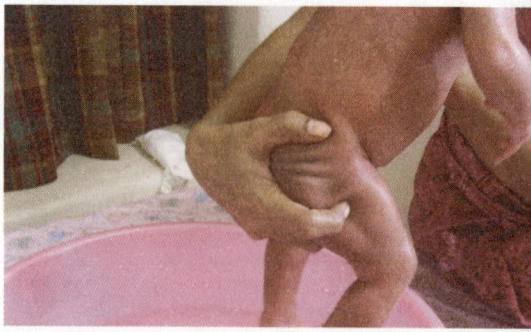

13 Remember, babies can be slippery so always keep a good grip on him. Don't worry; you will master the art of giving a baby bath very soon!

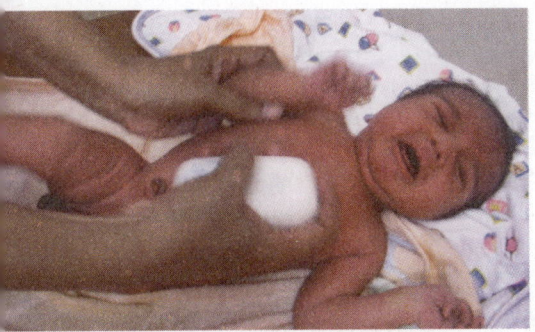 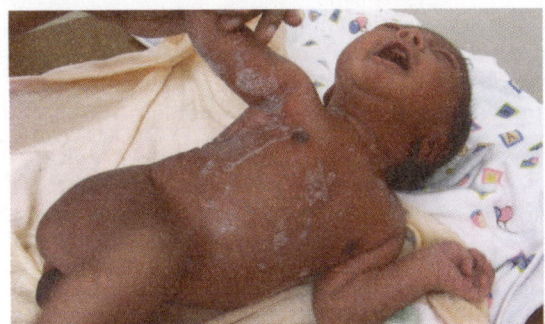

10 Now lay your baby on the table and unfold the towel that was wrapped around him. Rub soap on his body, and make sure that you don't forget to wipe all the folds.

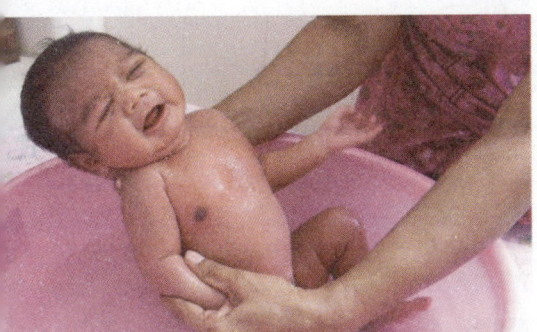 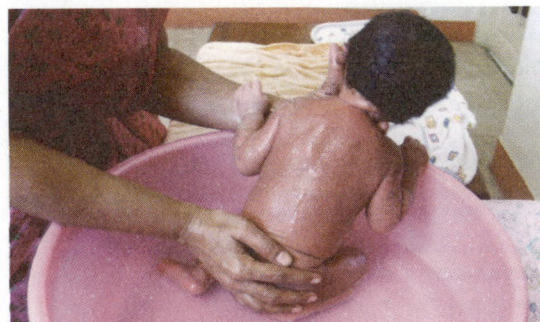

12 Place him back in the basin, making sure to hold him firmly. If you are worried that he will slip, you can place a folded terry towel in the bottom of the basin. This will provide traction for his bottom. Rinse the soap off the baby. You can use your cupped palm to pour water over the baby or use a mug.

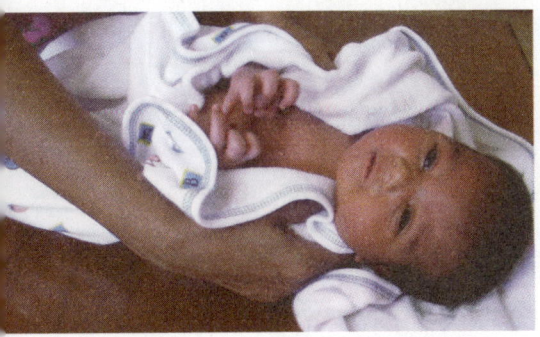 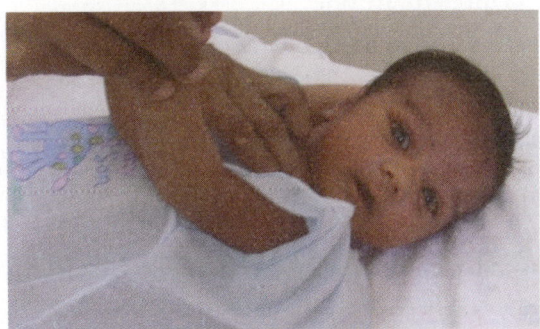

14 Gently rub your baby dry with a bath towel. Always keep him covered and warm when he is wet.

15 A fresh and clean baby!

The art of changing a diaper

New parents are usually apprehensive about changing diapers. Once you have done it a few times, you will become confident enough to do it fast and with the least amount of trouble!

When you are going to change the baby's diaper, make sure all the things that you need are right next to you.

- A fresh diaper: If using a cloth diaper, you will need diaper pins and waterproof panties. You can also use a cloth diaper which comes with ties
- Cotton and warm water in a mug for cleaning and a small towel for drying
- Zinc oxide ointment if needed (for diaper rash)
- Powder to apply over the baby's bottom
- A plastic bag or small plastic disposal basket to throw the used diaper in

Which diaper is best?

Most new parents dread changing diapers and worry that they may not be able to handle this chore! Diapering has become much more easier now with the availability of readymade cloth diapers and also disposable diapers. It does not matter which diapers you use. Just keep in mind that disposable diapers can be much more expensive. You can use cloth diapers for daily use and reserve disposable diapers for going out. Soiled cloth diapers are difficult to handle when you are out.

Tips for proper diapering

- Until the umbilical cord falls off, fold the diaper down to expose the raw area to the air and keep it from getting wet
- Make sure you wash the cloth diaper soon after it gets soiled otherwise it will be difficult to get rid of the stain
- There is no need to add an antiseptic solution to the water which is used to wash the diaper
- Dispose off plastic diapers by folding them over, retaping them and tying them in a plastic bag
- Wash your hands with soap and water after changing your baby

Diapering made easy

After unfastening the diaper, use it to wipe away most of a bowel movement, from front to back. Then clean away any urine and remaining faeces with wet cotton. Pat your baby dry with a towel. While changing a baby boy, keep a fresh diaper over his penis as much as you can otherwise he will spray you and himself too!

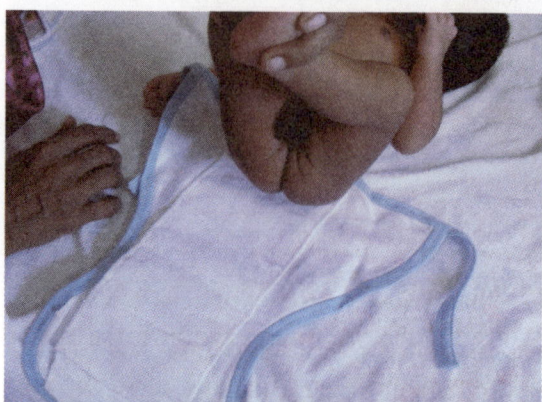

Put on the clean diaper. If you are using a **cloth diaper,** you may need to fold it to fit snugly around the baby. As your baby grows, the diaper will fit even without folding. Slide the diaper under your baby till the top edge is at the baby's waistline.

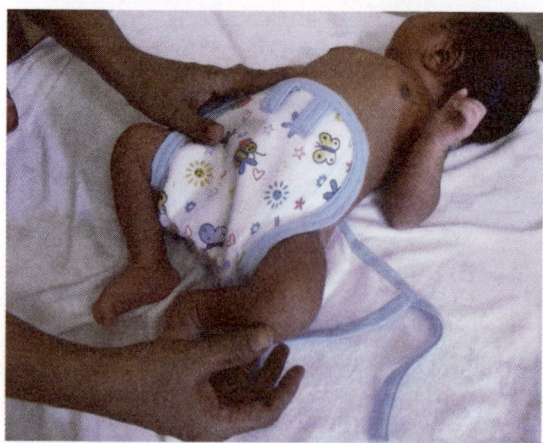

Bring the front up between his legs, and hold it in place while you fold the sides in toward the centre and fasten with a diaper pin. If the diaper comes with ties, you can knot them in front.

A pair of waterproof panties (available in all baby supply shops) can be pulled over the diaper. Waterproof pants should fit snugly but should not be too tight.

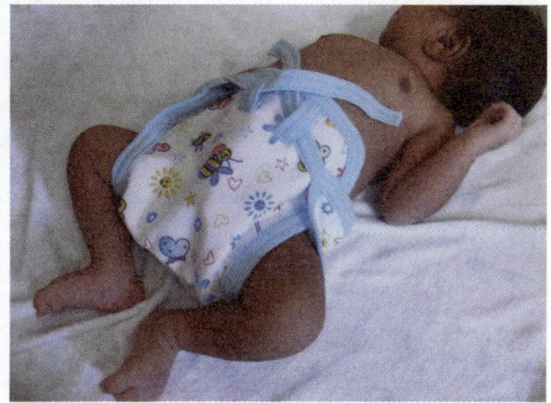

If you are using **disposable diapers,** lay the diaper flat, with the tabs at the back. Slide the diaper under your baby till the top edge is at the baby's waistline. Bring the front up between his legs and tuck it around his stomach. Unpeel the tabs, pull them firmly over the front flap and fasten the diaper. (Be sure not to fasten the tape to your baby's skin.) The diaper should fit snugly, but it shouldn't be tight.

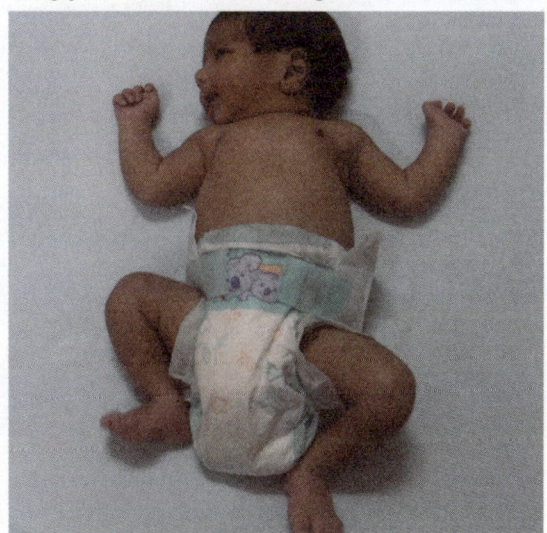

Diaper rash is common and can be treated by keeping the baby's bottom dry. You can use a zinc oxide based cream to help it heal.

What are the baby clothes you need?

Newborn baby clothes, first and foremost, need to be soft and comfortable. They do not have to be elaborate or expensive.

Before you decide to buy baby clothes for your newborn, keep the following factors in mind:

- What climate do you live in and what season of the year is it?
- Do you have help for washing the clothes or do you have a washing machine?
- Do you already have old clothes which you used for your first baby?
- Will your friends or relatives give or loan you clothes for the baby?

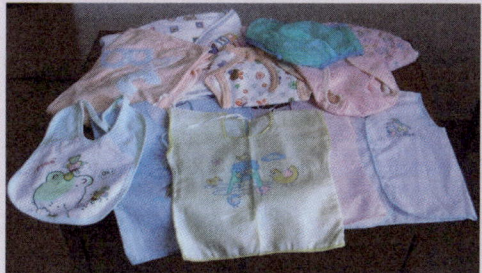

Do not go by the size given on baby clothes. The sizes given are often misleading. For example, a dress marked '2-6 months' may be too small for your newborn. You should buy clothes which are larger than needed because your baby will grow fast and will outgrow them.

In India, you will not go wrong if you buy or stitch cotton clothes, especially in the summer months. If you live in a colder area, you will need warmer clothes for the baby. Try to avoid synthetics which do not let the pores of the child breath.

When selecting newborn baby clothes, you must consider ease of wear and comfort of dressing. The clothing should be roomy and should not be restrictive. Most importantly, the clothes should be easy to put on and remove. In the beginning, jablas are uncomplicated to use and make it easy for a new parent to dress the baby.

Newborn jaundice

Most babies will have mild newborn or neonatal jaundice. Treatment is required when the jaundice is pronounced.

Jaundice is a yellow discolouration of the skin and the white part of the eyes. It results from having too much of a substance called **bilirubin** in the blood. Most babies are born with a high amount of red blood cells. Bilirubin is formed when the body breaks down old red blood cells.

The liver usually processes and removes the bilirubin from the blood. Jaundice in babies occurs because their immature livers are not efficient at removing bilirubin from the bloodstream.

Newborn babies will begin to appear jaundiced when they have more than 5 mg/dl of bilirubin in their blood. It is important to recognise and treat neonatal jaundice. The level of the bilirubin may be treated according to the baby's age. For example, a bilirubin level of 12 mg/dl needs to be treated if the baby is less than 48 hours old but is considered normal when the baby is more than 5 days old.

High levels of bilirubin can cause permanent damage to a baby's brain. This brain damage is called **kernicterus**. Today, because of increased awareness and effective treatment of neonatal jaundice, kernicterus is extremely rare. **Kernicterus will usually happen only when the bilirubin level crosses 20mg/dl in a baby born at full term.** A premature baby may have damage with a lower bilirubin level.

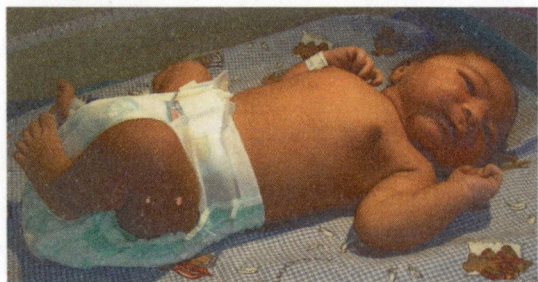

Newborn jaundice

The risk for newborn jaundice increases if:

- The mother's blood group is **O** and the baby's blood group is **A, AB** or **B**. This is called ABO incompatibility
- The mother is **Rh negative** and the baby is **Rh positive.** This is called Rh incompatibility
- The baby is premature
- The mother had diabetes during pregnancy

Treatment of newborn jaundice

Jaundice is most often treated with phototherapy. This involves placing the baby beneath special lights. Two factors help decide whether or not to start phototherapy: the age of the child and the level of bilirubin. If the baby develops jaundice within the first few days, phototherapy is definitely started. The level of bilirubin in the blood is assessed to decide when the phototherapy should be started and how long it should be continued. A premature baby will be started on phototherapy earlier than a full term baby.

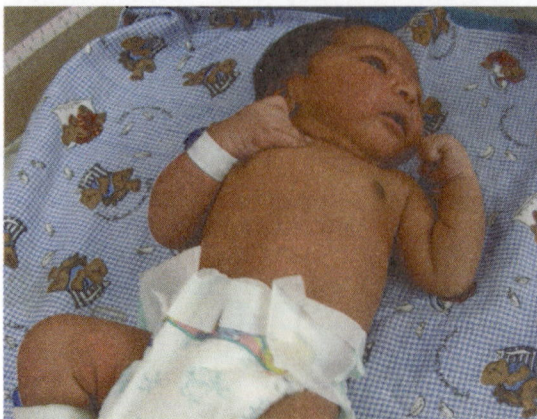

After phototherapy

The light used for phototherapy is able to penetrate a baby's skin. The light changes bilirubin into a soluble form which is easily handled by the baby's body.

Special eyeshades are placed over the baby's eyes to shield them from the lights.

When all other treatment has failed to reduce the bilirubin level enough, the last resort is an **exchange transfusion.** In this treatment, the baby's blood is exchanged with donated blood. This is a specialised procedure and is done only in centres where there are neonatologists who care for critically ill newborns.

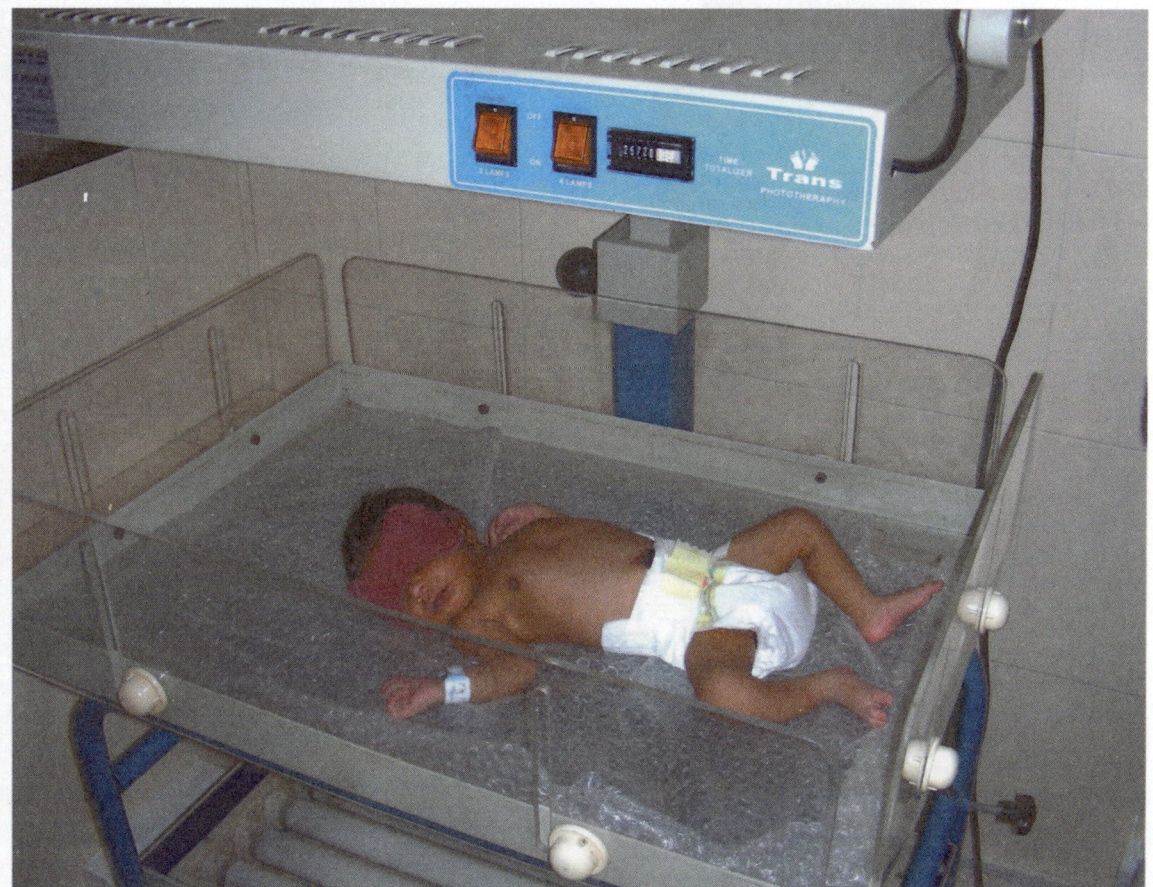
Baby under phototherapy

Warm clothes for the baby

If you live in a place where the temperatures are low, you will need some warm clothes like sweaters, woolen mittens and booties. Babies tend to lose body warmth from their heads so a woolen cap is essential to keep the baby's head warm.

Mittens

In cold weather, you can't do without them. Keep some cotton ones for the summers so that the baby doesn't scratch herself with her own nails.

Baby bibs

A bib is an essential baby requirement. Bibs soak up the baby's regurgitated milk. They can also be used to quickly clean up the area around the mouth. They help keep the area around the neck dry and this prevents rashes under the chin and in the neck folds. When the baby starts teething in a few months, she will drool a lot of saliva. A bib will soak up the saliva and prevent rashes around the neck.

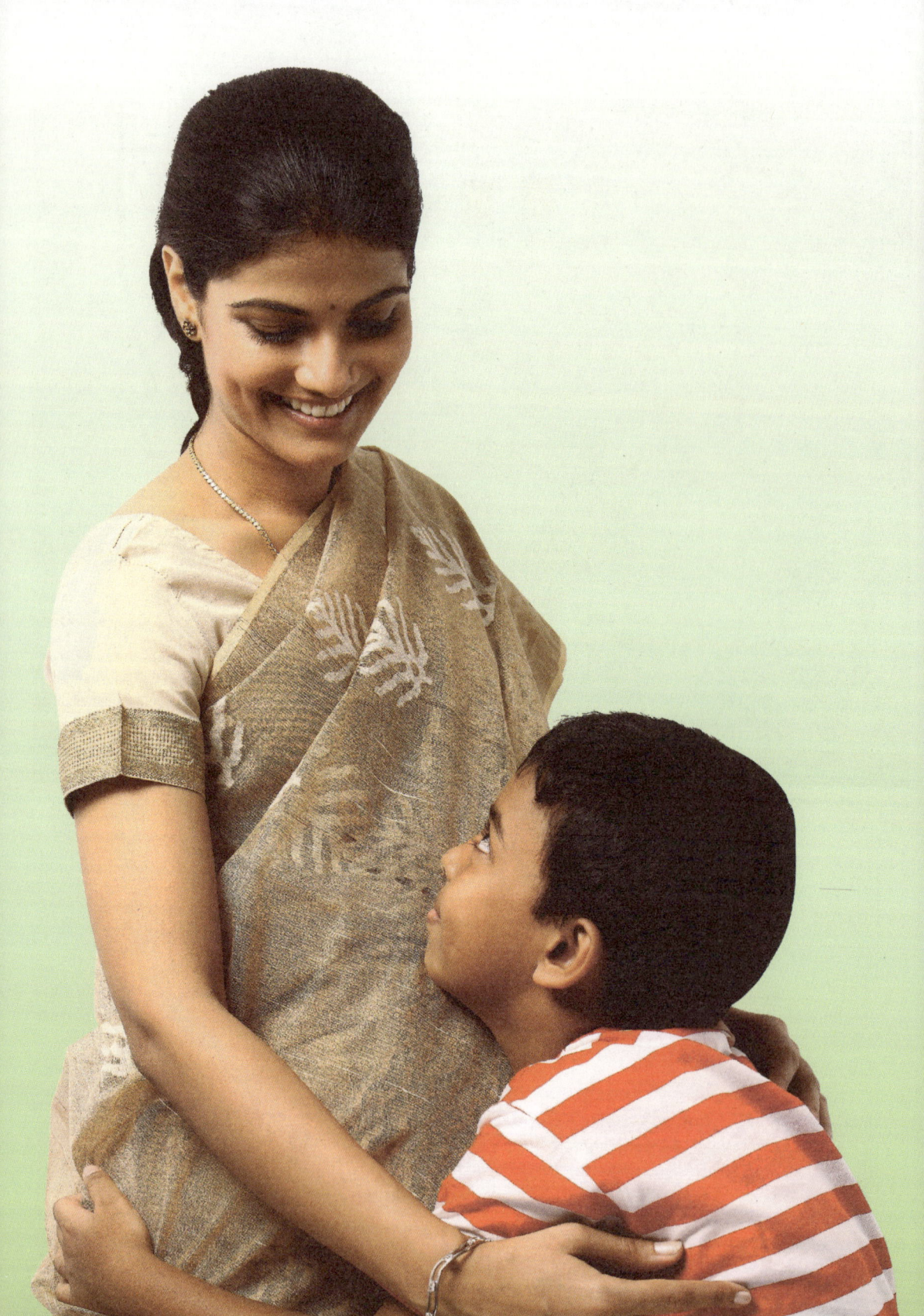

Birth control

CHAPTER 43

Methods of birth control

Sadhana is looking forward to her wedding with excitement. In the midst of the frenetic preparations, Sadhana has an appointment with her gynaecologist. She and her fiancé have decided to wait for a year before planning a family.

Sumangali has just had a baby. At her postnatal check-up, her obstetrician has discussed birth control with her. Sumangali wants to avoid a pregnancy for a few years.

Sandra has two children and wants a permanent method to avoid further pregnancies.

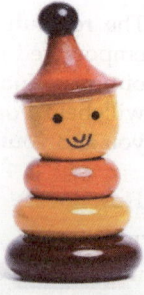

43 Methods of birth control

The need for contraception varies with each individual. It is important to choose the right method of avoiding a pregnancy. Today's woman has a variety of birth control options. Each method has its advantages and disadvantages. Birth control allows a woman to plan her family, not only allowing her to decide when she wants to have a baby, the number of children she wants, the spacing between children, but also allowing her to decide when she wants to permanently stop having children.

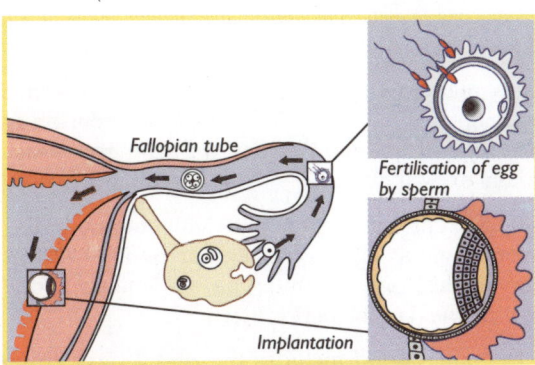

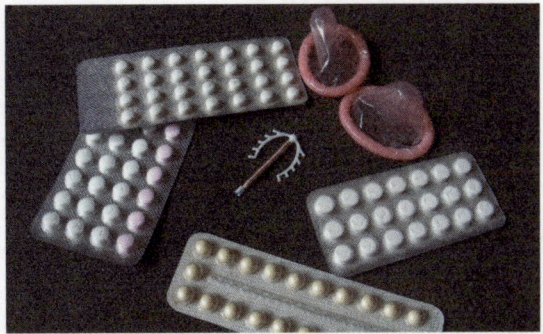

Process of fertilisation and implantation

All of methods are safe when used appropriately. Be sure to discuss the pros and cons of each method with your doctor so that you can choose the method best suited for you.

What is birth control or contraception?

Birth control or contraception is the term used for the prevention of pregnancy. There are many ways to prevent pregnancy. Some are much more effective than others. They include avoiding sex on certain days of the cycle (the so called 'safe period'), hormone medications, contraceptive devices (barriers) and surgery.

The revolution in contraceptive techniques has empowered women and given them several safe options. Knowing what methods are available will help you decide which option is right for you and your lifestyle.

How does birth control work?

To understand how birth control works, you must understand how a pregnancy occurs.

A woman has two ovaries, one on each side of the uterus. Each month, one of the ovaries releases an egg. This process is called **ovulation**. On an average, ovulation occurs about 12-14 days before the start of the next period.

If a woman has intercourse at the time of ovulation, fertilisation can occur. The sperm deposited into the vagina travels up through the cervix, through the uterus and into the fallopian tubes.

If a sperm encounters an egg in the Fallopian tube, **fertilisation** (union of egg and sperm) can occur (see figure above). The fertilised egg then moves down the Fallopian tube to the uterus where it attaches itself and starts growing **(implantation)**.

Birth control methods work by interfering with the process of reproduction in various ways. They may:

- Block the sperm from reaching the egg (male or female condoms, female diaphragm, sterilisation)
- Kill the sperm (spermicidals)
- Keep the eggs from being released each month (birth control pills, injections, implants)
- Change the lining of the uterus so that the fertilised egg cannot start growing (hormonal contraceptives, IUCD)
- Thicken the mucous in the cervix so the sperm cannot easily pass through it

'Natural' family planning

The 'natural' family planning methods of birth control do not depend on any devices or drugs.

The 'safe' period

This method depends on the regularity of the woman's ovulation. The so called 'safe' period is the time of the month when the woman is least likely to ovulate.

To prevent pregnancy with this method, the woman must have very regular periods (28-30 day cycles) and she must be meticulous about noting the day the period starts.

The 'safe' period includes the **first 7 days from the day the period starts (including the days of bleeding) and the last 7 days before the onset of the next period.**

The rigid adherence to certain dates when you can have sex, can take the spontaneity out of a normal marital relationship. It is also not a reliable form of contraception because mistakes can be made in calculating the dates.

Failure rate: The 'safe period' has a **high failure rate of 25 per cent** i.e. 1 out of 4 couples using this method will face an unplanned pregnancy.

The withdrawal method (coitus interruptus)

The withdrawal method involves removing the penis from the vagina just before semen is released (ejaculation). Often the sperms are deposited in the vagina before or during withdrawal, **making this method unreliable.**

Failure rate: The withdrawal method has a **high failure rate (20 per cent).**

Barrier methods

Barrier methods prevent the sperm from coming in contact with the egg by providing a chemical or physical barrier.

Barrier methods include spermicides, condoms (male and female), the diaphragm and the cervical cap. Male and female condoms are available in India.

- **Spermicides** are chemicals that kill the sperm. They are placed in the vagina close to the cervix. They include tablets, foam, cream or jelly. They are inserted into the vagina no earlier than 30 minutes before intercourse. Spermicides should not be used alone. They should be used with another contraceptive such as a condom, for increased effectiveness.
- **The male condom** is a thin sheath made of latex (rubber) or polyurethane (plastic). It is worn by the man over his erect penis.
- **The female condom** is a thin plastic pouch that lines the vagina. It is held in place by a closed inner ring at the cervix and an outer ring at the opening of the vagina. The female condoms are expensive as compared to male condoms.
- **The diaphragm** is a small, round rubber dome that fits inside the woman's vagina and covers her cervix. This is not available in India.
- **The cervical cap** is a small, thin rubber or plastic dome shaped like a thimble. It fits tightly over the cervix and stays in place by suction. This is not available in India.

Male condoms

Failure rate: Condoms have a **relatively high failure rate (15 per cent)** and should be used only if an unintended pregnancy will not pose a problem. If preventing a pregnancy is a high priority, some other form of contraception should be used.

The male condom is still the only reversible form of male contraception currently available. It is a tube of thin material that is rolled over the erect penis just before any contact of the penis is made with a woman's genitals.

The commonly available condoms are made of latex rubber. They are less likely to slip or break than those made of polyurethane, and they are contoured for a better fit which can provide fairly effective protection. Polyurethane condoms have a greater rate of tearing and failure.

The condom should be put on before intercourse when the penis is erect, long before ejaculation, since the male can discharge sufficient semen to cause pregnancy before ejaculation occurs.

If the woman has some discomfort because the vagina is dry, a pre-lubricated condom can be used. Water-based lubricants like K-Y jelly or Lubic gel can be used for extra lubrication. **Do not use white petroleum jelly (vaseline) or coconut oil because these can damage the condom and can cause failure of contraception.**

Prevention of sexually transmitted diseases

Condoms are important in the prevention of sexually transmitted disease in both male and female partners, but they have limitations. They are more protective in men against fluid-transmitted infections (gonorrhea, Chlamydia, trichomonasis and HIV) than in preventing infections transmitted by skin-to-skin contact (herpes simplex virus, human papilloma virus, syphilis and chancroid). Male condoms, in fact, offer better protection against herpes for women than they do for men.

Female condom

Failure rate: Female condoms have a **high failure rate (20 per cent)** and should be used only if an unintended pregnancy will not pose a problem.

The female condom is a lubricated, loose-fitting pouch that lines the vagina. It is designed to create a physical barrier against the sperm and sexually transmitted diseases by surrounding the penis during intercourse. The failure rate for the female condom is about the same as for the diaphragm and cervical cap. It is not yet easily available in India.

Prevention of sexually transmitted diseases

The female condom is an effective barrier to viruses, including HIV, and other sexually transmitted organisms, particularly since it covers a large area, including external genitals. However, no contraceptive device is foolproof.

Use and insertion of the female condom: The female condom is about three inches wide and 6-7 inches long (larger than a male condom), with a flexible ring at both ends. Current products are made of polyurethane.

- The ring at the closed end is used to insert the device into the vagina and hold it in place over the cervix.

- The ring at the open end remains outside the vagina and partly covers the labia.

Hormonal methods

Birth control pills (oral contraceptives) contain synthetic forms of the hormones estrogen and/or progesterone. The hormones stop a woman's ovaries from releasing an egg each month. They also cause the mucous in the cervix (mouth of the uterus) to thicken, which then acts as a barrier to sperm. Birth control pills are ideal for somebody who is recently married and wants to postpone a pregnancy for a while. The pills are taken according to a daily schedule prescribed by your gynaecologist or as given in the package insert.

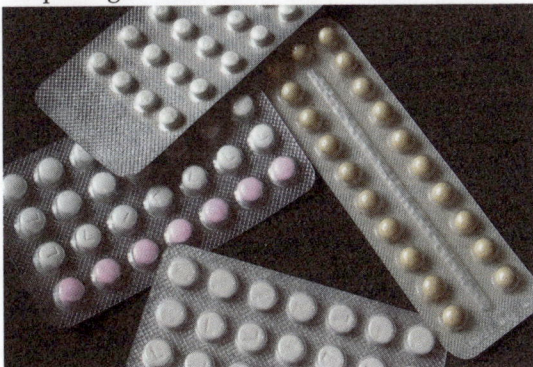

Combination estrogen-progestin contraceptive pills

Oral contraceptives that contain both estrogen and progestin are the more common type of oral contraceptive. **At least 100 million women worldwide use combination oral contraceptives.**

Low dosage: When they were first marketed in the early 1960s, oral contraceptives contained as much as five times the amount of estrogen and up to 10 times the amount of progestins currently used. The hormone amounts in currently available pills are significantly reduced.

Types of regimens: Combination pills are sold in 21-day or 28-day packs:

- Each pill in a 21-day pack contains estrogen and progestin. Women take a pill a day for 21 days, and then wait for seven days before starting a new 21-day pack.

- 28-day packs typically start with 21 hormone pills and add 7 placebo pills that do not contain hormones.

Taking the pill: A woman usually takes the first pill either on the Sunday after her period starts, on the fifth day of her period or on the first day of the period. The remaining pills are taken once a day, ideally at the same time of the day, until the pack is used up. If a woman has a 21-day pack, she waits for seven days before starting a new pack. The period starts in the period-free interval. **The contraceptive effect continues even on the days that you are not taking the pill.**

If you are on the 28-day pack, the period will occur during the days that you take the inactive pills.

Failure rate: Combination birth control pills have a **low failure rate of 3 per cent.** These low failure rates and the safety of birth control pills make them an ideal contraceptive method for couples looking for reversible contraception.

> **What if you miss a pill?**
> If you skip one or more pills, take the following precautions:
> - If you have missed the first pill in a new cycle, take a tablet as soon as you remember and the next one at the usual time. Two tablets can be taken in one day. Use condoms for seven days after the missed dose.
> - If you have missed a pill 2 days in a row, take 2 pills the next day. If you have forgotten more than two pills, continue the pills and also use condoms until the next pill cycle. Do not stop in the middle of the cycle, because you will start bleeding.

> **Getting married and want to be on the pill?**
> Try to see your doctor at least two months before the wedding so that you know how to take the pill properly. Do remember that the Pill is safe and will not prevent you from getting pregnant when you decide to.

Progestin-only birth control pills ("Mini-pills")

The progestin-only pill may contain desogestrol or norgestrel.

Progestin-only pills, which only contain progestins, are always sold in 28-day packs and all the pills are active. Progestin-only pill users will experience very scanty periods and some may not have periods at all. Progestin only pills have a **failure rate of 3-6 per cent.**

> Progestin-only pills must be taken at the same time each day to maintain top effectiveness. If there is a deviation of even three hours, back-up contraception (e.g. condoms) must be used for the next two days. These hormones should not be used by pre-menopausal women in their 40s, since they pose a higher risk for adverse effects in this group.

Continuous-dose birth control pills

These pills are not available in India yet. The continuous-dose pills available in the West are the kind that can cause a period to occur once every three months or once a year.

> **Old wives' tales**
> - Women are concerned that they will put on weight with birth control pills. This is **not true.** A minimal gain of one or two kilos may occur because of water retention.
> - The fear of cancer also worries women. It is interesting to note that birth control pills actually protect women against ovarian cancer.
> - Women worry about how long they need to wait before attempting a pregnancy after stopping the pills. Though it is recommended that you wait for three months before starting to try for a pregnancy, there is usually no problem even if you get pregnant the very next month after you stop birth control pills.

Advantages of birth control pills

- Worldwide, birth control pills continue to be a popular reversible contraceptive choice. Oral contraceptives are among the most effective contraceptives.
- Failure rates are very low and are usually due to noncompliance.

- In some women with heavy periods, they reduce heavy bleeding and so reduce the risk for anaemia.
- Birth control pills can be helpful in reducing the pain associated with periods.

Injectable contraception

Injectable contraceptives are given once every three months. The commonly used injection is depo-medroxy-progesterone acetate (Depo-Provera). Like other progestin contraceptives, Depo-Provera prevents pregnancy by halting ovulation, thickening the cervical mucous and stopping the implantation of fertilised eggs into the uterine lining.

Depo-Provera is effective in preventing pregnancies. However, Depo-Provera should not be used for more than two years because it can cause the thinning of bone (osteoporosis).

How are the injections taken?

After a physical examination, the doctor will give the injection into a muscle in the patient's arm or buttock. The hormone slowly diffuses out of the muscle into the bloodstream. The injection is repeated every three months.

While taking these injections, the periods can become scanty, irregular and may sometimes cease completely.

Once the injections are stopped, it may take 6 to 10 months for your periods to resume and fertility to be restored. This is one of the disadvantages of this method.

Depo-Provera should be avoided by women who have epilepsy, migraine, asthma, heart failure or kidney disease (due to the fact that the drug causes fluid retention). Depo-Provera can also cause a weight gain of 2 to 3 kilos.

Failure rate: Injectable contraceptives like Depo-Provera have a **low failure rate of 0.3 per cent.**

The intrauterine device (IUD):

The intrauterine device (IUD) is a small plastic device containing copper or hormones, which is placed inside the uterus and left there for 5 to 10 years. Instead of stopping a sperm from entering the uterus, the IUD changes the physical environment of the reproductive tract, which prevents the egg from being fertilised or implanting and growing in the uterus.

Over the years, several types of IUDs have been available. The ones most popularly available in India are the copper IUDs (Copper-T, Multiload) or the hormonal IUD (LNG-IUS).

The copper IUD is one of the safest, least expensive and most effective contraceptives available. The copper IUD constantly releases a small amount of copper into the uterus. This causes a reaction inside the uterus and Fallopian tubes which prevents the egg from being fertilised or attaching to the wall of the uterus. It also inactivates the sperm and reduces its ability to fertilise an egg. The Copper–T can be left in the uterus from five to 10 years, depending on the brand.

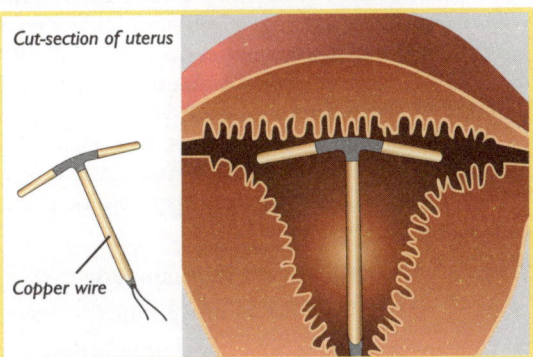

Intrauterine devices (IUDs) are molded plastic devices (some containing copper) which disrupt the normal uterine environment

The hormonal IUD releases a small amount of **progestin** into the uterus. This thickens the cervical mucous, which blocks the sperm from entering the cervix. It also thins the endometrium. This keeps a fertilised egg from attaching on to the lining of the uterus. The hormonal IUD can be left in the uterus for five years. Though the LNG-IUS is very effective, it is also very expensive.

Inserting an IUD

An intrauterine device (IUD) can be inserted at any time, but you might be asked to come immediately after a period. This ensures that you are not pregnant at the time of insertion. If you have just delivered a baby, the doctor will wait for your uterus to shrink back to its normal size before inserting the IUD. This usually happens about 6 to 8 weeks after the delivery.

You do not require any anaesthesia for the insertion. It is a simple procedure and is done on an out-patient basis.

Once the IUD is inserted, the doctor will instruct you on how to check the position of the IUD every month after the period. Attached to the IUD are two thin but strong nylon strings. These strings lie in the vagina and can be felt by inserting a finger into the vagina. They do not interfere with intercourse.

Who should choose the IUD?

An intrauterine device (IUD) is often an excellent choice for women who have had a child and want to postpone another pregnancy. It is also a good choice for women who do not want any more pregnancies but who do not want permanent sterilisation. Women who are unable to use hormonal contraceptives (for example, those with heart disease, epilepsy, migraines, hypertension or liver disease) may also be good candidates for the copper IUD.

Women who should avoid IUDs include

- Women with heavy or painful periods
- Current or recent history of pelvic infection
- A large uterus distorted by fibroids
- An abnormal uterus

Advantages of an intrauterine device

- The IUD is more effective than oral contraceptives in preventing pregnancy and it is reversible. Once it is removed, fertility returns.
- Unlike the birth control pill, there is no daily routine to follow.
- Unlike the barrier methods (spermicides, diaphragm, cervical cap, and the male or female condom), there is no insertion procedure to cope with before or during sex.
- Intercourse can resume at any time, and as long as the IUD is properly positioned, neither the user nor her partner typically feels the IUD or its strings during sexual activity.
- It is the least expensive form of contraception over the long term.

What to expect after inserting an intrauterine device

There might be some spotting or bleeding in the first few days after the insertion of the IUD. Some women may have cramps and backaches for 1-2 days after insertion, and others may suffer cramps and backaches with every period. Your doctor can prescribe a painkiller which will usually do away with this pain.

Some women never get used to the IUD and may have to have it removed to relieve the irregular bleeding and/or cramps. This happens in about 10 per cent of women.

Very rarely does infection set in after the insertion of an IUD. If there is severe lower abdominal pain along with fever and a foul smelling discharge from the vagina, an infection might be suspected. Removing the IUD immediately and treatment with antibiotics will usually alleviate the symptoms.

What happens if you get pregnant with an IUD?

If the strings attached to the IUD are still felt outside the cervix, then the IUD may be removed, with no harm to the pregnancy. If not, the pregnancy can be allowed to continue with the IUD in place. The IUD does not come into contact with the foetus and will not cause any abnormalities. If you do not want to go ahead with the pregnancy, an abortion can be performed.

If you do conceive with the IUD in place, your doctor will check to see if the pregnancy is inside the uterus or if there is an ectopic pregnancy i.e. the pregnancy is growing in the Fallopian tube.

There is also a slightly higher risk of miscarriage if the pregnancy is allowed to continue with the IUD still inside the uterus.

Expulsion: An estimated 2 to 8 per cent of IUDs are expelled from the uterus within the first year. Expulsion is most likely to occur during the first three months after insertion. The risk for expulsion is highest during menstruation, so women should be sure to check the strings after the period to make sure the IUD is in place.

Perforation is an extremely rare complication where the IUD punctures the uterus while being inserted or later on if the IUD shifts position.

Failure rate: Hormonal IUDs have a **failure rate of only 0.1 per cent.** The copper intrauterine device has a **failure rate of 0.8 per cent.** These low failure rates make the intrauterine device ideal for a woman who has already had a child.

Sterilisation

Sterilisation is the surgical closing of the tubes that normally carry the sperm or eggs. **A woman or man who undergoes sterilisation will no longer be able to conceive children.**

When a woman is sterilised, her Fallopian tubes, which carry the eggs from the ovaries to the uterus, are sealed.

In a **vasectomy,** which is the sterilisation procedure for a man, a surgeon cuts and seals the tubes that carry the sperm. A vasectomy is a more minor surgical procedure than female sterilisation.

Failure rate: The failure rate with a sterilisation procedure **is less than 1 per cent in both males and females.**

Female sterilisation

Female surgical sterilisation (also called tubal sterilisation or tubal ligation) is a low-risk, highly effective one-time procedure that offers lifelong protection against pregnancy.

How does female sterilisation work?

Every month, the ovary will produce an egg. The egg enters the Fallopian tube and when the sperm encounters the egg in the Fallopian tube, fertilisation can occur. Female surgical sterilisation procedures block the Fallopian tubes and thereby, prevent the sperm from reaching and fertilising the eggs. The ovaries continue to function normally, but the eggs they release break up and are harmlessly absorbed by the body. Tubal sterilisation is performed in a hospital.

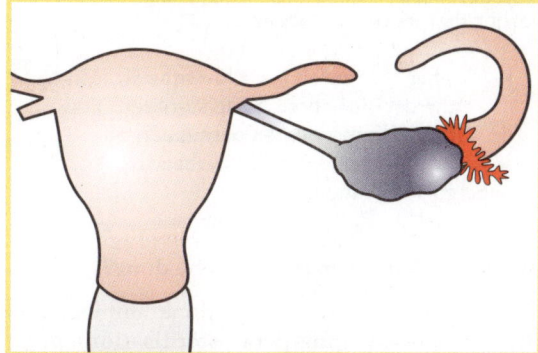

The Fallopian tube is cut so that fertilisation cannot occur in the tube

Periods are not affected by the sterilisation procedure. You will continue to have normal periods since the hormones in your body are not affected by the procedure.

Similarly, libido (sexual desire) is not affected by the procedure. In fact, many women feel so comfortable knowing they cannot get pregnant that they are able to enjoy their sex life better.

Old wives' tales

- Women are concerned that they will put on weight or lose weight after sterilisation. **Not true!** Getting sterilised does not have any effect on your weight.
- The eggs that are released every month accumulate inside the body and therefore will cause weight gain. **Not true!** Human eggs are microscopic and disintegrate within a few days of being produced.
- Sterilisation leads to back ache. **Not true!**
- Sterilisation causes problems with digestion. **Not true!**

Is female sterilisation reversible?

If a woman changes her mind and wants to become pregnant, a reversal procedure is available, but it is difficult to perform and requires an experienced surgeon. Subsequent pregnancy rates after reversal are between 20 to 30 per cent.

Nowadays, if a woman changes her mind or wants another pregnancy because of any adverse event, most gynaecologists would suggest undergoing an IVF pregnancy ('test-tube' baby) rather than reversal surgery.

> Remember that Indian law allows the woman to make the decision about being sterilised. You do not require the written permission of anybody else, including your husband, to undergo sterilisation.

When can female sterilisation be done?

Female sterilisation can be done immediately after a delivery **(puerperal sterilisation)** or at any time when the woman desires it **(interval sterilisation).**

> **Are you making the right decision?**
> Before undergoing sterilisation, you must be absolutely sure that you do not ever want to be pregnant again and bear children, even if the circumstances of your life change radically.
>
> Both you and your husband should be in complete agreement that you no longer want to have children. You should also discuss vasectomy for your husband because vasectomy is a simple procedure that has a lower failure rate than female surgical sterilisation and carries fewer risks.

Once you and your husband have made a decision to proceed with a permanent method of family planning, it is best to discuss this with your obstetrician during your antenatal visits. Your obstetrician will guide you in this regard and will discuss the options with you.

Puerperal sterilisation (done immediately after delivery)

When a woman chooses to undergo sterilisation immediately after childbirth, it is done on the second or third day following delivery. Because the uterus has still not contracted down completely after the delivery, the incision is made just below the umbilicus. Both tubes are tied and cut. Either spinal or general anaesthesia is used. This minor surgery only adds another two or three days to the hospital stay.

> If possible, it is better to have a paediatrician (child specialist) examine your baby before you go ahead with the sterilisation. This will ensure that sterilisation is not done if the baby has any major problem.

If you are undergoing a caesarean section, and you and your husband have decided to proceed with sterilisation, then the procedure will be carried out at the same time. The procedure adds another few minutes to the operation and does not in any way cause complications. If a paediatrician is available at the time of the caesarean section (most of the times there will be one in the operation theatre during the caesarean), he or she will examine the baby to make sure that it has no problems. Sterilisation is done after the paediatrician gives the go-ahead.

Interval sterilisation

Some women choose to wait for a while before they proceed with sterilisation. Some women find themselves unexpectedly pregnant and may want to undergo a sterilisation immediately following termination of pregnancy.

The two methods for interval sterilisation are by laparoscopy or by a minilaparotomy.

Laparoscopy

Laparoscopy is the most common surgical approach for tubal sterilisation. The procedure begins with a small incision in the abdomen in or just below the umbilicus. The gynaecologist inserts a narrow viewing scope called a laparoscope through the incision. A second small incision is made just above the pubic hairline, and a probe is inserted. After identifying the tubes, the gynaecologist blocks them using different methods. Tubal rings or electrocoagulation (using an electric current to block a portion of the tube) are the commonest methods used.

Laparoscopic sterilisation is considered a day surgery and you can be discharged on the same day of the surgery. You can resume normal work as soon the effects of the anaesthesia wear off. It is recommended that you avoid intercourse for two weeks after the procedure.

Myth: Laparoscopic sterilisation is a reversible and temporary form of contraception. **It is not!** It is as permanent a method of sterilisation as the other surgical procedures.

Minilaparotomy

Though this method is used less often now after the advent of the laparoscopic method, it may be performed for interval sterilisation. Minilaparotomy requires a small abdominal incision, usually just above the pubic hairline. The tubes are identified, tied and cut. Women who undergo minilaparotomy typically need a few days to recover.

Male sterilisation or vasectomy

A vasectomy is a permanent sterilisation technique for men. It requires minor surgery to cut the vas (the tubes that carry sperm). This operation keeps the sperm from being present in the semen when a man ejaculates. Without sperm, fertilisation of an egg cannot occur and pregnancy is prevented. Vasectomy is a much simpler procedure than female sterilisation.

Procedure

A vasectomy only requires local anaesthesia. The procedure itself takes about 15 minutes.

After the procedure, men are advised to take two days off and perform only light activities for a week. It may take a week for men to feel comfortable before resuming sexual activity.

Vasectomies are not effective right away. The sperms that were already in the tubes before the operation need to be ejaculated. This may take about a month or 10-30 ejaculations. **Using other forms of birth control is important until follow-up sperm counts show complete absence of sperms in the semen.**

Old wives' tales
- A man will become "weak" after having a vasectomy. **Not true!**
- Sexual desire and function will be affected. **Not true!**

How well do the various methods prevent pregnancy?

When a couple uses no contraception, the rate of pregnancy is 80 per cent in a year. Other than permanent sterilisation, the hormone medications and the IUD are the most effective methods of birth control. The least reliable methods are the 'safe period' and the withdrawal method.

Birth control method	Percentage of women who will get pregnant with the first year of typical use
Natural family planning ('Safe period')	25%
Withdrawal	20%
Female condom	21%
Male condom	14%
Combination birth control pills	3%
Progestin only pill ('mini pill')	3-6%
IUD-Copper T	0.8%
Injection(DMPA)	Less than1%
Female sterilisation	0.5%
Male sterilisation	0.15 %

CHAPTER 44

Emergency contraception

Sahana is extremely worried. She has miscalculated her dates and may have had intercourse during the fertile part of her cycle. She has not been using any contraceptive method to avoid a pregnancy. Her child is only six months old and she definitely does not want to be pregnant again.

Sucharita is newly married. During intercourse, the condom slipped, and she and her husband are anxious because they are not ready for a pregnancy yet. Both Sahana and Sucharita need emergency contraception.

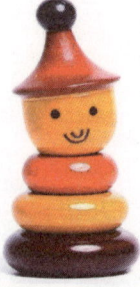

44 Emergency contraception

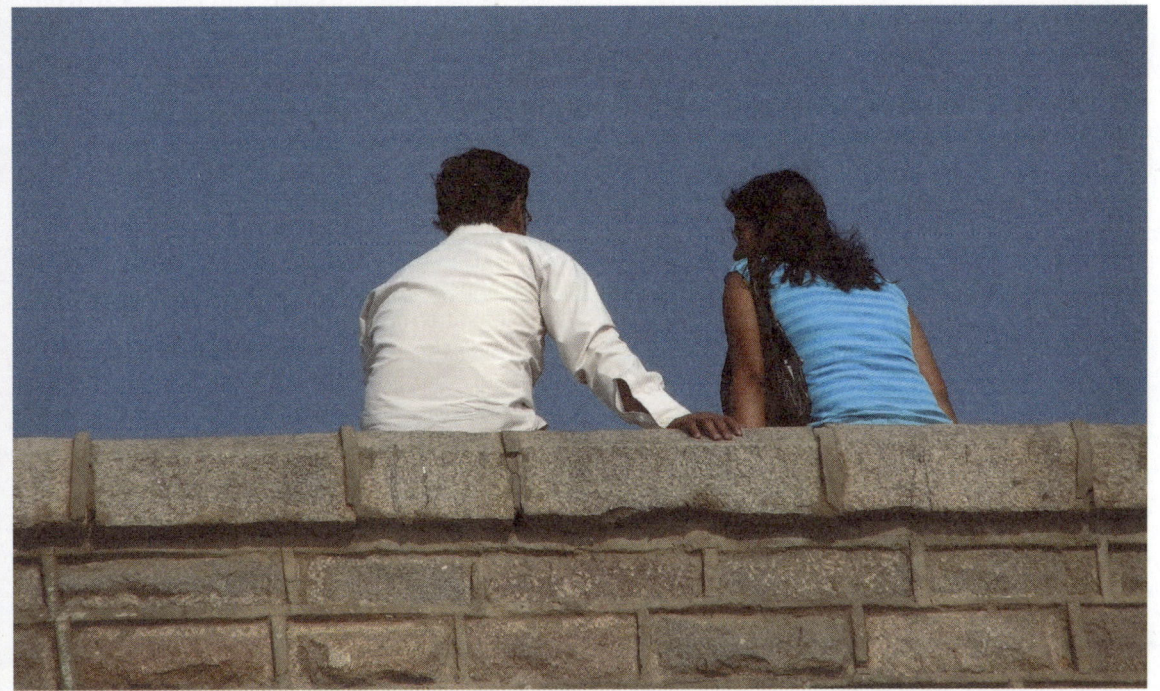

Emergency contraception

Emergency contraception (EC) is used to prevent pregnancy after a woman has had unprotected intercourse. In other words, she has not used any contraceptive method to avoid a pregnancy.

Emergency contraception can reduce the risk of pregnancy by at least 75 per cent. This means that only two out of 100 women will get pregnant, if emergency contraception is taken correctly within 72 hours after having unprotected intercourse.

Emergency birth control (also called "morning-after" contraception, emergency birth control or backup birth control) has been available for more than 30 years. It contains hormones found in birth control pills and must be started within 72 hours, and no later than 120 hours (5 days), after unprotected intercourse. The sooner it is started, the better the chances of preventing a pregnancy. EC prevents pregnancy by stopping ovulation or fertilisation.

Pills for emergency contraception

The two types of emergency contraception pills are **combined birth control pills** (containing estrogen and progestin hormones) and the **progestin-only pills.** The progestin-only method is more effective and is less likely to cause nausea. The hormones in both types of pills prevent pregnancy by preventing or delaying ovulation, blocking fertilisation or keeping a fertilised egg from implanting in the uterus.

Intrauterine device (IUD) for emergency contraception

An intrauterine device (IUD) can also be used for emergency contraception. The IUD works best if it is inserted within five days of having unprotected sex. The advantage of the IUD is that it can be left in place for the next five years and will continue to provide protection against pregnancy.

Taking emergency contraception pills

Emergency contraception pills may be prescribed in one of two forms:

- Regular birth control pills (containing estrogen and progestin): two pills must be taken orally within 72 hours (and no later than 120 hours) of unprotected intercourse and two more pills must be repeated 12 hours after the first dose. This dosage applies to pills containing 50 mcg of estrogen and not to low-dose birth control pills.
- A package with two pills (containing progestin only): both doses can be taken at the same time or 12–24 hours apart. These are most effective when taken immediately but should be taken no later than 120 hours (five days).

Side effects

Nausea and vomiting may occur after taking the pills. A medicine to prevent nausea may be required. If there is vomiting within two hours of taking either dose, that dose may need to be repeated. The next period may not occur at the expected time. There may be bleeding or spotting in the week or month after the treatment. Other side effects may include abdominal pain and cramps, breast tenderness, headache, dizziness and fatigue. These are the effects of the hormones in the pills. These side effects are temporary and will disappear within a few days.

Follow-up care

Emergency contraception can greatly reduce a woman's risk of getting pregnant after having unprotected sex. There is still a small chance of a pregnancy in spite of having taken emergency contraception. If the period is delayed and a pregnancy test is positive, an obstetrician must be consulted. It is important to remember that if you want to go ahead with the pregnancy, it is unlikely there will be any effect of the pills on the pregnancy or the health of the baby.

It must not be forgotten that other contraception will be needed till the next period unless an IUD has been inserted. **Although emergency contraception is a good option for preventing pregnancy when a woman has unprotected intercourse, it should not be used on a regular basis.** Regular use of a birth control method (such as birth control pills or an intrauterine device) is most effective.

Congratulations on your pregnancy!

We hope this book helps you handle the anxieties and fears that all pregnant couples face. We also hope that this book makes it all real for you. Knowing what is happening with your little one and knowing what is happening to you, will make it easier to cope with the enormous changes which occur in pregnancy.

For you

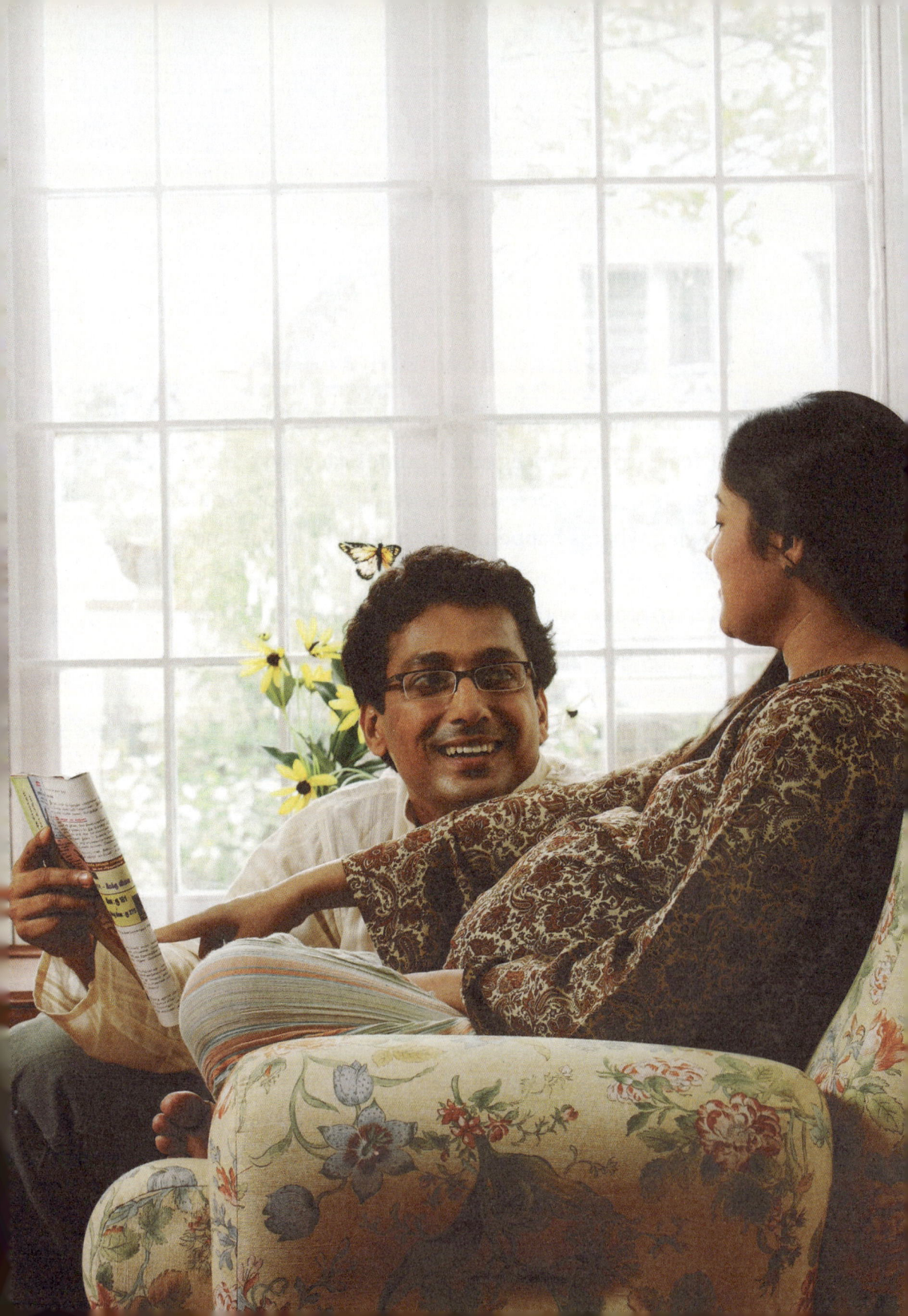

CHECKLIST FOR PREGNANCY

This is just a short checklist. Your obstetrician will guide you on everything else that is required especially for you.

First trimester

Blood tests

Ultrasound scan to look for age, growth and nuchal thickness

First trimester screening for Down syndrome

Second trimester

Second trimester screening for Down syndrome (if not done in first trimester)

Testing for diabetes in pregnancy

Ultrasound scan for foetal anomalies

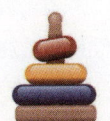

Third trimester

Immunisation for tetanus

Ultrasound scan, if recommended by obstetrician

Labour preparation class

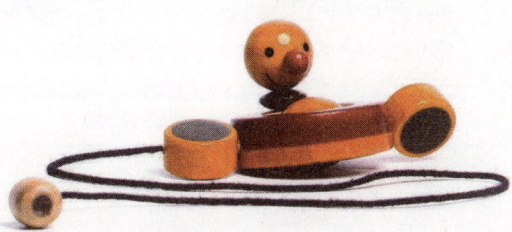

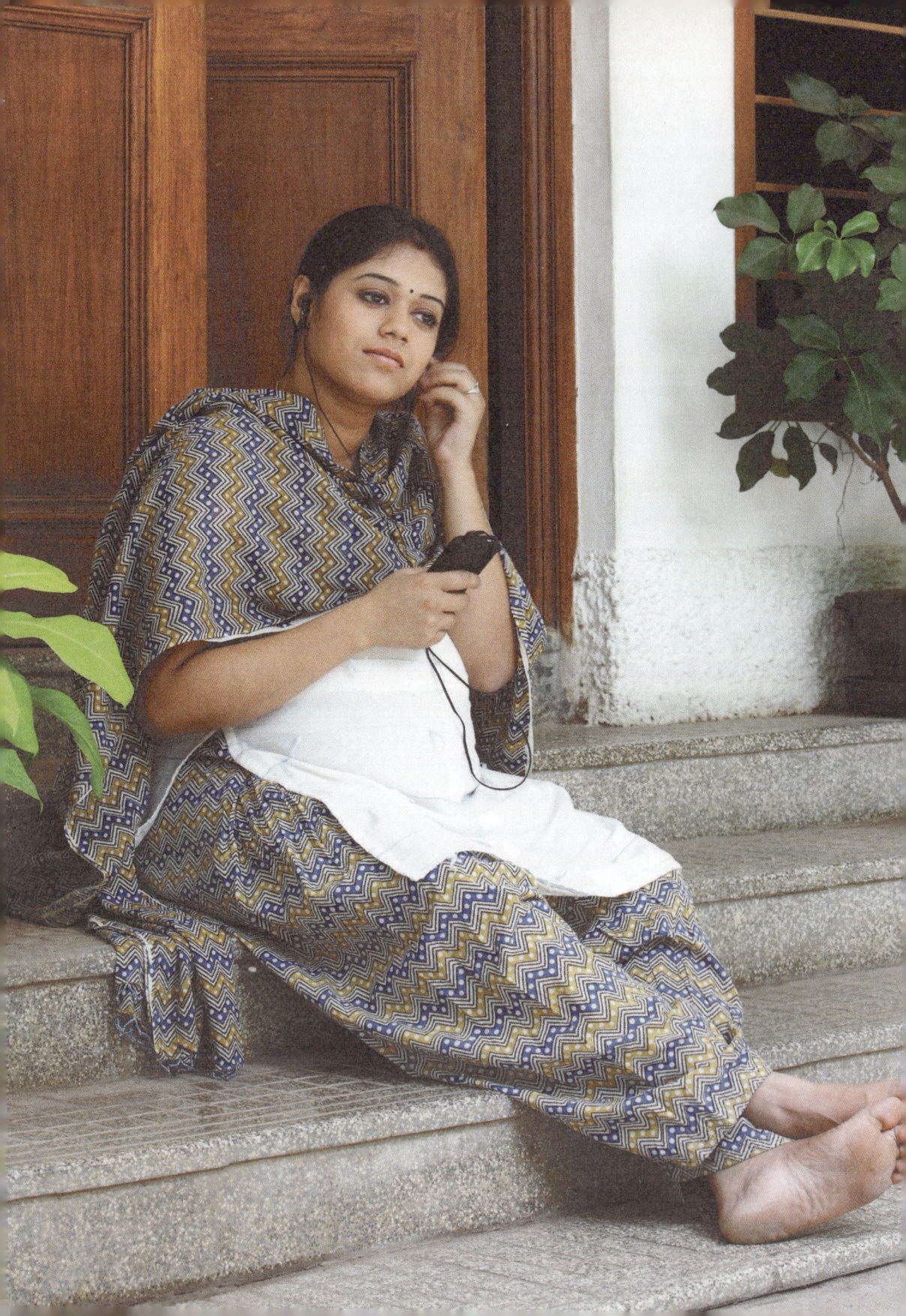

MY PERSONAL PREGNANCY CALENDAR

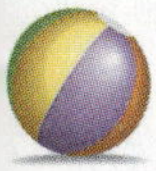

My pregnancy test was positive on: _____

My first visit to my obstetrician was on: _____

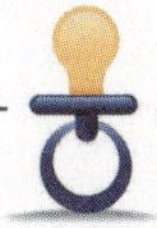

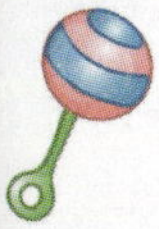

I felt the baby move on:

    Mom: _____

    Dad: _____

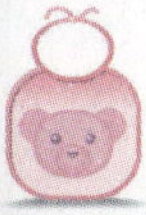

I had my first ultrasound scan on: _____

I had subsequent ultrasound scans on: _____

_____

_____

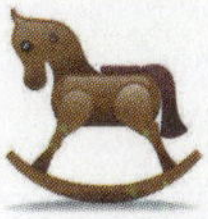

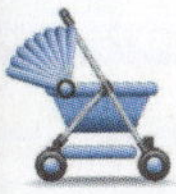

I first heard the baby's heartbeat on: _____

Shortlist of baby's name:

    Boy _____

_____

_____

    Girl _____

_____

_____

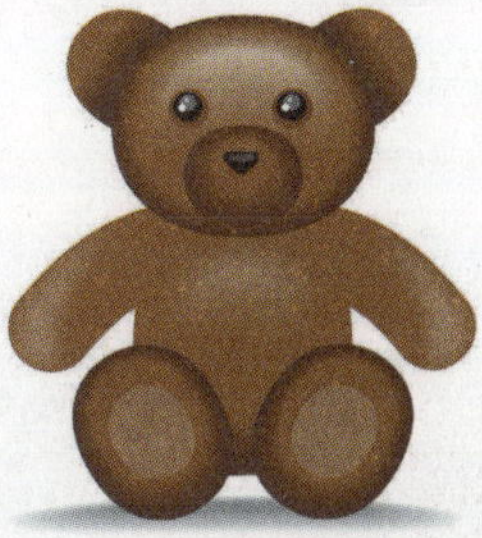

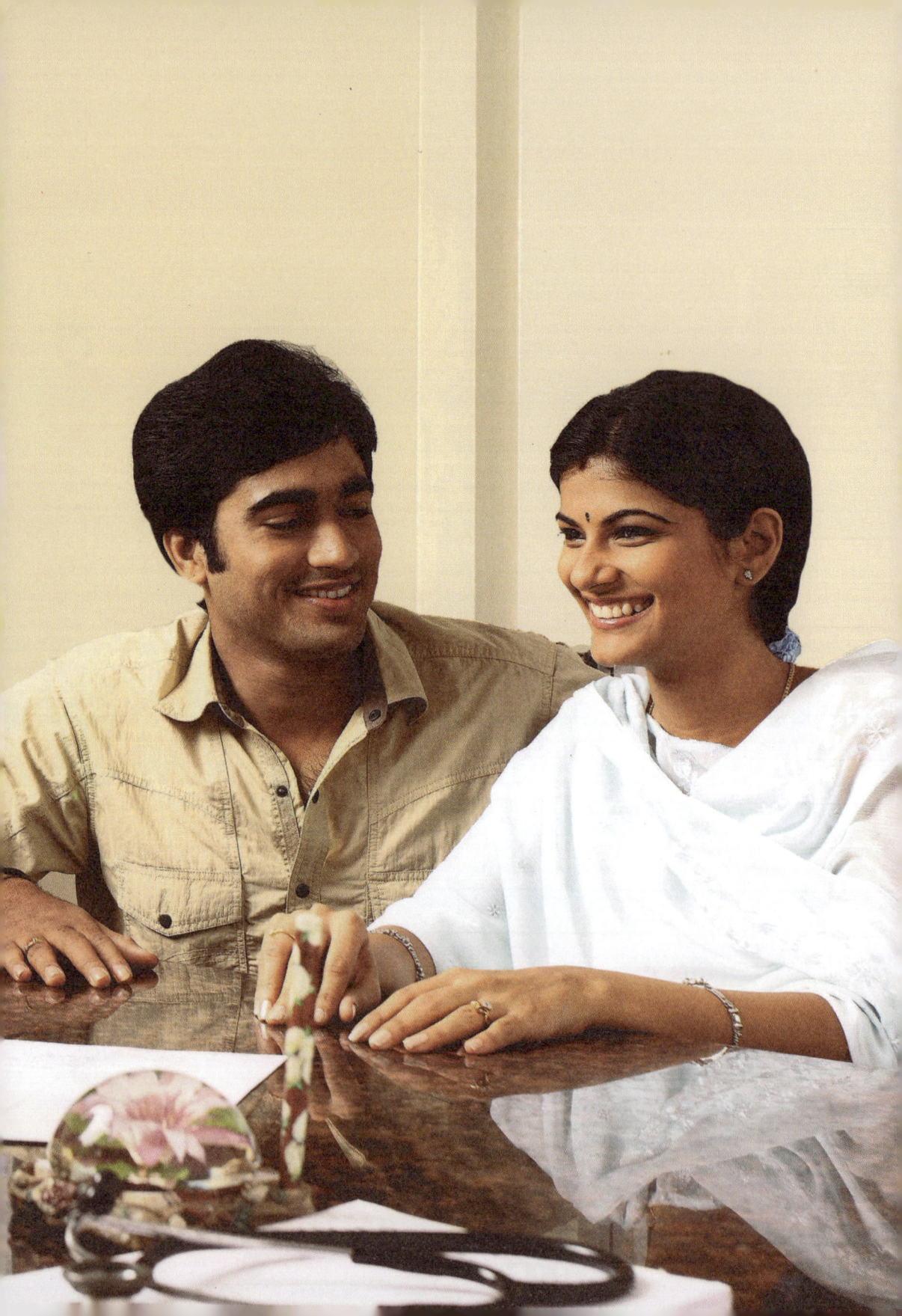

QUESTIONS FOR YOUR OBSTETRICIAN

YOUR OBSERVATIONS DURING YOUR PREGNANCY

YOUR OBSERVATIONS DURING YOUR PREGNANCY

Acknowledgements

This book has been a dream of mine for many years. It was Gautam Padmanabhan of Westland, who encouraged me and promised to support me in my endeavours. I would also like to thank Hemu Ramiah who was so instrumental in the initial design and concept of the book.

Savitha Gautam was my personal cheerleader, who egged me on and also helped in the editing of the book.

I would like to mention here that many of the chapters in the book were first published in a shorter version in my 'Women and Wellness' column in *The Hindu*. I thank the editorial staff for their support.

Malvika Mehra, and her able assistant Venu, of Art Works, typeset this book. Malvika's infectious enthusiasm carried me through the difficult final stages of putting this book together. If not for her, my energy would have floundered.

I have been lucky in being able to use the talents of people around me. My son Ashvin has guided me in many of the design elements in this book. Yuvaraj Vivek (yuvaraj@yuvarajvivek.com) a brilliant young photographer, is responsible for the great pictures in this book. I thank Alexander Zacharia and Elizabeth Jebaraj of Rubecon for their help.

My colleagues at E.V. Kalyani Medical Centre, Dr S. Rajasri and Dr Soumya Balakrishnan, have helped me by taking on a fair share of my clinical work so that I could write this book. To them I owe a big debt of gratitude.

I am particularly grateful to Dr S. Suresh, Director, Mediscan Systems, Chennai, for the ultrasound images.

M. Parimel Azhagan of Virtual Media (www.virtualmedia.in) provided the illustrations.

Arjun has always been the 'wind beneath my wings'. My love and thanks to Ashvin, Kavita and Sruti, for being there for me.

Gita Arjun

Index

A

Abdomen, 142, 189
    incision on, 71, 119, 139, 150, 266, 267
    of baby suffering from colic, 247
    sleeping on, 38, 42
Abdominal
    belt after delivery, 143, 151
    circumference (AC), 83
    discomfort and heaviness, 24, 41, 42, 69, 192
    exercises, 151, 161–63
    fat, 85
    muscles, 143, 150, 151, 162, 163
    pigmentation, 38
Abdominal pain
    after delivery, 151
    in ectopic pregnancy, 173
    false pains, 107
    after insertion of IUD, 264
    in miscarriage, 167, 169
    in pregnancy, 27, 38, 44, 50, 63, 174, 175, 177
    and preterm labour, 175, 178, 180
    in third trimester, 178, 180, 192, 199, 200
    in urinary tract infection, 227, 228
Abdominal wall defects, 75–76
Abortion, *See also miscarriage,* 24, 25, 39, 61, 166–71, 264
    causes, 167
    induced, 28
    missed, 82, 166, 167
    pregnancy after, 168
    sexual intercourse after, 168
    spontaneous, 167
Abruption of placenta, 116, 141, 175–76
Abscess, breast, 151, 156
Acidity, 24, 36, 41, 50, 58
Acupressure to relieve nausea, 36
Alcohol, 68
    and birth defects, 61
    preconception, 19
Amniotic fluid, 12, 45, 49, 78, 116, 119, 243
    assessment, 83–85, 88
    colour, 110, 115, 131 , 133
    decrease, 184
    excess, 180
    index, 185
    leaking, 65, 88, 117
    meconium, 42, 136
Amniotomy, 110, 115, 117
Anaemia, 19, 28, 29, 50
    before pregnancy, 17, 18
    in twin pregnancy, 192, 193

Anaesthesia, 97, 113, 142, 266
    epidural, 53, 111, 119, 121, 126, 142, 154
    spinal, 126, 142, 154
    general, 142
Anxiety, 96, 103, 104
    about labour, 128
    of loss of pregnancy, 219
APGAR score, 112
Areola, 22, 155
    darkening of, 36, 49
Aspirin, 231–32
    in high blood pressure, 201
    in thrombophilia, 170
Asthma, 18, 28, 230, 231–32
    before pregnancy, 17
    causes, 231
    medication in pregnancy, 231, 232

B

Baby, 242–55
    APGAR score, 112
    bed, crib and cradle, 99
    bibs, 255
    coping with loss of, 217–19
    oil and lotion, 250
    overweight or big, 204–05
    powder, 250
    premature, health problems, 179
    in first trimester, 33–39
    in second trimester, 41–45, 47
    in third trimester, 30, 49–55
Back
    pain, 45, 47, 50–51, 68, 161
    pimples on, 35
    sleeping on, 38, 42, 50, 55
    backache, 45, 107
    exercise for, 63
Bilirubin, 254
Birth control (contraception), 28, 149, 207
    after loss of pregnancy/miscarriage, 168, 219
    barrier methods of birth control, 260
    condoms, 262
        female condom, 259, 260, 261, 264
        male condom, 259, 260–61, 264
    diaphragm, 260
    emergency contraception (EC), 268–70
    injectable, 263
    intra-uterine device (IUD), 234, 259, 263–65, 267, 269–70

pills, 234, 259, 261–62, 264, 269–70
    advantages, 262–63
    spermicide, 259, 260, 264
    in women with epilepsy, 234
Birth defects, 74, 75–76, 87, 90–93, 217
    due to chromosomal abnormality, 75, 76, 77, 78, 83, 88, 89, 91
    combination of factors (multifactorial defects), 91
    diabetes and, 17, 76, 79, 204
    due to epilepsy, 233–34
    genetic disorders, 76, 77, 78, 79, 87, 89, 91, 93
    history in family, 28, 76, 79
    neural tube defects, 75, 77, 78, 91, 92, 234
    in pregnancy after 35, 76, 214
    prevention, 91–92
    previous child with, 18, 28, 76, 79
    tests for 76–77
    types, 91
Bladder and bowel function
    after delivery, 147–48
Blastocyst, 11, 13, 34
    development, 11–12
Bleeding in pregnancy, 65, 69, 82, 108, 112, 141, 147, 151, 172–77
    in early pregnancy, 27, 35, 37, 192
    during or after the caesarean section, 143
    after miscarriage, 167, 168, 169
    placentapraevia and, 175, 176
    postpartum, 71, 137
    in first trimester, 38, 82, 173
    in second trimester
    in third trimester, 175
    in twin pregnancy, 194
Blighted ovum, 82
Blood pressure, 30, 50, 142
    high, 17, 18, 29, 30, 65, 196–201, 205
    medications, 199–200
    in twin pregnancy,193
Blood tests, 23, 28–29, 31, 34, 39, 85
    for antiphospholipid syndrome, 170
    for birth defects, 77, 78, 82
    blood group and Rh type, 28–29, 49, 208–11
    for diabetes, 44, 204
Bra during pregnancy, 41, 156
Brain, 44
    development, 12, 13, 14, 18, 35, 36, 49, 50
Braxton-Hicks contractions, 45, 50, 107, 180
Breast(s) and/or nipples
    abscess, 151, 156
    discharge from, 49–50
    postpartum, 71
    swollen, tender or sore, 22, 27, 35, 36, 67
    engorgement, 155

Breastfeeding, 22, 33, 50, 71, 147, 149–50, 152ff, 246
    in asthma, 232
    after a caesarean section, 142, 154–55
    clothing for, 98
    in diabetes, 207
    diet and, 159
    in epilepsy, 234
    and missed period, 71
    positions, 155
    for twins, 195
Breast milk, 153–54, 234, 246
    adequacy of, 153
    leaking, 169
    medication and, 154
    mother's diet and, 154, 159, 160
Breathing and relaxation in labour, 126, 128
    techniques, 129, 134
Breathlessness, 37, 51, 65
Breech presentation, 119, 140–41, 186–89
    complete, incomplete and frank, 187–88
    external version, 188, 189
Burning urination, 151

C

Caesarean section, 18, 28, 54, 70, 71, 98, 105, 109, 117, 118, 119, 125, 126, 127, 131, 133, 135–37, 138–43
Calcium and calcium supplements, 19, 59–61, 159
    source of, 19, 59, 61
Calories
    in breastfeeding, 207
    extra in pregnancy, 18, 57–58
    need per day, 18
    restriction in diabetes, 206
Cephalo-pelvic disproportion (CPD), 119, 135, 140
Cervical
    dystocia, 135
Cervix, 52, 88, 170, 259, 260, 261
    changes, 108, 173, 175
    dilation and effacement, 30, 53, 105–11, 115–17, 119, 125, 127, 129, 135, 140, 168, 175, 180, 200, 228
    incompetence, 169–70, 175, 180
Check-ups, 19, 30
    antenatal, 39, 50, 66, 67, 68, 181, 197, 204, 208, 241
    monthly, 30, 58
    postnatal, 71, 207, 258
    in twin pregnancy, 192
    weekly, 30, 52
Children, spacing, 259
Chromosomal abnormalities
    and birth defects, 75, 76, 77, 78, 83, 88, 89, 91
    and miscarriage, 169
Cleft lip, 84
Cold and cough in pregnancy, 223
Colostrum, 153–54
Complications in labour, 134–37

Congenital disorder. *See birth defect*
Constipation
    in baby, 246
    in pregnancy, 25, 35, 41, 44, 58, 60, 63, 160
Contraception. *See birth control*
Contractions, 65, 105–06, 109–13, 117, 125, 127, 129, 131–32, 140, 181, 197
    Braxton-Hicks, 45, 50, 107, 180
    in false labour, 107
    irregular, 115
    premature, 193
    timing, 108, 112, 115
Cord, umbilical, 37, 42, 76, 89, 116, 211
    blood banking, 123
    clamping at birth, 245
    compression, 117, 140, 184
    around foetus's neck, 137
    prolapse, 118, 136
Cradle cap, 244
Cystic fibrosis, 18, 76, 78, 86, 87, 88, 93

D

Dairy products, 59, 60, 61, 159–60
Diabetes
    before pregnancy, 17, 18, 28, 79
    blood sugar control during pregnancy, 17, 44, 204, 205–06
    after delivery, 207
    family history, 18, 28
    managing pregnancy in , 206–07
    gestational, 29, 30, 92, 116, 135, 136, 141, 202–07
        after age 35, 215
        and birth defects, 17, 76, 79, 204
        and miscarriage, 170
        and premature labour, 180
        testing for, 29, 31, 44, 49, 203, 204
        at the time of conception, 17
        in twin pregnancy,193–94
        prevention, 207
Diaper, 252–53
    changing, 252
    cloth diaper, 252
    disposable diaper, 253
    proper diapering, 252
    rash, 244
Diet
    after caesarean, 142–43, 159
    calcium in, 19, 59–61
    after delivery, 146, 148, 158–63
    in diabetes, 205, 206
    during pregnancy, 24, 41, 47, 68, 154, 203
    during typhoid fever, 225
Dilation and effacement of cervix, 30, 53, 105–11, 115–17, 119, 125, 127, 129, 135, 140, 168, 175, 200, 228

Dizziness, 25, 35, 50
Down syndrome, 83, 85, 86, 88, 91
    age related risk (pregnancy after 35), 29, 77, 214
    and birth defects, 76, 77, 78, 83, 85
    test for, 29, 31, 39, 41
Due date (EDD), 15, 21–22, 27, 54, 101, 105, 135, 183, 185

E

Eclampsia, 199, 200
Ectopic pregnancy, 82, 85, 173
Effacement. *See Dilation and effacement of cervix*
Electronic foetal monitoring, 131, 132, 184, 185, 207
Endometriosis, 213
Endometrium, 21
Enema, in labour, 109
Entonox (pain relieving gas), 126, 127–28
Epidural
    analgesia, 53, 111, 119, 121, 126, 142, 154
    block, 126–27
Epilepsy
    and birth defect, 233
    before pregnancy, 17, 233
    in pregnancy, 18, 28, 92, 233
Episiotomy, 112
    after care, 113
    postpartum pain, 71, 113, 119, 148–49
Estimated date of delivery (EDD). *See due date*
Estrogen, 12, 21, 22, 24, 25, 33
Exercise, 207
    after caesarean section, 161
    after delivery, 146, 158–63
    in diabetes, 206
    after miscarriage, 169
    in pregnancy, 62–65, 150
    in twin pregnancy, 192
    after vaginal delivery, 161
Exhaustion or tiredness. *See fatigue*

F

Face
    brown patches on, 38
    darkening of skin, 47
    and Down syndrome, 76, 77
    pimples on, 35
Fallopian tubes, 11, 13, 33, 34, 259, 264, 265
    and ectopic pregnancy, 82, 173
False labour, 53, 107–08
Father, father-to-be, 66–71, 102, 110
    anxiety of, 39, 67
    and caesarean, 54, 70, 71, 154
    childbirth experience, 54, 67, 70
    and genetic disorders, 78, 79
    labour preparation classes, 54, 67, 69, 70, 128

Rh factor, 209, 210
   in first trimester, 39, 67–68
   in second trimester, 45, 68
   in third trimester, 54–55, 68–69
Fatigue, 22, 35, 150
Fever
   in newborn, 247
   in pregnancy, 222–25
Fibroids in pregnancy, 84, 118, 264
Fitness, 17, 48, 143, 150
Foetal
   abnormalities, 85; due to epilepsy, 18; due to Rubella (German measles), 19, 89
   anaemia, 89, 210
   asphyxia, 136
   blood sampling, 83, 87, 89
   complications in twin pregnancy, 193
   development, stages, 11
   distress, 117–18, 119, 132, 135–36, 140
   echocardiography, 84
   growth, 83
   heart beat, 29, 131–32, 136, 141, 177
   movement, 84, 116
   count, 184
   kicking, 14, 50–53; counting, 53; in first
Foetoscope, 131
Foetus 11–12, 13, 21, 33, 34, 35, 37, 82, 167, 264
   in breech position, 136, 187–89
   development, 12, 13, 14–15, 33
   effect on diabetes, 204
   embryo to foetus, 13
Folic acid supplementation, 33, 57, 59, 60–61, 233
   before a planned pregnancy, 18, 33, 57
   sources, 19
Food. *See diet*
Forceps delivery, 119, 120–23, 133

G

Gender or sex of baby, 41, 241
Genetic
   conditions in the family, 18
   counselling, 18, 76, 79, 87, 89, 93
   disorders and birth defects, 76–79, 87, 89, 91, 93
Glucometer, 206
Gum bleeding in first trimester, 37

H

Haemoglobin and haematocrit, 28
Haemophilia, 76, 78, 87, 88
Haemorrhoids (piles), 44, 148
Headache, 25, 36, 151, 224
Heart beat of foetus, 13, 29, 35, 36, 37, 40, 41, 43, 44, 75, 77, 81, 82, 84, 85, 112, 216, 241
   duringlabour, 115, 116, 119, 131–32, 134, 136

Heart defects, 76, 77, 78, 84, 91
   due to epilepsy, 234
Heart disease and miscarriage, 170
Heat rash, 244
HELLP syndrome, 200
Hepatitis B virus, 19, 29
Herpes, 141
Hiccups, in foetus 14, 247
High blood pressure. *See blood pressure*
Holding the baby, 243
Home pregnancy kit, 34, 35
Human chorionic gonadotropin (hCG), 11, 23, 24, 34, 35, 39, 41, 77, 78, 174
Human immunodeficiency virus (HIV), 29, 141, 229
Hyperbilirubinaemia (newborn jaundice), 206
Hyperemesis gravidarum, 24
Hypertension, 28, 135, 141
   antenatal care, 199
   chronic, 198, 199
   gestational, 197, 198, 201, 205
   medications, 199–200
   preconceptional counselling, 198
   and premature delivery, 198
Hypoglycaemia, 205, 206
Hypothyroidism in pregnancy, 28, 234

I

Immunisation, 30, 31, 45
In vitro fertilisation (IVF), 191
Indirect Coomb's test, 210
Infections, 28, 227
   in breast, 156
   in early pregnancy, 75
   intrauterine, 88
   due to intrauterine device, 264
   of kidney, 227
   maternal, 140, 141
   prevention, 19
   urinary tract (UTI), 29, 223, 226–29
Infertility, 34
Influenza; in pregnancy, 223, 224
Infra red lamps, 149
Insulin, 17, 44, 116, 203–07. *See also diabetes.*
Insurance and hospital payment, planning, 19, 71
Intrauterine demise, 84, 116, 216, 217
Intrauterine device (IUD), 259, 263–65, 269, 270
Intrauterine growth restriction (IUGR), 180, 198, 207
Intrauterine infections, 88
Iron and iron supplements, 18, 19, 25, 28, 33, 42, 47, 50, 60, 68. *See also diet*
Itching and burning
   due to vaginal discharge, 25, 43, 228
   all over body, 50

J
Jaundice to newborn, 253–54

K
Karyotyping test, 88, 169
Kegel's exercise, during pregnancy, 49, 149, 161
Kidney disease and miscarriage, 170

L
Labour, 54, 55, 68, 70, 185
    and delivery, 104–13
    and father-to-be, 54, 67, 68
    complications, 134–37
    failure to progress, 135, 140
    false, 107–08
    inducedlabour, 54, 114–19, 135, 184, 185, 207
    monitoring well-being of baby, 130–33
    pain relief, 124–29
    planning for, 100–03
    premature or preterm, 53, 105, 178–81, 192–93, 198, 201, 205, 208, 214–15
    preparing for, 53, 96–99, 101, 102
    preparation classes, 31, 51, 53, 54, 67, 69, 70, 111, 126, 128, 129, 134
    problems in pregnancy after 35, 215
    signs, 53
    three stages, 106, 109
Lactation, 153
Lactose intolerance, 61
Last menstrual period (LMP), 12, 15, 22, 27, 28, 33

M
Malaria in pregnancy, 223, 225
Marriage between close relatives and birth defects, 78, 79
Meconium, 42, 54, 119, 136, 184
Menstrual cycle, 11, 28, 150, 265
    and due date (EDD), 15, 21–22
    irregular, 15, 22, 183, 263
    missed periods, 20, 21, 23, 34
    painful, 264
Migraine, 25
Miscarriage, 18, 28, 35, 37, 41, 82, 88, 89, 166–71, 173, 216, 264
    causes, 167, 169, 171
    diagnosis, 167
    another pregnancy after, 168
    myths and misconceptions, 171
    recurrent or habitual, 168, 169
    sexual intercourse after, 168
    symptoms, 167
    threatened, 168, 174
    types, 168

Missed abortion, 82, 166, 167
Molar pregnancies, 85, 173
Morning sickness, 23–24, 38, 67
Multiple pregnancy, 141

N
Nausea and vomiting, 20, 23–24, 27, 35, 36, 37, 39, 42, 58, 67
Neonatal intensive care unit, 179
Non-stress test, 185

O
Obesity, 47
    risk for baby, 18
    and weight gain during pregnancy, 58, 68, 159
Oral contraceptives, 261, 262
Ovarian cysts, 84
Ovulation
    and conceiving, 11, 33–34, 259
    age, 12
    prevention, 263, 269
    safe period, 260

P
Pain
    abdominal. *See abdominal pain*
    in back. *See back pain*
    in breast, 22, 151
    due to breast engorgement, 155
    in breastfeeding, 155–56
    in ectopic pregnancy, 173
    false, 107
    of incision, 113, 149, 151
    after delivery, 148, 149
    in miscarriage, 167–69
    associated with periods, 263, 264
    and postnatal exercise, 161
    in preterm labour, 175, 178–81
    relief in labour and delivery, 119, 124–29, 232, 235
    during sexual intercourse, postpartum, 150
    under the ribs, 44, 50
    on urination, 227–29.
Paracetamol, 25, 36, 224
Pelvic
    examination, 21, 167, 174, 188
    infection, 264
    muscles, 49, 63, 161–62
    pressure on, 52, 125
Placenta, 11, 13, 34, 38, 42, 49, 57, 78, 89, 112, 119, 123, 128, 136, 137, 140, 168, 170, 177, 206
    abnormal, 174
    abruption, 116, 141, 175–76, 215
    position, 84, 85, 189